Partial Differential Equation Analysis in Biomedical Engineering

Case Studies with MATLAB

Aimed at graduates and researchers, and requiring only a basic knowledge of multi-variable calculus, this introduction to computer-based partial differential equation (PDE) modeling provides readers with the practical methods necessary to develop and use PDE mathematical models in biomedical engineering. Taking an applied approach, rather than using abstract mathematics, the reader is instructed through six biomedical example applications, each example characterized by step-by-step discussions of established numerical methods, and implemented in reliable computer routines. Adopting this technique, the reader will understand how PDE models are formulated, implemented and tested. Supported by a set of rigorously tested general purpose PDE routines online, and with enhanced understanding through animations, this book will be ideal for anyone faced with interpreting large experimental data sets that need to be analyzed with PDE models in biomedical engineering.

William E. Schiesser is Emeritus R.L. McCann Professor of Chemical Engineering and Professor of Mathematics at Lehigh University.

Partial Differential Equation Analysis in Biomedical Engineering

Case Studies with MATLAB

WILLIAM E. SCHIESSER
Lehigh University, Bethlehem, PA, USA

CAMBRIDGE
UNIVERSITY PRESS

CAMBRIDGE UNIVERSITY PRESS
Cambridge, New York, Melbourne, Madrid, Cape Town,
Singapore, São Paulo, Delhi, Mexico City

Cambridge University Press
The Edinburgh Building, Cambridge CB2 8RU, UK

Published in the United States of America by Cambridge University Press, New York

www.cambridge.org
Information on this title: www.cambridge.org/9781107022805

First published 2013

Printed and bound in the United Kingdom by the MPG Books Group

A catalog record for this publication is available from the British Library

Library of Congress Cataloging in Publication data
Schiesser, W. E.
Partial differential equation analysis in biomedical engineering : case studies with
MATLAB / William E. Schiesser.
p. ; cm.
Includes bibliographical references and index.
ISBN 978-1-107-02280-5 (hardback)
I. Title.
[DNLM: 1. MATLAB. 2. Mathematical Computing.
3. Biomedical Engineering – methods. 4. Models, Theoretical. QT 36]
610.28–dc23 2012008158

ISBN 978-1-107-02280-5 Hardback

To my parents
Laura Virginia Bauer
Edward Valentine Schiesser

Contents

Preface

This book is an introduction to the mathematical modeling of biomedical engineering systems. In particular, models based on partial differential equations (PDEs) are presented: antibody binding kinetics, acid-mediated tumor growth, retinal O_2 transport, hemodialyzer dynamics, epidermal wound healing, and polymer matrix drug delivery.

The numerical solution of the model equations is through a single, well-established method for PDEs, the method of lines (MOL), in which the spatial derivatives in the PDEs are replaced with algebraic approximations and a system of ordinary differential equations (ODEs) in an initial value variable, typically time, follows. The spatial approximations are finite differences (FDs), although other approximations could easily be accommodated within the MOL format, e.g., finite elements, finite volumes, spectral methods, Galerkin methods such as collocation, meshfree methods. The final result is a set of routines that numerically integrates the ODEs; the format of these routines is basically the same throughout the book.

To facilitate understanding of the PDE analysis, an introduction to the numerical methods and associated computational routines is presented in the first chapter. Then each application is cross referenced to this introduction in each step where some additional explanation is helpful.

In each example, we follow a combination of the following steps:

- Statement of the model PDE, along with the associated auxiliary (initial and boundary) conditions. This introduction to the model contains a reference to the original source and possibly related literature, and includes some discussion of the underlying biophysics, biochemistry, and physiology.
- Discussion of the numerical methods (algorithms) for the MOL solution of the model equations, principally by reference to the introduction in Chapter 1.
- List of MATLAB routines based on the MOL numerical solution of the PDEs, discussed in some detail, typically a few lines of code at a time. This discussion emphasizes how the associated mathematics of the model is programmed.
- Discussion of the numerical solution of the model equations, including the origin of any unusual features of the solution.
- Error analysis to establish if the numerical solution is reliable and has acceptable accuracy; typically techniques such as varying the MOL grid spacing and order of approximation are used to infer convergence of the numerical solution to an acceptable

level of accuracy. Also, physical constraints such as conservation of mass energy and energy are used to evaluate the solution.

- Concluding summary and discussion of extensions of the model and the MOL algorithms.

Our intention is not to provide a comprehensive treatise, but rather to provide a set of basic computational procedures that we hope readers can assimilate without becoming deeply involved in the details of numerical methods for PDEs and computer programming so that they can concentrate on the problem of interest with reasonable effort. This might take the form of extending the computer routines provided, or applying and extending the numerical methods that are presented through examples.

In summary, our intention is to provide a methodology for the PDE analysis of biomedical engineering systems. This includes the development of numerical methods and associated computer routines that can be used to study the characteristics and solutions of the model equations. The approach is not theoretical, e.g., limited theorems and no proofs; rather, the presentation is based on detailed example applications. The MOL analysis provides a general framework for the analysis of PDE models that we think can be broadly applied in biomedical engineering, and which can be applied to all of the major geometric classes of PDEs (parabolic, hyperbolic, elliptic). All of the MATLAB routines are available (gratis) as a download through a request to wes1@lehigh.edu.

We welcome comments from readers concerning this approach and will be pleased to answer questions to the extent possible by e-mail.

1 Introduction to partial differential equation integration in space and time

1.1 Introduction

The analysis of biomedical systems using mathematical models expressed as partial differential equations (PDEs) is the central theme of this book. This is done not with mathematical analysis such as theorems and proofs, but rather, through example applications to illustrate computational methods for the numerical solution of the model equations, and the details of implementing these numerical methods in computer codes. Example applications are taken from the recent literature: antibody binding kinetics, acid-mediated tumor growth, retinal O_2 transport, hemodialyzer dynamics, epidermal wound healing, drug distribution from a polymer matrix. Each chapter covers a self-contained example.

The numerical solution of the model equations is through a single, well-established procedure for PDEs, the method of lines (MOL), which has been applied to all of the major classes of PDE (parabolic, hyperbolic, and elliptic). Basically, the spatial derivatives in the PDEs are replaced with algebraic approximations; in the present book, the approximations are finite differences (FDs) although other approximations could easily be accommodated within the MOL format, e.g., finite elements, finite volumes, spectral methods, Galerkin methods such as collocation. The final result is a set of routines that implement the MOL calculations for each particular application; the format of these routines is the same throughout the set of applications.

In each example, we follow a series of steps:

- Statement of the mathematical model as a PDE system;
- Some background concerning the model and the original source (references);
- Discussion of the numerical methods (algorithms) for the MOL solution of the model equations;
- Listing of MATLAB routines that implement the MOL solution with a detailed discussion of the routines, a few lines at a time, to emphasize the connection of the programming to the model equations;
- Discussion of the numerical solution of the model equations, including the origin of any unusual features of the solution and an assessment of the accuracy of the solution;
- Concluding summary and discussion of extensions of the model and the MOL algorithms.

Since a common framework is used for all of the applications, we provide in this chapter an introductory discussion of MOL analysis and associated routines. Then, when additional explanation and clarification of computational details are required in the discussion of the applications, references back to Chapter 1 are included. We start with a discussion of hyperbolic PDEs that typically model convection.

1.2 Hyperbolic PDEs

We start the discussion of the numerical solution of PDEs with what is perhaps the simplest PDE, but which, somewhat ironically, is also one of the most difficult to integrate numerically, the linear advection equation (derived in Appendix 1):

$$\frac{\partial u}{\partial t} + v\frac{\partial u}{\partial z} = 0, \tag{1.1}$$

where

Variable	Definition
u	Dependent variable
z	Spatial (boundary value) independent variable
t	Temporal (initial value) independent variable
v	Constant, typically velocity

Equation (1.1) is a partial differential equation since it has more than one independent variable, that is, t and z. We mean by a solution to eq. (1.1), the dependent variable, u, as a function of the independent variables, t and z, that is, $u(z,t)$. The solution may be either a mathematical function, which is called an analytical, exact or closed form solution, or a numerical solution, in which case the solution $u(z,t)$ is in numerical form (as $u(z,t)$ in tabular numerical format or a graph of $u(z,t)$ plotted against t and z).

As a point of notation, we have adopted u as the designation of the dependent variable which is in accordance with much of the literature pertaining to PDEs. For a system of n simultaneous PDEs, we will use $u_1, u_2, ..., u_n$, that is, a vector of n dependent variables. However, in applications, the dependent variables can be, for example, concentrations of various chemical species, temperature, and velocity. Although different symbols for these chemical and physical entities would seem useful (for clarity), we will stay with u as a consistent representation of the PDE-dependent variable(s).

With regard to an application of eq. (1.1), u could represent a chemical composition or concentration for flow at velocity v through a circular channel or tube, which could represent, for example, an artery. z is the distance measured along the tube and t is time. Thus, in computing a numerical solution to eq. (1.1) ($u(z,t)$ in numerical format), we would obtain the concentration as a function of z and t.

Equation (1.1) is a hyperbolic PDE, one of three geometric classifications: hyperbolic, parabolic, and elliptic. Equation (1.1) has constant coefficients since the coefficient v is a constant.

Equation (1.1) is first order since both the derivative in t, $(\partial u/\partial t)$, and the derivative in z, $(\partial u/\partial z)$, are first order. Equation (1.1) is also first degree or linear since the dependent variable u and its derivatives are to the first power. If a PDE is not first degree, it is nonlinear. For example, the PDE $(\partial u/\partial t) + v(\partial u/\partial z)^2 = 0$ is nonlinear since the derivative in z is to the second power; it could also be termed second degree (the terms "order" and "power" are easily confused).

In summary, eq. (1.1) is a linear, first order, constant coefficient, hyperbolic PDE. This type of description with words is important not only to describe or classify the PDE, but also because it often suggests a method of analytical or numerical solution.

Since eq. (1.1) is first order in t, it requires one auxiliary condition in t, which is an initial condition (IC) (in general, the required number of ICs equals the order of the highest order derivative in the initial value independent variable; in this case, one IC for the first order derivative $(\partial u/\partial t)$). t is an initial value variable since it starts from an initial (prescribed) value and then proceeds indefinitely, that is, over the semi-infinite interval $0 \le t \le \infty$ or $-\infty \ge t \ge 0$, or the infinite interval $-\infty \ge t \ge \infty$. Another explanation for "initial" is that t usually represents time in an application.

Also, since eq. (1.1) is first order in z, it requires one auxiliary condition in z, which is a boundary condition (BC). z is a boundary value variable since it starts from a boundary (prescribed) value, z_l, and then proceeds to a second value, z_u usually over the finite interval $z_l \le t \le z_u$ (although either z_l or z_u can be ∞ or $-\infty$). Another explanation for "boundary" is that z usually represents space in an application with physical boundaries (z_l and z_u represent the locations of physical boundaries such as surfaces).

For the IC for eq. (1.1), we take

$$u(t=0,z) = f(z). \tag{1.2}$$

Note that eq. (1.2) is stated for $t = 0$ and $f(z)$ is a prescribed function of z.

For the BC for eq. (1.1), we take

$$u(t,z=0) = g(t). \tag{1.3}$$

Note that eq. (1.3) is stated for $z = 0$ and $g(t)$ is a prescribed function of t.

Equations (1.1) to (1.3) constitute a complete, well-posed PDE problem and we now seek a numerical solution for particular choices of $f(z)$ and $g(t)$. Many numerical methods for PDEs can be considered and we focus on one approach, the numerical method of lines (MOL). The basic idea in MOL analysis is to replace the boundary value (spatial) derivatives with algebraic approximations. This effectively removes these derivatives from the PDE and since only the initial value independent variable remains, e.g., t, the PDE has been converted to a system of approximating ordinary differential equations (ODEs) that can be integrated by standard, well-established numerical algorithms for initial value ODEs; this is the essence of MOL analysis. We next consider MOL analysis applied to eqs. (1.1) to (1.3) through a series of computer routines.

1.2.1 Spatial integration

To compute a numerical solution to eqs. (1.1) to (1.3), we have to express these equations in a way that a computer can accept or accommodate. Basically, a computer can only do arithmetic and store the results, but fortunately, it does these tasks with remarkable speed and reliability. A computer, however, cannot accept a PDE such as eq. (1.1) directly. In other words, a computer cannot integrate a PDE in the way a human being would, using rather sophisticated mathematical methods. Rather, we have to state the PDE in a way that requires only the operations a computer can do, namely arithmetic.

Therefore, the first challenge in computing a numerical solution is to state the PDE in an alternative form that can be programmed. In particular, integration in space and time (with respect to t and z in eq. (1.1)) is required. Thus, we now consider some numerical methods for temporal and spatial integration.

In the case of spatial integration, we can replace the derivative $(\partial u/\partial x)$ in eq. (1.1) with an algebraic approximation such as

$$\frac{\partial u_i}{\partial z} \approx \frac{u_i - u_{i-1}}{\Delta z}, \tag{1.4a}$$

where i is an index indicating position along a grid in z; Δz is the spacing between the grid points. $i = 1$ corresponds to $z = z_l = 0$ and $i = n$ corresponds to $z = z_u = z_L$ (note that we have selected the spatial interval $0 \leq z \leq z_L$, but any other interval could be considered, finite, semi-infinite, or infinite).

Since the approximation (RHS) of eq. (1.4a) is a ratio of a difference in u over a difference in z, it is termed a finite difference approximation. If eq. (1.4a) is substituted in eq. (1.1), we have

$$\frac{\mathrm{d}u_i(t)}{\mathrm{d}t} + v\frac{u_i(t) - u_{i-1}(t)}{\Delta z} = 0, \; i = 1, 2, ..., n. \tag{1.4b}$$

Note that the use of eq. (1.4a) eliminated the derivative in z in eq. (1.1) and thus only one independent variable, t, remains. Therefore, the derivative in eq. (1.4b) is an ordinary or total derivative in t. Also, eq. (1.4b) is an ODE at grid point i, and i is an index over the grid in z that ranges over the values $1 \leq i \leq n$. In other words, eq. (1.4b) is a system of n ODEs that approximates the PDE, eq. (1.1).

Equations (1.4b) require n ICs which follow from eq. (1.2) as

$$u_i(t = 0) = f(z(i)), \; i = 1, 2, ..., n. \tag{1.4c}$$

Also, BC (1.3) becomes

$$u_1(t) = g(t). \tag{1.4d}$$

Thus, we do not require the ODE of eqs. (1.4b) at $i = 1$ corresponding to $z = 0$ (because of BC (1.3)) and we therefore have to integrate only $n - 1$ ODEs. An alternative is to use at $i = 1$ the ODE

$$\frac{\mathrm{d}u_1(t)}{\mathrm{d}t} = 0, \tag{1.4e}$$

so that the integration in t does not move $u_1(t)$ away from its value prescribed by eq. (1.4d). Either approach, $n-1$ ODEs without eq. (1.4e) or n ODEs with eq. (1.4e), can be used in the numerical integration with respect to t.

At this point, we will assume that we have an algorithm programmed for the numerical integration of eqs. (1.4b) subject to the ICs of eqs. (1.4c) and BC (1.4d), and postpone temporarily a discussion of temporal integration (with respect to t). Equations (1.4b), (1.4c), and (1.4d) therefore constitute the MOL formulation of eqs. (1.1) to (1.3). After the MOL programming is discussed and some numerical results are reviewed, we will return to the matter of the temporal integration of eqs. (1.4b).

Finally, for the case $v < 0$ (flow right to left), eqs. (1.4b), (1.4d), and (1.4e) become,

$$\frac{\mathrm{d}u_i(t)}{\mathrm{d}t} + v\frac{u_{i+1}(t) - u_i(t)}{\Delta z} = 0,\ i = 1, 2, ..., n, \tag{1.4f}$$

$$u_n(t) = g(t), \tag{1.4g}$$

$$\frac{\mathrm{d}u_n(t)}{\mathrm{d}t} = 0. \tag{1.4h}$$

This form of the MOL approximation of eq. (1.1) is discussed subsequently.

1.2.2 A basic MOL format

We start the discussion of MOL programming with a basic format for the programming of eqs. (1.4b), (1.4c), (1.4d), and (1.4e) (or eqs. (1.4f), (1.4g), and (1.4h)). A main program follows.

```
  clc
  clear all
%
% Linear advection equation
%
% The linear advection equation
%
%   ut + v*uz = 0                                         (1)
%
% is integrated by the method of lines (MOL) subject to
% the IC
%
%   u(z,t=0) = f(z)                                       (2)
%
% BC
%
%   u(z=0,t) = g(t)                                       (3)
%
% We consider in particular f(z) = 0, g(t) = 1 corresponding
% to the Heaviside unit step function, h(t); the solution to
% eqs. (1) to (3) is
%
%   u(z,t)=h(t - z/v)                                     (4)
```

```
%
% which is used to evaluate the numerical (MOL) solution.
%
%  The numerical algorithms are:
%
%    z (spatial, boundary value) integration: Two point upwind
%      (2pu)
%
%    t (temporal, initial value) integration: Explicit Euler
%
  global z dz zL v n ncase ncall
%
% Grid (in z)
  zL=1; n=51; dz=0.02;
  z=[0:dz:zL];
%
% Level of output
%
%   Detailed output - ip = 1
%
%   Brief (IC) output - ip = 2
%
  ip=2;
%
% Step through cases
%
%   ncase = 1: v > 0
%
%   ncase = 2: v < 0
%
  for ncase=1:2
    if ncase==1 v= 1; end
    if ncase==2 v=-1; end
%
% Parameters for Euler integration
  nsteps=20;
  h=0.001;
%
% Initial condition
  for i=1:n
    u(i)=0;
  end
  t=0;
%
% Write ncase, h, v
  fprintf('\n\n ncase = %5d    h = %10.3e    v = %4.2f\n\n',ncase,h,v);
%
% Write heading
  if(ncase==1)
    fprintf('    t      zL     t-zL/|v|    u(zL,t)    ua(zL,t)    diff\n');
  end
```

```
%
% Write heading
  if(ncase==2)
    fprintf('    t       zL     t-zL/|v|     u(0,t)     ua(0,t)    diff\n');
  end
%
% Display numerical, analytical solutions at t = 0
  if(t <  zL/abs(v)) ua=0;   end
  if(t >  zL/abs(v)) ua=1;   end
  if(t == zL/abs(v)) ua=0.5; end
  if(ncase==1)
    diff=u(n)-ua;
    fprintf('%5.2f%7.2f%10.2f%10.3f%10.3f%10.4f\n',...
            t,zL,t-zL/abs(v),u(n),ua,diff);
  end
  if(ncase==2)
    diff=u(1)-ua;
    fprintf('%5.2f%7.2f%10.2f%10.3f%10.3f%10.4f\n',...
            t,zL,t-zL/abs(v),u(1),ua,diff);
  end
%
% Store solution for plotting
  if(ncase==1)
     uplot(1,1)=u(n);
    uaplot(1,1)=ua;
     tplot(1)=t;
  end
  if(ncase==2)
     uplot(2,1)=u(1);
    uaplot(2,1)=ua;
  end
%
% nout output points
  nout=101;
  ncall=0;
  for iout=2:nout
%
%   Euler integration
    u0=u; t0=t;
    [u,t]=euler(u0,t0,h,nsteps);
%
%   Numerical, analytical solutions
    if(t <  zL/abs(v)) ua=0;   end
    if(t >  zL/abs(v)) ua=1;   end
    if(t == zL/abs(v)) ua=0.5; end
    if(ip==1)
      if(ncase==1)
        diff=u(n)-ua;
        fprintf('%5.2f%7.2f%10.2f%10.3f%10.3f%10.4f\n',...
                t,zL,t-zL/abs(v),u(n),ua,diff);
      end
```

```
        if(ncase==2)
          diff=u(1)-ua;
          fprintf('%5.2f%7.2f%10.2f%10.3f%10.3f%10.4f\n',...
                  t,zL,t-zL/abs(v),u(1),ua,diff);
        end
      end
%
%     Store solution for plotting
      if(ncase==1)
         uplot(1,iout)=u(n);
        uaplot(1,iout)=ua;
         tplot(iout)=t;
      end
      if(ncase==2)
         uplot(2,iout)=u(1);
        uaplot(2,iout)=ua;
         tplot(iout)=t;
      end
%
% Next output
  end
%
% Plots for ncase = 1, 2
  if(ncase==1)
    figure(1);
    plot(tplot,uplot(1,:),'-o');
    axis([0 2 0 1]);
    ylabel('u(zL,t),ua(zL,t)');xlabel('t');
    title('ncase = 1; num - o; anal - line');
    hold on
    plot(tplot,uaplot(1,:),'-');
  end
  if(ncase==2)
    figure(2);
    plot(tplot,uplot(2,:),'-o');
    axis([0 2 0 1]);
    ylabel('u(0,t),ua(0,t)');xlabel('t');
    title('ncase = 2; num - o; anal - line');
    hold on
    plot(tplot,uaplot(2,:),'-');
  end
%
% Next case
fprintf ('\n ncall = %4d\n', ncall/);
  end
```

Listing 1.1 Main program pde_1_main for eqs. (1.1) to (1.3)

We can note the following details about this programming:

- Any previous files are cleared, the PDE problem is outlined as comments, and global variables are defined that can be shared with other routines.

```
  clc
  clear all
%
  Documentation comments are not repeated here to conserve space
%
  global z dz zL v n ncase ncall
```

- A grid of 51 points in z is defined over the interval $0 \leq z \leq 1$ with a uniform spacing of dz=0.02 ($= \Delta z$ in eqs. (1.4a),(1.4b)).

```
%
% Grid (in z)
  zL=1; n=51; dz=0.02;
  z=[0:dz:zL];
```

  Note that we used the MATLAB utility for the definition of a 1D vector, [], to define the grid z. n is not used here, but is defined numerically for later use. Also, a line of MATLAB code is usually terminated with a semicolon, ;, to suppress the result from that line. If the semicolon is not used, the resulting displayed result can be useful when debugging some associated code (but also, excessive output can result, particularly if the numerical content of a vector or array is not suppressed, or if the line is executed repeatedly in a loop). Fifty-one grid points were selected to give adequate resolution of the numerical solution with respect to z. This number is a compromise between too small a value (and thus inadequate resolution in z) and too large a value (and thus excessive calculations and run times).
- An integer index, ip, is used to select a level of output later. For ip=2, only the IC is displayed numerically, but plots of the solution are produced. A for loop is then used to step through two cases corresponding to a positive velocity, v=1 (with the solution traveling left to right) and a negative velocity, v=-1 (with the solution traveling right to left). This use of a positive and then a negative velocity tests if the code works as expected for both cases.

```
%
% Level of output
%
%   Detailed output - ip = 1
%
%   Brief (IC) output - ip = 2
%
  ip=2;
%
% Step through cases
%
%   ncase = 1: v > 0
```

```
%
%    ncase = 2: v < 0
%
  for ncase=1:2
    if ncase==1 v= 1; end
    if ncase==2 v=-1; end
```

- When eq. (1.1) is approximated as a system of ODEs based on the MOL approach, these ODEs must then be integrated numerically (with respect to t). There are many initial value ODE integration algorithms to choose from, and here we start with the most basic of all such algorithms, the explicit Euler method. Later, we will consider some other ODE integration algorithms. The explicit Euler method steps along the solution with respect to t using an integration step `h=0.001`. After `nsteps =20` such steps, the solution is displayed. Thus, the numerical solution is displayed at $(20)(0.001) = 0.02$ intervals in t. One hundred intervals are used in the subsequent programming so that t covers the interval $0 \leq t \leq 2$. As might be expected, these integration parameters are problem dependent and are usually selected from a knowledge of the problem and also by some trial and error.

```
%
% Parameters for Euler integration
  nsteps=20;
  h=0.001;
```

- The IC of eq. (1.2) is then defined numerically.

```
%
% Initial condition
  for i=1:n
    u(i)=0;
  end
  t=0;
```

We can note two points about this code:

- The function $f(z)$ in eq. (1.2) is taken as $u(z,t=0) = f(z) = 0$.
- This zero function has been defined numerically in a `for` loop. This could also be done somewhat more compactly by using the MATLAB `zeros` function, that is, `u=zeros(1,n)` for a row vector of n zeros or `u=zeros(n,1)` for a column vector of n zeros. Either format would work in the code that follows (but this is not necessarily the case, especially when using MATLAB utilities that require a particular vector format). Note also that `t=0`, corresponding to the IC of eq. (1.2).

- A heading is displayed at the start of the numerical solution for the two cases `ncase=1,2`.

```
%
% Write ncase, h, v
  fprintf('\n\n ncase = %5d    h = %10.3e    v = %4.2f\n\n',ncase,h,v);
%
% Write heading
```

```
  if(ncase==1)
    fprintf('    t      zL     t-zL/|v|    u(zL,t)    ua(zL,t)    diff\n');
  end
%
% Write heading
  if(ncase==2)
    fprintf('    t      zL     t-zL/|v|     u(0,t)     ua(0,t)    diff\n');
  end
```

These headings indicate that the numerical and analytical solutions to eqs. (1.1) to (1.3) will be displayed at `z=zL` for `ncase=1` and at `z=0` for `ncase = 2`.

- The numerical and analytical solutions, `u` and `ua`, are then displayed at $t = 0$ at grid point `n` (corresponding to `z=zL=1`) for `ncase=1` and at grid point `1` (corresponding to `z=0`) for `ncase=2`. The difference between the numerical and analytical solutions, `diff`, is also included in the output.

```
%
% Display numerical, analytical solutions at t = 0
  if(t <  zL/abs(v)) ua=0;   end
  if(t >  zL/abs(v)) ua=1;   end
  if(t == zL/abs(v)) ua=0.5; end
  if(ncase==1)
    diff=u(n)-ua;
    fprintf('%5.2f%7.2f%10.2f%10.3f%10.3f%10.4f\n',...
           t,zL,t-zL/abs(v),u(n),ua,diff);
  end
  if(ncase==2)
    diff=u(1)-ua;
    fprintf('%5.2f%7.2f%10.2f%10.3f%10.3f%10.4f\n',...
           t,zL,t-zL/abs(v),u(1),ua,diff);
  end
```

The numerical solution comes from the IC programmed previously; the analytical solution is explained next.

The analytical solution to eqs. (1.1) to (1.3) with $f(z) = 0$ and $g(t) = 1$ is

$$u(z,t) = \begin{cases} 0, & t < z/|v| \\ 1, & t > z/|v| \end{cases}. \tag{1.5}$$

Note that the absolute value of v is used in eq. (1.5) so that the analytical solution applies to both `ncase=1` ($v > 0$) and `2` ($v < 0$). Since eq. (1.5) corresponds to a unit finite jump (step, discontinuity), the value `ua=0.5` is used at the point of discontinuity, $t = z/|v|$, for the purposes of computation and displaying the analytical solution. These various properties of the analytical solution will become clear when considering the graphical output.

- The numerical and analytical solutions at $t = 0$ are stored in arrays `uplot` and `uaplot`, respectively, for subsequent plotting. Note for the numerical solution the use of grid point `n` for `ncase=1` (`u(n)`) and grid point `1` for `ncase=2` (`u(1)`).

```
%
% Store solution for plotting
  if(ncase==1)
     uplot(1,1)=u(n);
    uaplot(1,1)=ua;
     tplot(1)=t;
  end
  if(ncase==2)
     uplot(2,1)=u(1);
    uaplot(2,1)=ua;
  end
```

- One hundred and one output points (points in t) for the numerical and analytical solutions are then defined. This number was selected primarily to provide adequate resolution of the solution in t without excessive output; this property is seen in the graphical output that follows.

```
%
% nout output points
  nout=101;
  ncall=0;
  for iout=2:nout
```

A `for` loop then steps the calculations through 100 output points starting at `iout = 2` since `iout = 1` corresponds to the IC (starting point) of the solution that has already been programmed. The counter `ncall` is initialized, then passed as a global variable to the ODE integrator `euler` (discussed subsequently) where it is incremented as `ncall=ncall+1`; thus, each time `euler` is called, `ncall` is incremented by one, and at the end of the solution, the value of `ncall` is displayed as a measure of the total computational effort required to calculate the complete solution.

- The integration of the $n = 51$ ODEs of eqs. (1.4b) and (1.4f) from a starting value (`u0,t0`) to the next value along the solution at

```
t=t0+(h)(nsteps)=t0+(0.001)(20)=t0+0.02
```

is accomplished through a call to function `euler` that implements the explicit Euler method (discussed subsequently). Note that `u0,t0` are input arguments to `euler` and `u,t` are output arguments from `euler` (again, with `t=t0+0.02`).

```
%
%   Euler integration
    u0=u; t0=t;
    [u,t]=euler(u0,t0,h,nsteps);
```

In other words, each successive 100 pass through the `for` loop moves the solution of ODEs (1.4b) and (1.4f) in steps of 0.02 through the interval $0 \leq t \leq 2$.

- At each point along the solution, the analytical solution, eq. (1.5), is computed as discussed before and the numerical and analytical solutions and their difference are displayed.

```
%
%   Numerical, analytical solutions
    if(t <  zL/abs(v)) ua=0;   end
    if(t >  zL/abs(v)) ua=1;   end
    if(t == zL/abs(v)) ua=0.5; end
    if(ip==1)
      if(ncase==1)
        diff=u(n)-ua;
        fprintf('%5.2f%7.2f%10.2f%10.3f%10.3f%10.4f\n',...
                t,zL,t-zL/abs(v),u(n),ua,diff);
      end
      if(ncase==2)
        diff=u(1)-ua;
        fprintf('%5.2f%7.2f%10.2f%10.3f%10.3f%10.4f\n',...
                t,zL,t-zL/abs(v),u(1),ua,diff);
      end
    end
```

- For each pass through the `for` loop in `iout` the numerical and analytical solutions, and the corresponding value of t, are also stored for subsequent plotting.

```
%
%   Store solution for plotting
    if(ncase==1)
       uplot(1,iout)=u(n);
      uaplot(1,iout)=ua;
       tplot(iout)=t;
    end
    if(ncase==2)
       uplot(2,iout)=u(1);
      uaplot(2,iout)=ua;
       tplot(iout)=t;
    end
%
% Next output
  end
```

The `end` statement concludes the `for` loop with index `iout`.

- After the 100 passes through the `for loop`, the 101 values of the numerical and analytical solutions are plotted together with two calls to `plot`. The other plotting utilities (`axis, ylabel, xlabel, title`) are largely self-explanatory; `hold on` retains the plot of the numerical solution from the first call to `plots` (for the numerical solution in `uplot`) so that the second plot (for the analytical solution in `uaplot`) is superimposed; that is, the numerical and analytical solutions appear in the same plot.

```
%
% Plots for ncase = 1, 2
  if(ncase==1)
    figure(1);
    plot(tplot,uplot(1,:),'-o');
    axis([0 2 0 1]);
    ylabel('u(zL,t),ua(zL,t)');xlabel('t');
    title('ncase = 1; num - o; anal - line');
```

```
      hold on
      plot(tplot,uaplot(1,:),'-');
    end
    if(ncase==2)
      figure(2);
      plot(tplot,uplot(2,:),'-o');
      axis([0 2 0 1]);
      ylabel('u(0,t),ua(0,t)');xlabel('t');
      title('ncase = 2; num - o; anal - line');
      hold on
      plot(tplot,uaplot(2,:),'-');
    end
%
% Next case
  fprintf('\n ncall = %4d\n',ncall);
  end
```

The value of `ncall` for a complete solution is displayed and the `end` concludes the outer `for` loop for the two values `ncase=1,2`.

We will now consider the numerical and graphical output from `pde_1_main` of Listing 1.1. Then we will consider routine `euler` for the integration of eqs. (1.4b) and (1.4f).

For each case, `ncase=1,2`, 101 values of the numerical and analytical solutions are tabulated, starting at $t = 0$ and ending at $t = 2$, with an interval 0.02 (in Table 1.1, Figs. 1.1, 1.2).

Table 1.1. Selected output from `pde_1_main` of Listing 1.1

```
ncase =      1     h = 1.000e-003    v = 1.00

  t      zL     t-zL/|v|    u(zL,t)    ua(zL,t)    diff
0.00    1.00     -1.00       0.000      0.000     0.0000
0.02    1.00     -0.98       0.000      0.000     0.0000
0.04    1.00     -0.96       0.000      0.000     0.0000
0.06    1.00     -0.94       0.000      0.000     0.0000
0.08    1.00     -0.92       0.000      0.000     0.0000
0.10    1.00     -0.90       0.000      0.000     0.0000
         .                              .
         .                              .
         .                              .
       Output for t = 0.12 to 0.88 removed
         .                              .
         .                              .
         .                              .
0.90    1.00     -0.10       0.242      0.000     0.2418
0.92    1.00     -0.08       0.293      0.000     0.2926
0.94    1.00     -0.06       0.347      0.000     0.3470
0.96    1.00     -0.04       0.404      0.000     0.4039
0.98    1.00     -0.02       0.462      0.000     0.4621
1.00    1.00      0.00       0.520      1.000    -0.4797
```

```
1.02   1.00      0.02     0.577     1.000   -0.4228
1.04   1.00      0.04     0.632     1.000   -0.3681
1.06   1.00      0.06     0.683     1.000   -0.3167
1.08   1.00      0.08     0.731     1.000   -0.2691
1.10   1.00      0.10     0.774     1.000   -0.2260
         .                          .
         .                          .
         .                          .
      Output for t = 1.12 to 1.88 removed
         .                          .
         .                          .
         .                          .
1.90   1.00      0.90     1.000     1.000   -0.0000
1.92   1.00      0.92     1.000     1.000   -0.0000
1.94   1.00      0.94     1.000     1.000   -0.0000
1.96   1.00      0.96     1.000     1.000   -0.0000
1.98   1.00      0.98     1.000     1.000   -0.0000
2.00   1.00      1.00     1.000     1.000   -0.0000

ncall = 2000

ncase =     2    h = 1.000e-003    v = -1.00

  t     zL    t-zL/|v|   u(0,t)    ua(0,t)    diff
0.00   1.00    -1.00     0.000     0.000    0.0000
0.02   1.00    -0.98     0.000     0.000    0.0000
0.04   1.00    -0.96     0.000     0.000    0.0000
0.06   1.00    -0.94     0.000     0.000    0.0000
0.08   1.00    -0.92     0.000     0.000    0.0000
0.10   1.00    -0.90     0.000     0.000    0.0000
         .                          .
         .                          .
         .                          .
      Output for t = 0.12 to 0.88 removed
         .                          .
         .                          .
         .                          .
0.90   1.00    -0.10     0.242     0.000    0.2418
0.92   1.00    -0.08     0.293     0.000    0.2926
0.94   1.00    -0.06     0.347     0.000    0.3470
0.96   1.00    -0.04     0.404     0.000    0.4039
0.98   1.00    -0.02     0.462     0.000    0.4621
1.00   1.00     0.00     0.520     1.000   -0.4797
1.02   1.00     0.02     0.577     1.000   -0.4228
1.04   1.00     0.04     0.632     1.000   -0.3681
1.06   1.00     0.06     0.683     1.000   -0.3167
1.08   1.00     0.08     0.731     1.000   -0.2691
1.10   1.00     0.10     0.774     1.000   -0.2260
         .                          .
         .                          .
         .                          .
      Output for t = 1.12 to 1.88 removed
```

```
         .                              .
         .                              .
         .                              .
1.90   1.00      0.90      1.000      1.000    -0.0000
1.92   1.00      0.92      1.000      1.000    -0.0000
1.94   1.00      0.94      1.000      1.000    -0.0000
1.96   1.00      0.96      1.000      1.000    -0.0000
1.98   1.00      0.98      1.000      1.000    -0.0000
2.00   1.00      1.00      1.000      1.000    -0.0000

ncall = 2000
```

We can note the following details about this output:

- The two solutions for $v > 0$ and $v < 0$ are identical, which is to be expected since the problem is symmetric with respect to z and t.
- The numerical solution is inaccurate (particularly as demonstrated in Figs. 1.1 and 1.2). Specifically, the numerical solution has excessive numerical diffusion (rounding or smoothing), which results from the two point FD approximation of eqs. (1.4b) and (1.4f). This point will be discussed in more detail later, including the use of better approximations.
- The number of calls to the ODE routine is `ncall = 2000`, which reflects the previous parameters for the ODE integration, that is, `ncall = (nsteps)(nout-1) = (20)(100) = 2000`.

Although the agreement between the numerical and analytical solutions is not satisfactory, we should also recognize that the problem based on eq. (1.1) is essentially

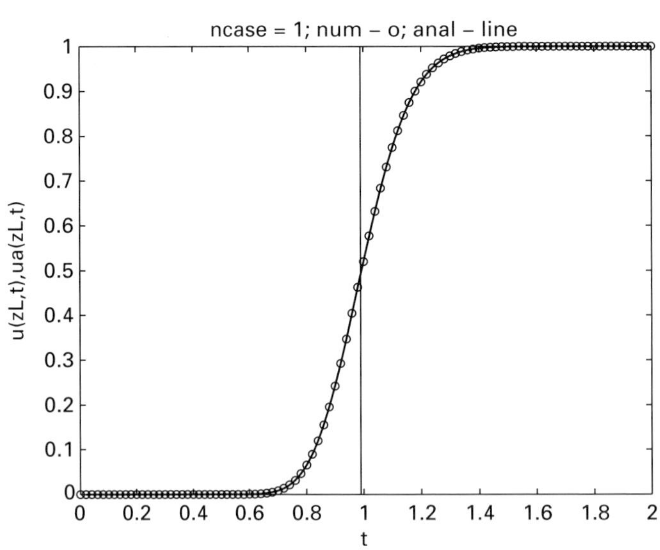

Figure 1.1 Numerical and analytical solutions of eq. (1.1), $v > 0$

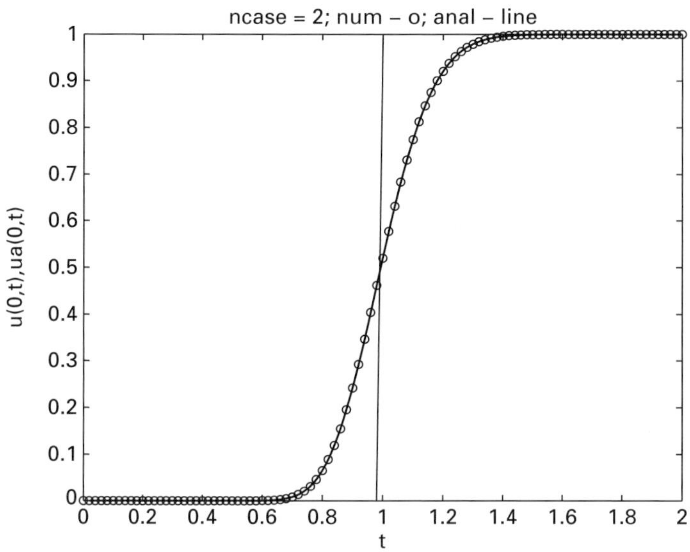

Figure 1.2 Numerical and analytical solutions of eq. (1.1), $v < 0$

impossible to solve numerically. This follows from a consideration of the analytical solution in Figs. 1.1 and 1.2. Note that at $t = z/v$, the analytical solution is a finite discontinuity of magnitude one (the Heaviside unit step function). Thus, the derivative $(\partial u/\partial z)$ in eq. (1.1) is a Dirac delta function (derivative of the Heaviside function), which is undefined numerically and cannot be represented with computer arithmetic. In other words, when numerically integrating eq. (1.1), we are attempting to compute an undefined derivative in z and t at $t = z/v$.

This impossible computation is suggested in the plot of the analytical solution, which is not a vertical line at $t = z/v = 1/1 = 1$, but rather has an offset from a vertical line (essentially due to the limited spatial resolution corresponding to `dz = 0.02`). The vertical line could be plotted correctly (just for the purpose of plotting) but this does not come about automatically because of the offset or finite increment in z and t.

The previous discussion suggests that a smoother problem with a finite slope should be more tractable numerically, and this is in fact the case. We can also add that the problem with a finite discontinuity is not realistic physically; that is, physical systems generally do not produce discontinuities, owing to inherent smoothing processes such as diffusion. This point will be discussed further in subsequent examples.

As another point of terminology, eq. (1.1) with IC (1.2) is an example of a Cauchy problem (an initial value problem). If the IC has a discontinuity (which is essentially the situation because of the change in the IC of eq. (1.2) from zero to one in BC (1.3)), is termed a Riemann problem (an initial value problem with a discontinuity). An extensive literature has developed pertaining to the Riemann problem; later we will consider some numerical approximations for the Riemann problem that perform better than the FD of eq. (1.4a).

Euler method

As discussed previously, computers do not naturally integrate ODEs as a human being would, e.g., to arrive at exponential solutions for linear, constant coefficient ODEs. Rather, to compute a solution to an ODE system, we must first develop an integration algorithm that can be programmed for a computer and basically does not require anything more than arithmetic. We start with the simplest of all algorithms for initial value ODEs, the explicit Euler method.

ODE numerical integration algorithms are generally based on the use of the Taylor series. These algorithms typically step along the solution from point i to point $i+1$, where i is an index for the integration and $u_i(t), t_i$ are the dependent and independent variables at $t = t_i$, respectively. Note that eqs. (1.4b) and (1.4f) are an ODE system with index i that refers to a grid point or location in z; here we briefly use i as an index for t, but when considering stepping along the solution in both z and t, we will use two indices, i and j, respectively.

To take a step in t from i to $i+1$ using the Taylor series, we can write

$$u_{i+1} = u_i + \frac{\mathrm{d}u_i}{\mathrm{d}t}(t_{i+1} - t_i) + \frac{\mathrm{d}^2 u_i}{\mathrm{d}t^2}(t_{i+1} - t_i)^2/2! \cdots \tag{1.6a}$$

If the series in eq. (1.6a) is truncated after the linear (first derivative) term and we assume a uniform grid spacing in t, written as $h = t_{i+1} - t_i$, eq. (1.6a) gives as an approximate stepping algorithm along the solution from i to $i+1$

$$u_{i+1} = u_i + \frac{\mathrm{d}u_i}{\mathrm{d}t}h + O(h), \tag{1.6b}$$

where $O(h)$ denotes a truncation error of order h (the error is proportional to h).

This latter point requires some additional explanation since the second order (second derivative) term in eq. (1.6a) includes h^2 (the one-step error is $O(h^2)$). However, as we shall see in the subsequent discussion, eq. (1.6b) is applied repetitively at a series of points along the solution, and the one-step error accumulates over these successive steps; as a result, the total or global error (after a series of steps) is proportional to h (i.e., $O(h)$).

We can apply eq. (1.6b) to eqs. (1.4b) (or eqs. (1.4f)). However, we have to change the index for one of the independent variables (i cannot be used for both z as in eqs. (1.4b) and eqs. (1.4f) and t as in eq. (1.6b)); therefore, we will use j as a superscript for t in eq. (1.6b). Then eqs. (1.4b) become at $t = t^j$

$$\frac{\mathrm{d}u_i^j}{\mathrm{d}t} = -v\frac{u_i^j - u_{i-1}^j}{\Delta z} \tag{1.6c}$$

and application of eq. (1.6b) to take a step h in t from j to $j+1$ (t^j to t^{j+1}) gives

$$u_i^{j+1} = u_i^j + \frac{\mathrm{d}u_i^j}{\mathrm{d}t}h = u_i^j - \left[v\frac{u_i^j - u_{i-1}^j}{\Delta z}\right]h. \tag{1.6d}$$

A similar argument applies to eqs. (1.4f). Note that eq. (1.6d) can be used to step along the solution with respect to t directly or explicitly, from j to $j+1$ (since $j+1$ does not appear in the RHS of eq. (1.6d)), and it is therefore termed the explicit Euler method. Equation (1.6d) can be applied to a system of ODEs such as eqs. (1.4b) or (1.4f), that is, for $i = 1, 2, ...n$ and that is in fact what is done in the ODE integrator `euler` called from `pde_1_main` of Listing 1.1: `euler` is listed next.

```
  function [u,t]=euler(u0,t0,h,nsteps)
%
% nsteps Euler steps
  for i=1:nsteps
%
%   Euler integration
%     ut=pde_1(u0,t0);
%     u=u0+ut*h;
%     t=t0+h;
%
%   Runge Kutta format - 1
%     k1=pde_1(u0,t0);
%     u=u0+k1*h;
%     t=t0+h;
%
%   Runge Kutta format - 2
      k1=pde_1(u0,t0)*h;
      u=u0+k1;
      t=t0+h;
%
% Next Euler step
  u0=u; t0=t;
  end
```

Listing 1.2 Routine `euler` called by the main program `pde_1_main` of Listing 1.1

We can note the following points about `euler`:

- The function is defined.

  ```
  function [u,t]=euler(u0,t0,h,nsteps)
  ```

  The arguments are

  Input:

  - `u0`: initial (starting) values of the `n` dependent variables (u_i^j in eq. (1.6d) with $j = 0$).
  - `t0`: initial (starting) value of the independent variable (t^j with $j = 0$ corresponding to u_i^j).

  - h: length of one Euler step (h in eq. (1.6d)).
  - nsteps: number of Euler steps (number of steps of eq. (1.6d)).

  Output:

  - u: values of the n dependent variables after nsteps Euler steps.
  - t: value of the independent variable corresponding to u.

  Note that u0 and u are n-vectors.

- Three variants of the explicit Euler method are programmed (at any time, only one is used and the other two are commented). These three forms are discussed briefly.

  - Form 1:

```
%
%   Euler integration
%     ut=pde_1(u0,t0);
%     u=u0+ut*h;
%     t=t0+h;
```

    A straightforward application of eq. (1.6b). The function pde_1 computes the RHS of the ODEs, in this case eq. (1.6c). We use the pde designation in pde_1 because of the MOL application even though ODEs are programmed in pde_1. pde_1 is discussed subsequently.

  - Form 2: A minor variation of Form 1 to put the explicit Euler integration in Runge Kutta format expressed in terms of k1.

```
%
%   Runge Kutta format - 1
%     k1=pde_1(u0,t0);
%     u=u0+k1*h;
%     t=t0+h;
```

    The use of k1 indicates that the explicit Euler method is the first order Runge Kutta method. The use of multiple ks for higher order Runge Kutta algorithms will be discussed subsequently.

  - Form 3: A minor variation of Form 2.

```
%
%   Runge Kutta format - 2
      k1=pde_1(u0,t0)*h;
      u=u0+k1;
      t=t0+h;
```

    The only difference between Form 2 and Form 3 is the placement of the h multiplication. Both forms are used in the literature and the intention here is just to point out this different format for the Runge Kutta method.

- The for loop is terminated and the numerical solution, u,t, is returned after nsteps Euler steps.

```
%
% Next Euler step
  u0=u; t0=t;
  end
```

euler is general purpose in the sense that it can, in principle, be applied to any set of ODEs. The particular ODEs are then programmed in pde_1, which for eq. (1.6c) is discussed next.

ODE MOL routine

pde_1 follows in Listing 1.3.

```
  function ut=pde_1(u,t)
%
% Function pde_1 computes the t derivative vector of the u vector
%
  global z dz zL v n ncase ncall
%
% Boundary condition
  if(ncase==1) u(1)=1; end
  if(ncase==2) u(n)=1; end
%
% Temporal derivative
  if(ncase==1)
    for i=2:n
      ut(i)=-v*(u(i)-u(i-1))/dz;
    end
    ut(1)=0;
  end
  if(ncase==2)
    for i=1:n-1
      ut(i)=-v*(u(i+1)-u(i))/dz;
    end
    ut(n)=0;
  end
%
% Increment calls to pde_1
  ncall=ncall+1;
```

Listing 1.3 Function pde_1 to define the RHS of eq. (1.6c)

We can note the following details about pde_1.

- The function is first defined and a series of variables is declared global.

```
  function ut=pde_1(u,t)
%
% Function pde_1 computes the t derivative vector of the u vector
%
  global z dz zL v n ncase ncall
```

The arguments for `pde_1` are

Input:

- `u`: dependent variable vector at t
- `t`: independent variable corresponding to `u`.

Output:

- `ut`: derivative vector, i.e., the RHS of eq. (1.6c).

Note that `u` and `ut` are n-vectors.

- The BC for eq. (1.1) is defined with $g(0) = 1$ in eq. (1.3).

```
%
% Boundary condition

  if(ncase==1) u(1)=1; end
  if(ncase==2) u(n)=1; end
```

Note the use of the subscript `1` and `n` corresponding to $u(z=0,t)$ and $u(z=z_L,t)$ for $v > 0$ and $v < 0$, respectively. That is, the BC is set at the left and right ends, respectively, corresponding to the entering values of $u(z,t)$.

- For the left end ($z = 0$), $v > 0$ and the flow is left to right. Thus, an upwind FD approximation for the derivative $(\partial u/\partial z)$ in eq. (1.1) is used based on the points `u(i)` and `u(i-1)` (according to eq. (1.4b)).

```
%
% Temporal derivative
  if(ncase==1)
    for i=2:n
      ut(i)=-v*(u(i)-u(i-1))/dz;
    end
    ut(1)=0;
  end
```

The grid spacing `dz` is defined in `pde_1_main` of Listing 1.1 and passed to `pde_1` as a global variable. Also, since `u(1)` is defined through BC (1.4d), the `for` loop starts at `i=2` and the derivative `ut(1)` is set to zero so the integrator does not move `u(1)` away from the value prescribed by the BC (eq. 1.4e)).

As some additional explanation of the upwind FD of eq. (1.4d), what is happening at grid point `i` is determined by what is happening at the upwind (or upstream if the reader is not a sailor) point `i-1` with flow left to right ($v > 0$). What is happening at `i` is not determined by what is happening at the downwind or downstream point at `i+1`. In fact, if downwinding is used (`u(i+1)` used in place of `u(i-1)` in the preceding code), the numerical solution will be unstable.

- For flow right to left ($v < 0$), the upwind point `i+1` is used in the FD approximation (according to eq. (1.4f)).

```
if(ncase==2)
  for i=1:n-1
    ut(i)=-v*(u(i+1)-u(i))/dz;
  end
  ut(n)=0;
end
```

Note that the `for` loop has the upper limit `n-1` since at `n`, `u(n)` is defined by BC (1.4g) and the derivative `ut(n)` is set to zero (eq. (1.4h)).

In general what is required in `pde_1` is for all `n` values of `ut` to be defined numerically before the return to the calling program `euler`.

- The counter for the calls to `pde_1` is incremented and passed back to `pde_1_main` as a global variable.

```
%
% Increment calls to pde_1
  ncall=ncall+1;
```

This statement is what gives `ncall` a value of `2000` in Table 1.1, and serves as a measure of the total effort required to compute the numerical solution. Choosing `2000` calls to `pde_1` is modest and the routines produce a complete numerical solution over $0 \le t \le 2$ within a few seconds on a modest computer for `ncase=1,2`.

This completes the MATLAB program for eqs. (1.1) to (1.3) (or eq. (1.6c)). We have used a modular approach with the main program to set up the `n` ODEs with their IC and to provide a display of the solution after the call to `euler`. The ODE integrator, `euler`, is called separately since it is a general purpose routine that does not have to be changed for each new application. In turn, `euler` calls the ODE routine `pde_1` that is specific to the application, in this case, eq. (1.6c). By using this modular format based on functions, the general purpose and problem-specific routines can be separated, thus facilitating an understanding of the computational steps and the coding.

1.2.3 Temporal integration

We now consider some additional details about the temporal integration (in the initial value variable t). First, with regard to the use of the explicit Euler method, here are some advantages and disadvantages.

Advantages:

- The explicit Euler method is the simplest initial value integration algorithm and it is therefore the easiest to understand. Note that in `euler` of Listing 1.2, only about seven lines of executable code are required to integrate the system of $n = 51$ ODEs.
- Because of this simplicity, we can easily follow the numerical integration step-by-step, which could be useful in understanding how the integration is proceeding.
- Using a fixed-step integration (with constant h), we can specify precisely how many steps will be taken (in contrast to a variable step integrator for which the number of steps is largely uncontrolled). For example, we observed that `ncall = 2000` in

the preceding example and we could set this total number of calls to whatever value we think will produce a solution of acceptable accuracy (by varying `nsteps` and the integration step h in eq. (1.6d)).

Disadvantages:

- Because the explicit Euler method is the simplest initial value integration algorithm, it also has the lowest accuracy or order, that is, first order (see eq. 1.6b)). The consequence of this low order is the requirement to use a relatively small integration step to produce a solution of acceptable accuracy. This limitation of the order is circumvented by the higher order integration algorithms to be discussed next.
- The explicit Euler method has a stability limit that is a characteristic of all explicit integration algorithms. Specifically, for the Euler method, the step h is constrained to a value below $|h\lambda| < 2$ where λ is the ODE eigenvalue with the largest magnitude (note the use of the absolute value in the sense of the magnitude of a complex number, since an ODE eigenvalue can be complex). Although the eigenvalues of the 51-ODE system of the preceding example were not computed to check the stability constraint, the practical effect of this constraint is easily recognized since the solution will eventually become unstable as h is increased (perhaps to try to reduce the computational effort in producing a numerical solution by taking a larger integration step).

In summary, the choice of the integration step h is a balance between producing a numerical solution with reasonable computational effort and a solution that is stable and has an acceptable accuracy. Choosing the integration step is usually a trial-and-error process. Also, if the ODE system is stiff, that is, has widely separated eigenvalues, then an integration step that balances stability and reasonable computational effort may not be possible with an explicit algorithm such as the explicit Euler method. In this case, a stiff or implicit integrator must be used that will generally require additional computational effort for each integration step, but that also allows integration steps that are much larger than can be used with a nonstiff or explicit integrator. The net effect of using a stiff integrator is the calculation of a complete ODE solution with substantially less effort than with a nonstiff integrator. We will consider one such integrator subsequently. Additional discussion of stiff systems is given in [8,11]. A detailed analysis of the stability of the Euler method applied to PDEs is given in [7].

Modified Euler method

The preceding discussion indicates that the explicit Euler method is first order and therefore has relatively low accuracy for a given integration step. To improve on the accuracy of this algorithm, we now consider some integration algorithms of higher order. The first is the modified Euler method, which is second order correct (also termed a second order Runge Kutta method, the modified trapezoidal method [5] or the Heun method [5]).

We will not derive the modified Euler method from the Taylor series, but rather, just present the final result. A derivation and discussion is given in [5].

$$u_{i+1}^{\mathrm{p}} = u_i + \frac{du_i}{dt}h + O(h) \tag{1.7a}$$

$$u_{i+1}^{c} = u_i + \frac{\left[\frac{du_i}{dt} + \frac{du_{i+1}^{p}}{dt}\right]}{2} h + O(h^2). \tag{1.7b}$$

We can note the following points about eqs. (1.7).

- Eq. (1.7a) is just the explicit Euler method (eq. (1.6b)). It is used to take a step along the solution and the result is u_{i+1}^{p}. The superscript "p" indicates a predicted value.
- The result of eq. (1.7a), u_{i+1}^{p} is then used in the ODE

$$\frac{du}{dt} = f(u,t) \tag{1.7c}$$

to calculate the derivative corresponding to the predicted value, that is

$$\frac{du_{i+1}^{p}}{dt} = f(u_{i+1}^{p}, t_{i+1}). \tag{1.7d}$$

- The derivatives at u_i and u_{i+1}^{p}, (du_i/dt) and (du_{i+1}^{p}/dt), respectively, are averaged in the RHS of eq. (1.7b). This averaged derivative is then used to step along the solution with the result u_{i+1}^{c}. The superscript "c" designates a corrected value.
- Thus, the combination of eqs. (1.7a) and (1.7b) is a predictor–corrector pair (designated with the superscripts "p" and "c", respectively). Note in particular that the result from eq. (1.7b) is second order correct.

Equations (1.7a) and (1.7b) can be expressed in Runge Kutta format ([1]) as

$$\begin{aligned}
k_1 &= \frac{du_i}{dt} = f(u_i, t_i) \\
u_{i+1} &= u_i + k_1 h;\ t_{i+1} = t_i + h \\
k_2 &= \frac{du_{i+1}}{dt} = f(u_{i+1}, t_{i+1}) \\
u_{i+1} &= u_i + \frac{k_1 + k_2}{2} h + O(h^2),
\end{aligned} \tag{1.8}$$

where u_{i+1} from the last equation is the numerical solution at $t_{i+1} = t_i + h$. Note again that this result is second order correct. Also, k_1 and k_2 are the ODE derivatives evaluated at different points along the solution. This idea is the essence of the Runge Kutta method and will be illustrated subsequently by a fourth order Runge Kutta method.

The improved accuracy (first order for the explicit Euler method, second order for the modified Euler method) is achieved through additional computations. Specifically, the explicit Euler method of eq. (1.6b) requires one derivative evaluation, (du_i/dt), while the modified Euler method of eqs. (1.7) requires two derivative evaluations, (du_i/dt) and (du_{i+1}^{p}/dt). Since the derivative evaluations constitute a significant part of the total computation, this increase from one to two derivative evaluations is a direct indication of how the higher order of the modified Euler method is achieved. In general, higher

Table 1.2. Comparison of the numerical and analytical solutions for eq. (1.9a) from `euler` of Listing 1.2 for $\lambda = 1$, $t = 1$

h	`numer - anal`
0.1	-1.9201e-002
0.01	-1.8471e-003
0.001	-1.8402e-004

order or accuracy is achieved through additional computations, as will be illustrated by the fourth order method discussed subsequently.

We now illustrate the importance of the second order condition with the following single ODE test problem:

$$\frac{\mathrm{d}u}{\mathrm{d}t} = \lambda u;\ u(0) = 1 \tag{1.9a}$$

where λ is a constant termed an eigenvalue. The analytical solution to eq. (1.8a) is

$$u(t) = \mathrm{e}^{\lambda t}, \tag{1.9b}$$

which can be used to evaluate the numerical solution.

If function `euler` is used to numerically integrate eq. (1.9a) for $h = 0.001, 0.01, 0.1$, the following differences between the numerical solution and the exact solution of eq. (1.9b) result (for $t = 1$):

Note in particular the nearly linear variation of the difference (or error) with the integration step h (the variation is not exact since the order condition for the Euler method, $O(h)$, is only approximate). $h = 0.01$ can be considered adequate (small enough) for most practical purposes since the error in the solution (at $t = 1$) is -0.001847 compared with the solution (with $\lambda = 1$) $\mathrm{e}^{-(1)(1)} = 0.368$ (from eq. (1.9b), that is, about 0.5% of the exact solution).

As another feature of the numerical solution, $h = 2$ would correspond to the stability limit $|h\lambda| = (2)(1)$ (discussed previously). If h were increased above 2, the solution would become unstable. However, it is clear that the accuracy for $h = 2$ would be unacceptable (from Table 1.2). Thus, in this case, the largest acceptable value of h is determined by accuracy and not stability. This will, however, not always be the case. In particular, for stiff ODEs, stability will determine the largest usable value of h.

The preceding discussion also illustrates how the integration step might be selected. Generally when integrating a system of ODEs, an analytical solution such as eq. (1.9b) will not be available (if an analytical solution is available, there is no need to compute a numerical solution). Thus, there is no direct way to determine the accuracy of the numerical solution for a particular h, at least with what we now have available for an error analysis.

However, Table 1.2 suggests an indirect method for an error analysis, that is, vary h and observe the effect on the numerical solution. For $h = 0.001$ the numerical solution is 0.368 and for $h = 0.01$ it is 0.366. Thus the observed variation in the numerical solution is $0.368 - 0.366 = 0.002$, which could be considered small enough that $h = 0.01$ could also be considered small enough. Note that this procedure does not require an analytical solution, but rather, just repetitive calculation of the numerical solution at different values of h. This procedure for varying the integration step is termed h refinement since it involves refining h until the numerical solution does not change by more than a prescribed tolerance. Note also that the result is an implicit error estimate since the integration error is not computed directly or explicitly, but rather, is inferred.

This line of reasoning also suggests that the acceptable variation in the solution could be considered an error tolerance (such as 0.002) and that h could be varied until the tolerance is satisfied. In other words, the computer code could vary h and estimate the error in the solution (by monitoring changes in the numerical solution); once the observed variation drops below the tolerance, the solution could be considered to have the required accuracy (to satisfy the error tolerance). Viewed this way, the code can adjust the integration step in accordance with a user-specified tolerance. In fact, this is one way that variable step integrators work.

Another approach is to use an explicit error estimate, that is, the estimated error is calculated directly or explicitly. Calculating the error suggests a knowledge of the exact solution, but we should note the word estimate since the exact error is actually unknown (if it were known, this would imply that the exact solution is known, which generally will not be the case). The efficacy of this approach then depends on the reliability of the error estimate. An example of an explicit error estimate is discussed next; this approach has been thoroughly studied and is implemented in available ODE integration codes.

This second approach to selecting h (in addition to h refinement) is to compare the numerical solutions from two integration algorithms of different order. For example, for a given h, we could compare the solutions from the Euler method (eq. (1.6b)) and the modified Euler method (eqs. (1.7)). If the solutions agree to within a prescribed tolerance, we could infer the solution from either method to be sufficiently accurate. Going a step further, we could take the difference in the two solutions to be an explicit estimate of the error (as mentioned previously), and depending on the magnitude of this estimate, h could be considered small enough or in need of further reduction. Since in the numerical analysis literature the order of an algorithm is usually designated as p in $O(h^p)$ (for example, $p = 1$ for the Euler method and $p = 2$ for the modified Euler method), this procedure of comparing the solutions and adjusting the integration step is termed p refinement.

We now consider the improved accuracy of the numerical solution of eq. (1.9a) from the modified Euler method as produced by `meuler` of Listing 1.4 (which closely follows `euler` of Listing 1.2).

```
  function [u,t]=meuler(u0,t0,h,nsteps)
%
% nsteps modified Euler steps
  for i=1:nsteps
%
%   Modified Euler integration
```

```
%        ut=pde_1(u0,t0);
%        u1=u0+ut*h;
%        t=t0+h;
%        u1t=pde_1(u1,t);
%        u=u0+(ut+u1t)*h/2;
%
%     Runge Kutta format
         k1=pde_1(u0,t0);
         u1=u0+k1*h;
         t=t0+h;
         k2=pde_1(u1,t);
         u=u0+(k1+k2)*h/2;
%
% Next modified Euler step
  u0=u; t0=t;
  end
```

Listing 1.4 Routine `meuler` for the modified Euler method of eqs. (1.8)

We can note the following details about `meuler`.

- The function is defined.

  ```
  function [u,t]=meuler(u0,t0,h,nsteps)
  ```

  The arguments are the same as for `euler` of Listing 1.2 and therefore are not discussed here.
- Two forms of the modified Euler method are programmed. The first is based on eqs. (1.7) (and is deactivated as comments).

  ```
  %
  %   Modified Euler integration
  %     ut=pde_1(u0,t0);
  %     u1=u0+ut*h;
  %     t=t0+h;
  %     u1t=pde_1(u1,t);
  %     u=u0+(ut+u1t)*h/2;
  ```

  The individual steps are from eqs. (1.7).

  - An explicit Euler step is first taken in accordance with eq. (1.7a) to give the predicted solution at $t_{i+1} = t_i + h$ (`u1`).

    ```
    %     ut=pde_1(u0,t0);
    %     u1=u0+ut*h;
    %     t=t0+h;
    ```

    Note the call to the ODE routine `pde_1` which is the same as in Listing 1.3.
  - The derivative is then evaluated at $t_{i+1} = t_i + h$ (`ut1`) and the corrected solution at t_{i+1} (`u`) is computed based on the averaging of the two derivatives according to eq. (1.7b).

Table 1.3. Comparison of the numerical and analytical solutions for eq. (1.9a) from `meuler` of Listing 1.4 for $\lambda = 1, t = 1$

h	numer - anal
0.001	6.1359e-008
0.01	6.1775e-006
0.1	6.6154e-004

```
%       u1t=pde_1(u1,t);
%       u=u0+(ut+u1t)*h/2;
```

- These calculations are also performed in Runge Kutta format according to eqs. (1.8):
  - k_1 computed by a call to `pde_1` (first of eqs. (1.8)).

```
%
%   Runge Kutta format
      k1=pde_1(u0,t0);
```

  - An explicit Euler step that gives the predicted solution at $t_{i+1} = t_i + h$ (second of eqs. (1.8)).

```
      u1=u0+k1*h;
      t=t0+h;
```

  - k_2 computed by a second call to `pde_1` (third of eqs. (1.8)).

```
      k2=pde_1(u1,t);
```

  - Averaging of the two derivatives expressed as k_1 and k_2 (fourth of eqs. (1.8)).

```
      u=u0+(k1+k2)*h/2;
```

- After the solution is computed at t_{i+1}, the calculation is repeated by the `for` loop for a total of `nsteps` steps along the solution. The final result is the solution returned as the LHS (output) arguments of `meuler`.

```
%
% Next modified Euler step
  u0=u; t0=t;
  end
```

We now consider the numerical output from `meuler` of Listing 1.4 for $h = 0.001, 0.01, 0.1$. We can note the following details about this output.

- For each order of magnitude (factor of 10) reduction in h, the error decreases by two orders of magnitude (factor of 10^2), which demonstrates the second order characteristic of the modified Euler method.
- The errors are substantially less than those of the explicit Euler method in Table 1.2. For example, for $h = 0.001$, the errors are -1.8402×10^{-4} for the explicit Euler method and 6.1359×10^{-8} for the modified Euler method, a reduction of more than 10^3 (and achieved with just one additional derivative evaluation (call to

pde_1) per step along the solution; clearly this additional derivative evaluation was worthwhile).

These reduced errors also suggest that a larger h could be used for a given error. This is true, but the previous stability constraint, $|h\lambda| < 2$, for the explicit Euler method applies to the modified Euler method as well ([1], p94, Fig. 238(i)). In other words, greater accuracy (higher order) does not mean greater stability so that if h is extended (increased) beyond the stability constraint, the modified Euler method will be unstable in the same way as the explicit Euler method.

Fourth order Runge Kutta method

We now consider a fourth order Runge Kutta method, a classical formulation dating back more than 100 years. The basic idea in stepping along the solution from t_i to t_{i+1} is to evaluate the ODE derivative at a series of intermediate points, then take a linear combination of these derivatives to advance to t_{i+1}. The derivatives at the intermediate points will be designated as k_1, k_2, k_3, k_4, that is, four stages, which are defined next in terms of the RHS derivative function of eq. (1.7c) ([1], p91).

$$k_1 = f(u_i, t_i), \tag{1.10a}$$

$$k_2 = f(u_i + (1/2)k_1, t_i + (1/2)h), \tag{1.10b}$$

$$k_3 = f(u_i + (1/2)k_2, t_i + (1/2)h), \tag{1.10c}$$

$$k_4 = f(u_i + k_3, t_i + h), \tag{1.10d}$$

$$u_{i+1} = u_i + \frac{h}{6}(k_1 + 2k_2 + 2k_3 + k_4). \tag{1.10e}$$

Note that this algorithm is explicit in the sense that the calculation of each k requires only the previous ks. The main limitation is the usual one for explicit algorithms, that is, a limited stability region that can be expressed as $|h\lambda| < 2.7$. Note that the constant (2.7) is only slightly greater than for the explicit Euler and modified Euler methods (constant $= 2$) so that again, higher order explicit methods do not have significantly better stability than lower order methods (they have only better accuracy, which is achieved in this case by using four stages).

Equations (1.10) are implemented in the following routine, rk4.

```
  function [u,t]=rk4(u0,t0,h,nsteps)
%
% nsteps Runge Kutta steps
  for i=1:nsteps
%
%   Runge Kutta integration
    k1=pde_1(u0,t0);
    u1=u0+k1*h/2;
    t=t0+h/2;
    k2=pde_1(u1,t);
    u1=u0+k2*h/2;
    k3=pde_1(u1,t);
```

```
        u1=u0+k3*h;
        t=t0+h;
        k4=pde_1(u1,t);
        u=u0+(1/6)*(k1+2*k2+2*k3+k4)*h;
%
% Next Runge Kutta step
  u0=u; t0=t;
  end
```

Listing 1.5 Routine rk4 for the fourth order Runge Kutta method of eqs. (1.10)

We can note the following details about rk4.

- The function is defined.

```
function [u,t]=rk4(u0,t0,h,nsteps)
```

  The arguments are the same as for euler of Listing 1.2 and therefore are not discussed here.
- The calculations are performed in Runge Kutta format according to eqs. (1.10).
  - k_1 is computed by a call to pde_1 (from eq. (1.10a)).

```
%
%   Runge Kutta integration
      k1=pde_1(u0,t0);
      u1=u0+k1*h/2;
      t=t0+h/2;
```

    The dependent and independent variables are then incremented to new values, u1 and t, for use in the next stage.
  - k_2 is computed by a second call to pde_1 (from eq. (1.10b)).

```
      k2=pde_1(u1,t);
      u1=u0+k2*h/2;
```

    The dependent variable is incremented to a new value, u1, for use in the next stage. The independent variable does not have to be incremented since it has the same value for k_2 and k_3.
  - k_3 is computed by a third call to pde_1 (from eq. (1.10c)).

```
      k3=pde_1(u1,t);
      u1=u0+k3*h;
      t=t0+h;
```

    The dependent and independent variables are then incremented to new values, u1 and t, for use in the next stage.
  - k_4 is computed by a fourth call to pde_1 (from eq. (1.10d)).

```
      k4=pde_1(u1,t);
```

  - The solution is advanced from u_i, t_i (u0,t0) to u_{i+1}, t_{i+1} (u,t) by a linear combination of the ks according to eq. (1.10e).

Table 1.4. Comparison of the numerical and analytical solutions for eq. (1.9a) from `rk4` of Listing 1.5 for $\lambda = 1, t = 1$

h	numer - anal
0.1	3.3324e-007
0.01	3.0913e-011
0.001	4.2188e-015

```
u=u0+(1/6)*(k1+2*k2+2*k3+k4)*h;
```

- After the solution is computed at t_{i+1}, the calculation is repeated by the `for` loop for a total of `nsteps` steps along the solution. The final result is the solution returned as the LHS (output) arguments of `euler` and `meuler`.

```
%
% Next Runge Kutta step
  u0=u; t0=t;
  end
```

We now consider the numerical output from `rk4` of Listing 1.5 for $h = 0.1, 0.01, 0.001$. We note the following details about this output.

- For each order of magnitude (factor of 10) reduction in h, the error decreases by four orders of magnitude (factor of 10^4), which demonstrates the fourth order characteristic of the Runge Kutta method.
- The error for $h = 0.001$ is at the level of the machine epsilon or unit roundoff,[1] i.e., 10^{-15} for MATLAB, so that a further reduction in h would not produce still greater accuracy. This conclusion is confirmed by using $h = 0.0001$, for which the error in the numerical solution at $t = 1$ is -3.1863×10^{-14}. This increase in the error (compared with the error in Table 1.4 for $h = 0.001$) can be attributed to the use of `nsteps=1000` for $h = 0.0001$, which is a ten-fold increase in the number of steps compared with `nsteps=100` for $h = 0.001$. In other words, the increased number of steps at the level of the computer arithmetic adds additional roundoff error, but not improved accuracy.
- The errors are substantially smaller than those of the explicit Euler method in Table 1.2 and the modified Euler method of Table 1.3. Clearly the additional derivative evaluations for the calculation of k_1 to k_4 were worthwhile. In general, this is a valid

[1] The machine epsilon, *eps*, is the smallest number for which the computer will consider $1 + eps$ greater than 1. In other words, it is a measure of the precision of the computer arithmetic. In the case of MATLAB, $eps \approx 10^{-15}$ so that the calculations can be performed with a maximum precision of about 1 part in 10^{15}. The machine epsilon is determined by how the computer arithmetic is performed, e.g., 32-bits or 64-bits per word are common formats. The value of the machine epsilon can be controlled by the analyst to some extent, for example, by using double or quadruple precision arithmetic. Also, multiple precision arithmetic is available in some computing systems, such as Maple, for which the machine epsilon can be set by the analyst. Our experience has been generally that $eps \approx 10^{-15}$ is adequate, although certainly there could be requirements for greater precision depending on the application.

conclusion, that is, higher order methods give much improved accuracy if stability is not a constraint.

As a few concluding points about the Runge Kutta algorithms,

- The explicit Euler method can be considered as the first order Runge Kutta method (this is suggested by the dual programming in `euler` of Listing 1.2).
- The modified Euler method can be considered as a second order Runge Kutta method (this is suggested by the dual programming in `meuler` of Listing 1.4).
- The Runge Kutta methods step from the solution at t_i to the solution at t_{i+1}; that is, they take one step along the solution and are therefore termed *one-step methods* (of course, the stepping can be repeated to generate a complete solution). This is in contrast to multistep or multivalue methods, to be considered briefly in the next section.
- The number of stages (derivative evaluations) does not necessarily equal the order of the method ([2]). For example, the explicit Euler method has one stage and is first order, the modified Euler method has two stages and is second order, and the fourth order Runge Kutta method has four stages. However, above fourth order, the number of stages generally exceeds the order so, for example, a fifth order Runge Kutta method requires six stages.

Further discussion of Runge Kutta methods is available in [2].

Stiff integration

The previous example of the MOL analysis of eqs. (1.1) to (1.3) resulted in a system of ODEs, eqs. (1.6c), that were then integrated by explicit methods, that is, the explicit Euler method, the modified Euler method and the fourth order Runge Kutta method. The integration step, h was determined by accuracy, as reflected in the numerical results of Tables 1.2, 1.3, and 1.4, and was not determined by stability. However, as was discussed, stability can limit the step through a stability constraint of the form $|h\lambda| < c$ where c is a constant, typically in the range $2 \leq c \leq 3$ ([2]). This stability constraint will be most restrictive for the ODE eigenvalue with the largest real part[2] (and thus the smallest h to satisfy the constraint). But the eigenvalue with the smallest real part will determine how far the integration in t must proceed to produce a complete numerical solution, that is, the time scale of the ODE system. This is suggested by eq. (1.9b), for which a small value of λ will require a large value of t to produce a complete solution (in order for the exponential to decay to a small value starting at unity).

The combination of the eigenvalue with the largest real part determining the maximum step size for stability and the eigenvalue with the smallest real part determining the total range in t to define a complete solution is the principal characteristic of a system of stiff,

[2] A system of n linear, constant coefficient ODEs will have n eigenvalues. Thus, in the case of eqs. (1.1) to (1.3), a 51 point grid in z produced 51 ODEs with 51 eigenvalues. These eigenvalues were not computed as part of the MOL analysis, but for our discussion, all we require is an understanding that when the eigenvalues are widely separated with respect to their real parts (a stiff system), many small steps are required to compute a complete solution.

constant coefficient ODEs. The reason why this combination presents a computational problem is the requirement of a small h (for stability) and a large problem time scale so that many small steps are required to compute a complete solution.

We therefore consider briefly two stiff (implicit) ODE integrators that circumvent the stability constraint of explicit methods.

The first is an implicit Runge Kutta (one-step) method ([1], p 92; [2]; [5], pp 37–39).

$$k_1 = f\left(u_i + \frac{1}{4}k_1 + \left(\frac{1}{4} - \frac{\sqrt{3}}{6}\right)k_2, t_i + \left(\frac{1}{2} - \frac{\sqrt{3}}{6}\right)h\right), \tag{1.11a}$$

$$k_2 = f\left(u_i + \left(\frac{1}{4} + \frac{\sqrt{3}}{6}\right)k_1 + \frac{1}{4}k_2, t_i + \left(\frac{1}{2} + \frac{\sqrt{3}}{6}\right)h\right), \tag{1.11b}$$

$$u_{i+1} = u_i + \frac{h}{2}(k_1 + k_2) + O(h^4). \tag{1.11c}$$

We can note the following details about eqs. (1.11).

- Equations (1.11a) and (1.11b) are implicit in k_1 and k_2. If the derivative function $f(u,t)$ of eq. (1.7c) is nonlinear in u, eqs. (1.11a) and (1.11b) will be nonlinear in k_1 and k_2; typically a variant of Newton's method is used to solve the nonlinear equations.
- Equations (1.11) are A-stable ([2, 5], p 43) which practically means that the stability constraint of the explicit methods is circumvented. This improved stability is achieved through the additional computation required to solve nonlinear equations. Although the computation at each step is greater than for an explicit method, much larger steps can be used (because the stability constraint is lifted) and therefore overall, a complete solution can be computed by an implicit method with substantially less calculation than with an explicit method (provided the ODE system is stiff). A more detailed discussion of stiffness is given in [11]. Also, Appendix 2 includes the analysis of a 2×2 constant coefficient ODE system[3] for which the stiffness can be set arbitrarily; computer programming for this 2×2 stiff ODE integrators is given in [8], Appendix C.
- Equations (1.11) are $O(h^4)$ so have both good accuracy and good stability.

A more detailed discussion of ODE integration of initial value ODEs is given in [8], [12].

Equations (1.11) are an example of an implicit Runge Kutta method (again, a one-step method, since the solution at $i+1$ requires only the solution at i). We can also consider multistep or multivalue methods for initial value ODEs that require more than one past

[3] A 2×2 (two linear constant coefficient ODEs in two unknowns) will have two eigenvalues, $\lambda_1 = a_1 + ib_1$ and $\lambda_2 = a_2 + ib_2$. If these two eigenvalues are real ($b_1 = b_2 = 0$), the analytical solution will consist of two real exponentials, $e^{a_1 t}, e^{a_2 t}$ which produce a stable solution if $a_1 < 0, a_2 < 0$. If $|a_1| >> |a_2|$, a_1 will require small integration steps with an explicit integrator for stability, and a_2 will require a large interval in t to compute a complete solution. It is this combination that requires many steps when integrating the ODEs numerically with an explicit algorithm. In the test problem in Appendix 2, a_1, a_2 can be set arbitrarily and thus the stiffness ratio a_1/a_2 can be made arbitrarily large, so this problem is a good test of an implicit (stiff) integrator.

value to go to the next point along the numerical solution. A well-known example is the backward differentiation formula (BDF) [5]. We will not go into the details of the BDF methods, but rather, just indicate that they are the basis of some of the MATLAB library stiff integrators, and in particular `ode15s` ([13]). We conclude this section on stiff integration with the MOL solution of eqs. (1.1) to (1.3) (or eqs. (1.4b) and (1.4f)). A main program that calls `ode15s` follows.

```
  clc
  clear all
%
%  Linear advection equation
%
%  The linear advection equation
%
%    ut + v*uz = 0                                        (1)
%
%  is integrated by the method of lines (MOL) subject to
%  the IC
%
%    u(z,t=0) = f(z)                                      (2)
%
%  BC
%
%    u(z=0,t) = g(t)                                      (3)
%
%  We consider in particular f(z) = 0, g(t) = 1 corresponding
%  to the Heaviside unit step function, h(t); the solution to
%  eqs. (1) to (3) is
%
%    u(z,t)=h(t - z/v)                                    (4)
%
% which is used to evaluate the numerical (MOL) solution.
%
%  The numerical algorithms are:
%
%    z (spatial, boundary value) integration: Two point upwind
%      (2pu)
%
%    t (temporal, initial value) integration: ode45 or ode15s
%
  global dz zL v n ncase ncall
%
% Grid (in z)
  zL=1; n=51; dz=0.02;
%
% Level of output
%
%   Detailed output - ip = 1
%
%   Brief (IC) output - ip = 2
%
```

```
  ip=1;
%
% Step through cases
%
%   ncase = 1: v > 0
%
%   ncase = 2: v < 0
%
  for ncase=1:2
    if ncase==1 v= 1; end
    if ncase==2 v=-1; end
%
% Write ncase, v
  fprintf('\n\n ncase = %5d  v = %4.2f\n\n',ncase,v);
%
% Write heading
  if(ncase==1)
    fprintf('   t     zL    t-zL/|v|   u(zL,t)   ua(zL,t)    diff\n');
  end
%
% Write heading
  if(ncase==2)
    fprintf('   t     zL    t-zL/|v|    u(0,t)    ua(0,t)    diff\n');
  end
%
% Initial condition
  for i=1:n
    u0(i)=0;
  end
  t=0;
%
% Independent variable for ODE integration
  t0=0;
  tf=2;
  tout=[t0:0.02:tf];
  nout=101;
  ncall=0;
%
% ODE integration
  mf=2;
  reltol=1.0e-06; abstol=1.0e-06;
  options=odeset('RelTol',reltol,'AbsTol',abstol);
%
% Explicit (nonstiff) integration
  if(mf==1)[t,u]=ode45(@pde_1,tout,u0,options); end
%
% Implicit (sparse stiff) integration
  if(mf==2)
    S=jpattern_num;
    options=odeset(options,'JPattern',S)
    [t,u]=ode15s(@pde_1,tout,u0,options);
```

```
  end
%
% nout output points
  for iout=1:nout
%
%   Numerical, analytical solutions
    if(t(iout) <  zL/abs(v)) ua=0;   end
    if(t(iout) >  zL/abs(v)) ua=1;   end
    if(t(iout) == zL/abs(v)) ua=0.5; end
    if(ip==1)
      if(ncase==1)
        diff=u(iout,n)-ua;
        fprintf('%5.2f%7.2f%10.2f%10.3f%10.3f%10.4f\n',...
                t(iout),zL,t(iout)-zL/abs(v),u(iout,n),ua,diff);
      end
      if(ncase==2)
        diff=u(iout,1)-ua;
        fprintf('%5.2f%7.2f%10.2f%10.3f%10.3f%10.4f\n',...
                t(iout),zL,t(iout)-zL/abs(v),u(iout,1),ua,diff);
      end
    end
%
%   Store solution for plotting
    if(ncase==1)
       uplot(1,iout)=u(iout,n);
      uaplot(1,iout)=ua;
       tplot(iout)=t(iout);
    end
    if(ncase==2)
       uplot(2,iout)=u(iout,1);
      uaplot(2,iout)=ua;
       tplot(iout)=t(iout);
    end
%
% Next output
  end
%
% Plots for ncase = 1, 2
  if(ncase==1)
    figure(1);
    plot(tplot,uplot(1,:),'-o');
    axis([0 2 0 1]);
    ylabel('u(zL,t),ua(zL,t)');xlabel('t');
    title('ncase = 1; num - o; anal - line');
    hold on
    plot(tplot,uaplot(1,:),'-');
  end
  if(ncase==2)
    figure(2);
    plot(tplot,uplot(2,:),'-o');
    axis([0 2 0 1]);
```

```
      ylabel('u(0,t),ua(0,t)');xlabel('t');
      title('ncase = 2; num - o; anal - line');
      hold on
      plot(tplot,uaplot(2,:),'-');
    end
  %
  % Next case
  fprintf ('\n ncall = %4d\n', ncall/);
    end
```

Listing 1.6 Main program `pde_1_main` for eqs. (1.1) to (1.3) with ODE integration by `ode45` and `ode15s`

`pde_1_main` of Listing 1.6 is sufficiently different from that of Listing 1.1 that we will discuss it some detail. These differences are due mainly to the ODE integration by `euler`, `meuler`, and `rk4` in Listing 1.1 and by `ode45` and `ode15s` in Listing 1.6.

We can note the following details about Listing 1.6.

- Any previous files are cleared, the PDE problem is outlined as comments, and global variables are defined that can be shared with other routines.

```
    clc
    clear all
  %
    Documentation comments are not repeated here to conserve space
  %
    global dz zL v n ncase ncall
```

- A grid of 51 points in z is defined over the interval $0 \leq z \leq 1$ with a uniform spacing of `dz=0.02`.

```
  %
  % Grid (in z)
    zL=1; n=51; dz=0.02;
```

  These parameters are the same as for the z grid in Listing 1.1 so that the solutions from these two main programs can be compared.

- Again, as in Listing 1.1, a level of output is selected and two cases are programmed for $v > 0$ and $v < 0$.

```
  %
  % Level of output
  %
  %   Detailed output - ip = 1
  %
  %   Brief (IC) output - ip = 2
  %
    ip=1;
  %
  % Step through cases
  %
  %   ncase = 1: v > 0
```

```
%
%    ncase = 2: v < 0
%
  for ncase=1:2
    if ncase==1 v= 1; end
    if ncase==2 v=-1; end
```

- A heading for the two cases includes the numerical and analytical solutions and their difference.

```
%
% Write ncase, v
  fprintf('\n\n ncase = %5d  v = %4.2f\n\n',ncase,v);
%
% Write heading
  if(ncase==1)
    fprintf('   t      zL     t-zL/|v|    u(zL,t)    ua(zL,t)    diff\n');
  end
%
% Write heading
  if(ncase==2)
    fprintf('   t      zL     t-zL/|v|     u(0,t)     ua(0,t)    diff\n');
  end
```

These headings indicate that the numerical and analytical solutions to eqs. (1.1) to (1.3) will be displayed at `z = zL` for `ncase=1` and at `z = 0` for `ncase = 2`.

- The IC is set and a time scale for t is defined as $0 \le t \le 2$ with an output interval of `0.02` (`101` output points including the IC). The function $f(z)$ in eq. (1.2) is taken as $u(z, t = 0) = f(z) = 0$.

```
%
% Initial condition
  for i=1:n
    u0(i)=0;
  end
  t=0;
%
% Independent variable for ODE integration
  t0=0;
  tf=2;
  tout=[t0:0.02:tf];
  nout=101;
  ncall=0;
```

The counter for the calls to the ODE routine, `ncall`, is also initialized.

- The ODE integration with `ode45, mf=1` (nonstiff) or `ode15s, mf=2` (stiff) is specified. The MATLAB integrators first require the specification of some options through a call to the utility `odeset`. Here, two error tolerances are set for a relative error, `reltol=1.0e-06` and an absolute error, `abstol=1.0e-06`. The use of error tolerances indicates that the integrators are variable step, that is, they adjust the integration step internally to attempt to meet the error tolerances.

```
%
% ODE integration
  mf=2;
  reltol=1.0e-06; abstol=1.0e-06;
  options=odeset('RelTol',reltol,'AbsTol',abstol);
```

Note that the names of the options are specified with `' '`, in this case `'RelTol'` and `'AbsTol'`, and the numerical values associated with these options are set separately, in this case, `reltol=1.0e-06` and `abstol=1.0e-06`. Thus, in this case `odeset` has four input (RHS) arguments, and returns `options`, which is then an input to `ode45` or `ode15s`. Also, the format `' '` defines a character string that is case sensitive (so that, for example, `'reltol'` should not be used).

- For `mf=1`, the nonstiff integrator `ode45` is called.

```
%
% Explicit (nonstiff) integration
  if(mf==1)[t,u]=ode45(@pde_1,tout,u0,options); end
```

The arguments for this call to `ode45` are briefly explained next.

Input:

- `@pde_1`: As before, `pde_1` is the ODE routine (discussed subsequently). In this, case, it is passed as an argument, specified by the `@` (to designate a function (`pde_1`) as an argument for another function (`ode45`)). Thus, `ode45` is expecting `pde_1` with certain format requirements as explained subsequently.
- `tout`: A vector of 101 values of t at which `ode45` will return the solution to the `n=51` ODEs. Recall that `tout` was defined previously and is therefore available as an input to `ode45`.
- `u0`: The ICs for the 51 ODEs, also defined previously. Note that `ode45` does not have the number of ODEs ($n = 51$) as an input argument. The way `ode45` knows how many ODEs to integrate is through the length of `u0` (which is 51).
- `options`: The options defined through `odeset` that specify the operation of `ode45`.

Output:

- `t`: A vector of 101 values of t at which the solution is returned (which should be the same as `tout`).
- `u`: A 2D array containing the solution of dimension 101×51, that is 101 rows corresponding to the values of t in array `t`, with each row having 51 numerical solution values of the 51 ODEs. Thus, `u` has $101 \times 51 = 5151$ values. While this may seem complicated, `u` is actually straightforward to use, as will be illustrated with the subsequent programming for numerical and graphical display of the ODE solution.

- For `mf=2`, the stiff integrator `ode15s` is called.

```
%
% Implicit (sparse stiff) integration
  if(mf==2)
```

```
  S=jpattern_num;
  options=odeset(options,'JPattern',S)
  [t,u]=ode15s(@pde_1,tout,u0,options);
end
```

The arguments for this call to ode15s are the same as for the previous call to ode45. However, a second option is used in a call to odeset as explained next.

- Since ode15s is an implicit integrator, in general it requires the solution of a system of nonlinear algebraic equations as was discussed previously for the implicit Runge Kutta algorithm of eqs. (1.11). If a system of n ODEs is to be integrated

$$\frac{du_1}{dt} = f_1(u_1, u_2, \cdots, u_n, t)$$

$$\frac{du_2}{dt} = f_2(u_1, u_2, \cdots, u_n, t)$$

$$\vdots$$

$$\frac{du_n}{dt} = f_n(u_1, u_2, \cdots, u_n, t) \tag{1.12a}$$

the Jacobian matrix, $\mathbf{J}$, of eqs. (1.12a) is required[4] for the solution of the nonlinear equations

$$\mathbf{J} = \begin{bmatrix} \frac{\partial f_1}{\partial u_1} & \frac{\partial f_1}{\partial u_2} & \cdots & \frac{\partial f_1}{\partial u_n} \\ \frac{\partial f_2}{\partial u_1} & \frac{\partial f_2}{\partial u_2} & \cdots & \frac{\partial f_2}{\partial u_n} \\ \vdots & \vdots & \ddots & \vdots \\ \frac{\partial f_n}{\partial u_1} & \frac{\partial f_n}{\partial u_2} & \cdots & \frac{\partial f_n}{\partial u_n} \end{bmatrix} = \begin{bmatrix} J_{11} & J_{12} & \cdots & J_{1n} \\ J_{21} & J_{22} & \cdots & J_{2n} \\ \vdots & \vdots & \ddots & \vdots \\ J_{n1} & J_{n2} & \cdots & J_{nn} \end{bmatrix}. \tag{1.12b}$$

$\mathbf{J}$ is the $n \times n$ Jacobian matrix, consisting of all first order partial derivatives of the functions, $[f_1\, f_2 \cdots f_i \cdots f_n]^T$ with respect to the dependent variables $[u_1\, u_2 \cdots u_j \cdots u_n]^T$, i.e.,

$$J_{ij} = \frac{\partial f_i}{\partial u_j}. \tag{1.12c}$$

An important detail of $\mathbf{J}$ is that its size, $n \times n$, increases rapidly with n. For example, with $n = 51$, $\mathbf{J}$ is $51 \times 51 = 2601$

- The Jacobian matrix of eq. (1.12b) is usually sparse (many zero elements) because the functions $[f_1\, f_2 \cdots f_i \cdots f_n]^T$ of eq. (1.12a) usually depend on only a few of the

[4] Recall that Newton's method for a single equation ($n = 1$), $f(u) = 0$, requires the derivative $(df/d)u$ in the equation $u^{k+1} = u^k - (f(u^k)/df(u^k)/du)$ where k is an iteration number or index. For Newton's method applied to n simultaneous equations, the requirement of the derivative becomes the requirement for all of the first order partial derivatives in the $n \times n$ Jacobian matrix of eq. (1.12b).

$[u_1\ u_2 \cdots u_j \cdots u_n]^T$. For example, in the MOL ODEs of eqs. (1.4b) and (1.4f), each derivative (du_i/dt) is a function of only u_i, u_{i-1} or u_i, u_{i+1} (two of the dependent variables out of the full set of $[u_1\ u_2 \cdots u_j \cdots u_n]^T$). Because of this sparsity, any algorithm that works with the full Jacobian matrix of $n \times n$ elements will process mostly zeros (which are do-nothing operations). To avoid the processing of mostly zeros, or in other words, to work with only the nonzero elements, a special sparse matrix algorithm is used in `ode15s`. In order for the sparse matrix algorithm to work on only the nonzero elements of the Jacobian matrix, it must first locate these nonzero elements. This is accomplished through the call to `ode15s` as explained next.

- The $n \times n$ partial derivatives in the Jacobian matrix of eq. (1.12b) are generally not evaluated analytically by differentiating the RHS functions of eqs. (1.12a); this is a matter of having to differentiate the n functions $[f_1 f_2 \cdots f_i \cdots f_n]^T$ with respect to the n variables $[u_1\ u_2 \cdots u_j \cdots u_n]^T$, which can be impractical with typical values of n (such as $n = 51$ in the case of eqs. (1.4b) and (1.4f)). Rather, the partial derivatives of eq. (1.12b) are evaluated numerically, typically by FDs. The numerical approximation to the Jacobian matrix is demonstrated in the following discussion of the call to `ode15s`.
- The first step in using the sparse option of `ode15s` is to locate the elements of the Jacobian matrix and assign a numerical value by FD approximations. This is done by a call to `jpattern_num`.

```
S=jpattern_num;
```

  This call produces a map of the Jacobian matrix that is then plotted; the plot includes the percentage of nonzero elements of the Jacobian matrix, which is usually below 10% and often below 1%, thereby validating the use of the sparse matrix algorithms in `ode15s`. The plot of the Jacobian map is discussed subsequently.
- The preceding call to `S=jpattern_num` produces the string `S` that is then included in this second call to `odeset` to specify the sparse matrix option in the call to `ode15s`.

```
options=odeset(options,'JPattern',S)
[t,u]=ode15s(@pde_1,tout,u0,options);
```

  Note that the call to `odeset` includes the input argument `options`, which is for the error tolerance specification discussed previously. The output from `odeset` then includes both options (for the error tolerance and the sparse matrix algorithm).
- The input and output arguments for `ode15s` are the same as for `ode45` discussed previously.

• The numerical and analytical solutions, `u` and `ua`, are then displayed at $t = 0$ at grid point `n` (corresponding to `z = zL = 1`) for `ncase=1` and at grid point `1` (corresponding to `z = 0` for `ncase=2`. The difference between the numerical and analytical solutions, `diff`, is also included in the output (this code is repeated from Listing 1.1).

```
%
% nout output points
  for iout=1:nout
```

```
%
%   Numerical, analytical solutions
    if(t(iout) <  zL/abs(v)) ua=0;    end
    if(t(iout) >  zL/abs(v)) ua=1;    end
    if(t(iout) == zL/abs(v)) ua=0.5; end
    if(ip==1)
      if(ncase==1)
        diff=u(iout,n)-ua;
        fprintf('%5.2f%7.2f%10.2f%10.3f%10.3f%10.4f\n',...
                t(iout),zL,t(iout)-zL/abs(v),u(iout,n),ua,diff);
      end
      if(ncase==2)
        diff=u(iout,1)-ua;
        fprintf('%5.2f%7.2f%10.2f%10.3f%10.3f%10.4f\n',...
                t(iout),zL,t(iout)-zL/abs(v),u(iout,1),ua,diff);
      end
    end
```

The derivation of the analytical solution, eq. (1.5), was discussed previously.

- The numerical and analytical solutions at $t = 0$ are stored in arrays `uplot` and `uaplot`, respectively, for subsequent plotting. Note for the numerical solution the use of grid point `n` for `ncase=1` (`u(n)`) and grid point `1` for `ncase=2` (`u(1)`); this code is the same as in Listing 1.1.

```
%
% Store solution for plotting
  if(ncase==1)
     uplot(1,1)=u(n);
    uaplot(1,1)=ua;
     tplot(1)=t;
  end
  if(ncase==2)
     uplot(2,1)=u(1);
    uaplot(2,1)=ua;
  end
%
% Next output
  end
```

The end terminates the `for` loop for `iout` (programmed after the call to `ode15s` for the 101 values of t).

- The solution for the 101 output points in t is then plotted by a call to `plots` for `ncase=1,2`.

```
%
% Plots for ncase = 1, 2
  if(ncase==1)
    figure(1);
    plot(tplot,uplot(1,:),'-o');
    axis([0 2 0 1]);
    ylabel('u(zL,t),ua(zL,t)');xlabel('t');
    title('ncase = 1; num - o; anal - line');
```

```
      hold on
      plot(tplot,uaplot(1,:),'-');
    end
    if(ncase==2)
      figure(2);
      plot(tplot,uplot(2,:),'-o');
      axis([0 2 0 1]);
      ylabel('u(0,t),ua(0,t)');xlabel('t');
      title('ncase = 2; num - o; anal - line');
      hold on
      plot(tplot,uaplot(2,:),'-');
    end
  %
  % Next case
    fprintf('\n ncall = %4d\n',ncall);
    end
```

The value of `ncall` for a complete solution is displayed and the `end` concludes the outer `for` loop for the two values `ncase=1,2`.

`jpattern_num` for the evaluation of the Jacobian matrix of ODE system (1.4b) and (1.4f) is listed next.

```
  function S=jpattern_num
%
  global n
%
% Sparsity pattern of the Jacobian matrix based on a
% numerical evaluation.  Note: the reference to the ODE
% routine (two places below) should be edited to specify
% the current ODE routine.
%
% Set independent, dependent variables for the calculation
% of the sparsity pattern
  tbase=0;
  for i=1:n
    ybase(i)=0.5;
  end
  ybase=ybase';
%
% Compute the corresponding derivative vector
  ytbase=pde_1(tbase,ybase);
  fac=[];
  thresh=1e-16;
  vectorized='on';
  [Jac,fac]=numjac(@pde_1,tbase,ybase,ytbase,thresh,fac,vectorized);
%
% Replace nonzero elements by "1" (so as to create a "0-1" map of the
% Jacobian matrix)
  S=spones(sparse(Jac));
%
% Plot the map
```

```
  figure(3)
  spy(S);
  xlabel('dependent variables');
  ylabel('semi-discrete equations');
%
% Compute the percentage of nonzero elements
  [njac,mjac]=size(S);
  ntotjac=njac*mjac;
  non_zero=nnz(S);
  non_zero_percent=non_zero/ntotjac*100;
  stat=sprintf('Jacobian sparsity pattern - nonzeros %d (%.3f%%)',...
       non_zero,non_zero_percent);
  title(stat);
```

Listing 1.7 jpattern_num called in pde_1_main of Listing 1.6

We can note the following details about jpattern_num (Listing 1.7).

- The function is defined with no arguments.

```
  function S=jpattern_num
%
  global n
```

  The only input to jpattern_num is the number of ODEs passed as a global variable.
- The dependent variable vector, ybase, is defined at a base value of 0.5. This gives the first of two values to the dependent variables in forming a FD approximation to the partial derivatives of the Jacobian matrix.

```
%
% Sparsity pattern of the Jacobian matrix based on a
% numerical evaluation.  Note: the reference to the ODE
% routine (two places below) should be edited to specify
% the current ODE routine.
%
% Set independent, dependent variables for the calculation
% of the sparsity pattern
  tbase=0;
  for i=1:n
    ybase(i)=0.5;
  end
  ybase=ybase';
```

- The derivative vector at this base value is computed by a call to the ODE routine pde_1

```
%
% Compute the corresponding derivative vector
  ytbase=pde_1(tbase,ybase);
```

- The numerical (FD) approximation of the Jacobian matrix is then computed by a call to the utility numjac.

```
fac=[];
thresh=1e-16;
vectorized='on';
[Jac,fac]=numjac(@pde_1,tbase,ybase,ytbase,thresh,fac,vectorized);
```

The Jacobian approximation is returned as Jac. A brief explanation of the operation of numjac follows.

- The FD approximation of a Jacobian partial derivative used in numjac is

$$\frac{\partial f_i}{\partial u_j} \approx \frac{f_i(u_1,u_2,\cdots,u_j+\delta,\cdots,u_n) - f_i(u_1,u_2,\cdots,u_j,\cdots,u_n)}{(u_j+\delta)-u_j}, \tag{1.13}$$

  where δ is an increment in dependent variable u_j (defined and used internally in numjac). In other words, since u_j is incremented, the partial derivative is with respect to u_j, that is, $(\partial f_i/\partial u_j)$.
- u_j is the base value of dependent variable j in eq. (1.13) (component j in ybase). $f_i(u_j)$ is RHS function i in eqs. (1.12a) evaluated at u_j and computed by the first call to pde_1 (component i in ytbase).
- u_j is then incremented by δ (internally in numjac, according to eq. (1.13)), and the corresponding derivative vector is computed by pde_1 (passed as the first argument of numjac). The result is $f_i(u_1,u_2,\cdots,u_j+\delta,\cdots,u_n), i=1,2,\cdots,n$. Note that all of the other dependent variables (other than u_j) remain at the same values for the first and second calls to pde_1 as required in the partial derivative of eq. (1.13), i.e., only dependent variable u_j is incremented to form the partial derivative with respect to u_j in eq. (1.13), that is, $(\partial f_i/\partial u_j)$.
- The partial derivative is then computed by eq. (1.13) (internally in numjac) and returned as component (i,j) of the $n \times n$ components of Jac.
- As discussed previously, two calls to ODE function pde_1 return vectors of RHS functions, $f_i(u_1,u_2,\cdots,u_j,\cdots,u_n), i = 1,2,\cdots,n$ and $f_i(u_1,u_2,\cdots,u_j+\delta,\cdots,u_n), i = 1,2,\cdots,n$ for each incremented $u_j, j = 1,2,\cdots,n$. Thus, n calls to pde_1, each with a different incremented u_j, gives the $n \times n$ partial derivatives of the Jacobian matrix from eq. (1.13).
- The other arguments for numjac briefly are:

  thresh: Threshold that any component u_j must exceed to be used in the calculation of a Jacobian partial derivative. Here thresh is set to approximately the machine epsilon.

  fac: A work array passed into and out of numjac, but not used in the user programming.

  vectorized: Flag for vectorized operations within numjac.

Jac as returned from numjac is a full $n \times n$ matrix and is subsequently used as a sparse matrix in ode15s after its structure is determined by the remaining programming in jpattern_num.

- The map of the Jacobian matrix is constructed with ones to represent the nonzero elements of S.

```
%
% Replace nonzero elements by "1"
  S=spones(sparse(Jac));
```

  sparse is a utility that converts a sparse or full matrix to sparse form by squeezing out any zero elements. spones is a utility that generates a matrix (S) with the same sparsity structure as the input matrix (sparse(Jac)), but with ones in the nonzero positions.
- The Jacobian map is then plotted by a call to spy (note the figure(3) numbering since two figures numbered 1,2 are produced by the main program of Listing 1.6 for ncase=1,2.

```
%
% Plot the map
  figure(3)
  spy(S);
  xlabel('dependent variables');
  ylabel('semi-discrete equations');
```

  spy is a utility for visualizing a sparse matrix (S). The significance of the two labels will be discussed when the map of the 51×51 Jacobian is discussed subsequently.
- A line is included in the Jacobian map indicating the percent of nonzero elements.

```
%
% Compute the percentage of nonzero elements
  [njac,mjac]=size(S);
  ntotjac=njac*mjac;
  non_zero=nnz(S);
  non_zero_percent=non_zero/ntotjac*100;
  stat=sprintf('Jacobian sparsity pattern - nonzeros %d (%.3f%%)',...
       non_zero,non_zero_percent);
  title(stat);
```

  size is a utility to determine the dimensions of a 2D array (for S, njac = mjac = 51). Then the total number of elements of S is the product of the two dimensions ncaj,mjac or $51 \times 51 = 2601$. nnz is a utility to determine the number of nonzero elements in a matrix (S). The percent nonzero elements is then computed and displayed by sprintf as part of a string; s in the name sprintf designates that a string (stat) is produced. This string is displayed by the utility title.
- Finally, once the structure of the sparse matrix S has been determined, it is returned as the output (LHS) argument of jpattern_num. S is then used as an option in the call to ode15s, as discussed previously. In other words, the structure of S controls the sparse matrix ODE integration performed by ode15s.

```
  S=jpattern_num;
   options=odeset(options,'JPattern',S)
   [t,u]=ode15s(@pde_1,tout,u0,options);
```

We have one additional routine to consider, pde_1, which defines the $n = 51$ ODE of the MOL solution of eqs. (1.1) to (1.3).

```
  function ut=pde_1(t,u)
%
% Function pde_1 computes the t derivative vector of the u vector
%
  global dz zL v n ncase ncall
%
% Boundary condition
  if(ncase==1) u(1)=1; end
  if(ncase==2) u(n)=1; end
%
% Temporal derivative
  if(ncase==1)
    for i=2:n
      ut(i)=-v*(u(i)-u(i-1))/dz;
    end
    ut(1)=0;
  end
  if(ncase==2)
    for i=1:n-1
      ut(i)=-v*(u(i+1)-u(i))/dz;
    end
    ut(n)=0;
  end
  ut=ut';
%
% Increment calls to pde_1
  ncall=ncall+1;
```

Listing 1.8 ODE routine pde_1 called by jpattern_num and ode15s

pde_1 of Listing 1.8 is very similar to pde_1 of Listing 1.3. There are the following differences.

- The input arguments for pde_1 of Listing 1.8 are given in the first line as t,u

  ```
  function ut=pde_1(t,u)
  ```

  while in Listing 1.3 they are given as

  ```
  function ut=pde_1(u,t)
  ```

  The first choice (t,u) was made in accordance with the requirements of ode15s. The second choice was made in accordance with the calls to euler, meuler, rk4, as discussed previously (see, for example, the call to pde_1 by euler in Listing 1.2).
- Similarly, the solution dependent and independent variables are returned by ode15s in the order (t,u) (from Listing 1.6)

  ```
  [t,u]=ode15s(@pde_1,tout,u0,options);
  ```

  while they return in the order (u,t) from euler, meuler, rk4, e.g., from Listing 1.1

```
[u,t]=euler(u0,t0,h,nsteps);
```

This may seem like a trivial difference, but it must be observed; if not, the ODE integration will not be done correctly by a particular integrator.

- `ut` computed by `pde_1` of Listing 1.8 must be transposed at the end

```
ut=ut';
```

because `ode15s` requires a column derivative vector. However, this transpose is not used in `pde_1` of Listing 1.3 since `euler` (and `meuler`, `rk4`) can accept a row derivative vector. The `size` utility can be used to determine whether a vector is in row or column format. For example, `size(u)` would indicate either `51 1` (a column vector with `51` rows and one column) or `1 51` (a row vector with one row and `51` `columns`). Since MATLAB processes vectors and matrices with scalar-like operations, knowing the dimensions of the vectors and matrices at various stages of the calculations is essential; `size` provides a way for monitoring the dimensions at each stage.
- These same differences apply to `ode45` as well as to `ode15s`. We emphasize these differences as illustrative of the attention to detail generally required in using library routines such as `euler` and `ode15s`, that is, the requirements for the input and output arguments must be carefully observed and implemented.

This completes the discussion of programming for the 51×51 ODE system of eqs. (1.1) to (1.3) with the integration by `ode45` (`mf=1` in Listing 1.6) or `ode15s` (`mf=2` in Listing 1.6). We conclude this section with a discussion of the output from `pde_1_m` from Listing 1.6.

Table 1.5. Selected output from `pde_1_main` of Listing 1.6

```
options =

          AbsTol: 1.0000e-006
             BDF: []
          Events: []
     InitialStep: []
        Jacobian: []
       JConstant: []
        JPattern: [51x51 double]
            Mass: []
    MassConstant: []
    MassSingular: []
        MaxOrder: []
         MaxStep: []
     NormControl: []
       OutputFcn: []
       OutputSel: []
          Refine: []
          RelTol: 1.0000e-006
           Stats: []
      Vectorized: []
```

```
   MStateDependence: []
          MvPattern: []
       InitialSlope: []


ncase =      1  v = 1.00

  t      zL    t-zL/|v|   u(zL,t)   ua(zL,t)    diff

0.00   1.00     -1.00     0.000     0.000     0.0000
0.02   1.00     -0.98     0.000     0.000     0.0000
0.04   1.00     -0.96     0.000     0.000     0.0000
0.06   1.00     -0.94     0.000     0.000     0.0000
0.08   1.00     -0.92     0.000     0.000     0.0000
0.10   1.00     -0.90     0.000     0.000     0.0000
         .                                    .
         .                                    .
         .                                    .
      Output for t = 0.12 to 0.88 removed
         .                                    .
         .                                    .
         .                                    .
0.90   1.00     -0.10     0.247     0.000     0.2468
0.92   1.00     -0.08     0.297     0.000     0.2967
0.94   1.00     -0.06     0.350     0.000     0.3499
0.96   1.00     -0.04     0.405     0.000     0.4054
0.98   1.00     -0.02     0.462     0.000     0.4621
1.00   1.00      0.00     0.519     0.500     0.0188
1.02   1.00      0.02     0.574     1.000    -0.4256
1.04   1.00      0.04     0.628     1.000    -0.3722
1.06   1.00      0.06     0.678     1.000    -0.3217
1.08   1.00      0.08     0.725     1.000    -0.2749
1.10   1.00      0.10     0.768     1.000    -0.2322
         .                                    .
         .                                    .
         .                                    .
      Output for t = 1.12 to 1.88 removed
         .                                    .
         .                                    .
         .                                    .
1.90   1.00      0.90     1.000     1.000    -0.0000
1.92   1.00      0.92     1.000     1.000    -0.0000
1.94   1.00      0.94     1.000     1.000    -0.0000
1.96   1.00      0.96     1.000     1.000    -0.0000
1.98   1.00      0.98     1.000     1.000     0.0000
2.00   1.00      1.00     1.000     1.000    -0.0000

ncall =   406


ncase =      2  v = -1.00
```

```
   t      zL    t-zL/|v|    u(0,t)    ua(0,t)     diff
 0.00   1.00     -1.00      0.000      0.000     0.0000
 0.02   1.00     -0.98      0.000      0.000     0.0000
 0.04   1.00     -0.96      0.000      0.000     0.0000
 0.06   1.00     -0.94      0.000      0.000     0.0000
 0.08   1.00     -0.92      0.000      0.000     0.0000
 0.10   1.00     -0.90      0.000      0.000     0.0000
          .                            .
          .                            .
          .                            .
       Output for t = 0.12 to 0.88 removed
          .                            .
          .                            .
          .                            .
 0.90   1.00     -0.10      0.247      0.000     0.2468
 0.92   1.00     -0.08      0.297      0.000     0.2967
 0.94   1.00     -0.06      0.350      0.000     0.3499
 0.96   1.00     -0.04      0.405      0.000     0.4054
 0.98   1.00     -0.02      0.462      0.000     0.4621
 1.00   1.00      0.00      0.519      0.500     0.0188
 1.02   1.00      0.02      0.574      1.000    -0.4256
 1.04   1.00      0.04      0.628      1.000    -0.3722
 1.06   1.00      0.06      0.678      1.000    -0.3217
 1.08   1.00      0.08      0.725      1.000    -0.2749
 1.10   1.00      0.10      0.768      1.000    -0.2322
          .                            .
          .                            .
          .                            .
       Output for t = 1.12 to 1.88 removed
          .                            .
          .                            .
          .                            .
 1.90   1.00      0.90      1.000      1.000    -0.0000
 1.92   1.00      0.92      1.000      1.000    -0.0000
 1.94   1.00      0.94      1.000      1.000    -0.0000
 1.96   1.00      0.96      1.000      1.000    -0.0000
 1.98   1.00      0.98      1.000      1.000     0.0000
 2.00   1.00      1.00      1.000      1.000    -0.0000

 ncall =   406
```

We can note the following details about this output:

- `ode15s` provides a summary of the options that were selected with the `options` utility.

```
options =

             AbsTol: 1.0000e-006
                BDF: []
             Events: []
        InitialStep: []
```

```
        Jacobian: []
       JConstant: []
        JPattern: [51x51 double]
            Mass: []
    MassConstant: []
    MassSingular: []
        MaxOrder: []
         MaxStep: []
     NormControl: []
       OutputFcn: []
       OutputSel: []
          Refine: []
          RelTol: 1.0000e-006
           Stats: []
      Vectorized: []
MStateDependence: []

       MvPattern: []
    InitialSlope: []
```

We can note two details about this table.

- The selected options are the absolute error tolerance, `AbsTol: 1.0000e-006`, the relative error tolerance, `RelTol: 1.0000e-006`, and the mapping of the ODE Jacobian matrix, `JPattern: [51x51 double]`.
- `ode15s` provides several other options that will not be considered here, but are explained in the documentation for `odeset` (enter `help odeset` at the MATLAB prompt).

- The numerical solutions from `euler` and `ode15s` are in close agreement. Part of these solutions (from Tables 1.1 and 1.5) around `t-zL/|v|=0` are listed below.

```
Table 1.1

0.98   1.00    -0.02    0.462    0.000    0.4621
1.00   1.00     0.00    0.520    1.000   -0.4797
1.02   1.00     0.02    0.577    1.000   -0.4228

Table 1.5

0.98   1.00    -0.02    0.462    0.000    0.4621
1.00   1.00     0.00    0.519    0.500    0.0188
1.02   1.00     0.02    0.574    1.000   -0.4256
```

The large difference in the solutions at `t-zL/|v|=0` is a result of the difference in the analytical solutions, not the numerical solutions. Specifically, the analytical solution of eq. (1.5) is undefined at `t-zL/|v|=0`, owing to the unit finite discontinuity. For the solution in Table 1.1, the analytical solution was set to one. In Table 1.5, it was set to the average value 0.5. Of course, there is no specific value at `t-zL/|v|=0`, and a value of zero could have been used just as well.

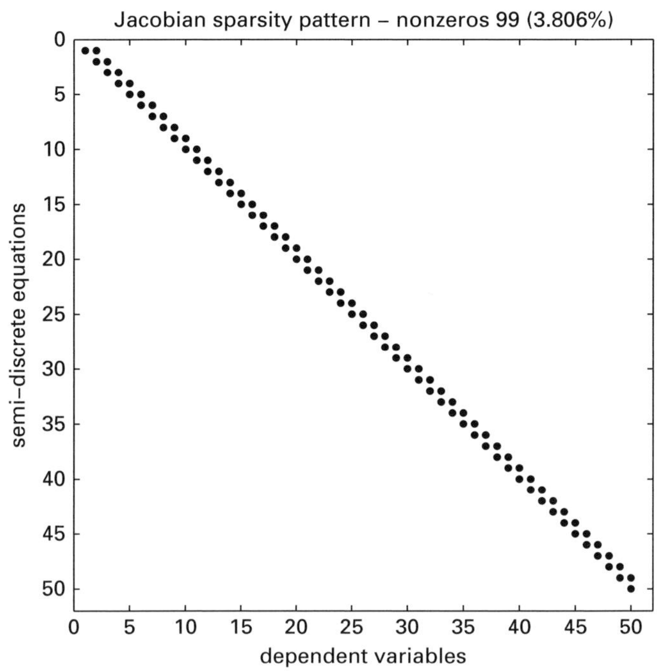

Figure 1.3 Map of the Jacobian matrix from `ode15s` called in `pde_1_main` of Listing 1.6

In any case, the numerical solutions are in good agreement. This suggests a method for evaluating a numerical solution; that is, use two different algorithms, such as `euler` and `ode15s`, and compare the solutions. This approach can be considered as a form of p refinement in which the order of the algorithm (generally designated as p) is changed ($O(h)$ for `euler` and $O(h)$ to $O(h^5)$ for `ode15s`. Note that `ode15s` is a variable order method with the order varying from one to five (and thus the use of `15` in the name `ode15s`); the order varies as the solution is calculated, starting with $O(h)$, which is self-starting (one step).

- The plots produced by `pde_1_main` are not reproduced here since they are essentially identical to Figs. 1.1 and 1.2. Again, the numerical solution has excessive numerical diffusion (rounding or smoothing), which results from the two point FD approximation of eq. (1.4a). This point will be discussed in more detail later, including the use of better approximations.
- The number of calls to the ODE routine (Table 1.5) is `ncall = 406`, which compares with `ncall = 2000` for `euler` (Table 1.1). Thus, `ode15s` was about five times more efficient than `euler` in terms of calls to the ODE routine, `pde_1`. This lower number of calls results from the variable step feature of `ode15s`, that is, it takes steps according to the error tolerances and not fixed steps as `euler`.

`pde_1_main` of Listing 1.6 produces the map of the Jacobian matrix in Fig. 1.3. We can note the following details about this map.

- The labels for the axes originate from `jpattern_num` of Listing 1.7. Specifically,
  - The abscissa (horizontal) label `dependent variables` designates the 51 $u_i, i = 1, 2, \cdots, 51$ in eqs. (1.4b) and (1.4f).
  - The ordinate (vertical) label `semidiscrete equations` designates the 51 derivatives $(du_i/dt), i = 1, 2, \cdots, 51$ in eqs. (1.4b) and (1.4f). The term semidiscrete is an alternative name for the method of lines. Basically, it refers to the replacement of the derivative $(\partial u/\partial z)$ in eq. (1.1) with a FD (a discrete approximation) and the remaining derivative $(\partial u/\partial t)$, which is represented by (du_i/dt) in eqs. (1.4b) and (1.4f), so that eq. (1.1) is only partly discretized or semidiscretized.
  - The map has two diagonals and is therefore termed bidiagonal. The main diagonal indicates that derivative (du_i/dt) depends on u_i according to eqs. (1.4b) and (1.4f). The superdiagonal above the main diagonal indicates that (du_i/dt) depends on u_{i+1} according to eqs. (1.4f); for eqs. (1.4b), a subdiagonal would indicate the use of u_{i-1}. Note that the map for eqs. (1.4f) appears in Fig. 1.3 since it is produced for `ncase=2` in `pde_1_main` of Listing 1.6 (after completion of the solution for `ncase=1`).
  - The number of nonzero elements is 99 out of a total of $51 \times 51 = 2601$ elements, or 3.8% of the total. This small fraction is not usual, and comes from the structure of eqs. (1.4b) and (1.4f), that is, each (du_i/dt) depends on only two values of u_i, and the remaining 49 are not used in the ODE. This low number of nonzero elements clearly indicates the advantage of the sparse matrix integration by `ode15s` in which only the nonzero elements are used. In other words, the sparse matrix structure determination by `jpattern_num` in Listing 1.7, which is then used by `ode15s`, is very worthwhile.
  - Generally, the map has two elements in each row (for each (du_i/dt)). However, for row 50, (lower right corner), there is only one element. This is due to BC (1.4g) so that (du_{50}/dt) depends only on u_{50} and not on u_{51} from an ODE. In other words, u_{51} is set by BC (1.4g) and an ODE at $i = 51$ is not used to set u_{51}. Thus, u_{51} does not appear along the horizontal axis of the map and (du_{51}/dt) does not appear along the vertical axis of the map. In summary, this reflects the entering (inflow) condition at $z = z_L$ with flow right to left ($v < 0$).
  - At the top left corner of the map, (du_1/dt) depends on u_1 and u_2 according to eq. (1.4f) for $i = 1$. This reflects the exit (outflow) condition at $z = 0$ for $v < 0$.

In summary, the Jacobian map gives a complete picture of the MOL ODE structure.

1.2.4 Front resolution

The disagreement between the numerical and analytical solutions of Tables 1.1 and 1.5, and Figs. 1.1 and 1.2, is due in part to the two point upwind FD approximations in `pde_1` of Listings 1.3 and 1.8 (generally, the difference is also due to the impossibility of calculating a discontinuous numerical solution as discussed previously after Table 1.1 using the FD MOL approach to eq. (1.1)). We now consider some other approximations for eq. (1.1), which will in some cases give numerical solutions that are in much better agreement with the analytical solution of eq. (1.5). That is, they will give better resolution of the moving step or front of eq. (1.5). Since moving fronts are of importance in a variety of applications involving first order hyperbolic PDEs, the front resolution methods to be discussed are of general interest and are the subject of an extensive literature.

To provide an introductory survey for a series of front resolution methods, we consider six methods all programmed with a single set of routines that closely parallel those of Listings 1.1 to 1.5 for explicit (nonstiff) integration in t. Although we will focus on explicit integration, the discussion is readily extended to implicit (stiff) integration through straightforward modification of Listings 1.6 to 1.8 (based on the use of `ode15s`).

Also, to give a clearer picture of the propagation of a steep front, that is, rather than consider just the solution at $z = z_u = z_L$ for $v > 0$ or at $z = z_l = 0$ for $v < 0$, we will plot the spatial profiles at a few values of t. For example, for the case of the unit step between a zero IC for eq. (1.2) ($f(z) = 0$) and a unit BC for eq. (1.3) ($g(t) = 1$), we would have as an ideal solution the propagation of the unit step according to eq. (1.5). This will not be achieved (again, numerically, this is basically an impossible problem, at least within the FD MOL format considered previously), but we can observe how closely the various methods approach this ideal.

We start with a main program that is based on the explicit Euler integrator, `euler`.

```
  clc
  clear all
%
% Linear advection equation
%
% The linear advection equation
%
%   ut + v*uz = 0                                          (1)
%
% is integrated by the method of lines (MOL) subject to
% the IC
%
%   u(z,t=0) = f(z)                                        (2)
%
% BC
%
%   u(z=0,t) = g(t)                                        (3)
%
% We consider in particular f(z) = 0, g(t) = 1 corresponding
% to the Heaviside unit step function, h(t); the solution to
% eqs. (1) to (3) is
%
%   u(z,t)=h(t - z/v)                                      (4)
%
% which is used to evaluate the numerical (MOL) solution.
%
% The numerical algorithms are:
%
%   z (spatial, boundary value) integration: Two point upwind
%     (2pu)
```

```
%
%    t (temporal, initial value) integration: Explicit Euler
%
  global z dz zL v ifd n ncase ncall
%
% Select an approximation for the convective derivative uz
%
%   ifd = 1: Two point upwind approximation
%
%   ifd = 2: Centered approximation
%
%   ifd = 3: Five point, biased upwind approximation
%
%   ifd = 4: van Leer flux limiter
%
%   ifd = 5: Superbee flux limiter
%
%   ifd = 6: Smart flux limiter
%
  ifd=1;
%
% Grid (in z)
  zL=1; n=51; dz=0.02;
  z =[0:dz:zL];
%
% Step through cases
%
%   ncase = 1: v > 0
%
%   ncase = 2: v < 0
%
  for ncase=1:2
    if ncase==1 v= 1; end
    if ncase==2 v=-1; end
%
% Parameters for Euler integration
  nsteps=250;
  h=0.001;
%
% Initial condition
  if(ncase==1)
    for i=2:n
      u(i)=0;
    end
    u(1)=1;
  end
  if(ncase==2)
    for i=1:n-1
      u(i)=0;
    end
    u(n)=1;
```

```
  end
  t=0;
%
% Write ncase, h, v
  fprintf('\n\n ncase = %5d    h = %10.3e    v = %4.2f\n\n',ncase,h,v);
%
% nout output points
  nout=3;
  ncall=0;
  for iout=1:nout
%
%   Euler integration
    u0=u; t0=t;
    [u,t]=euler(u0,t0,h,nsteps);
%
%   Store solution for plotting at t = 0.25, 0.5, 0.75
    if(ncase==1)
      for i=1:n
        if(z(i)>= v*t) ua(i)=0;   end
        if(z(i)<  v*t) ua(i)=1;   end
         uplot(iout,i)=u(i);
        uaplot(iout,i)=ua(i);
      end
    end
    if(ncase==2)
      for i=1:n
        if(z(i)>=z(n)-abs(v)*t) ua(i)=0;   end
        if(z(i)< z(n)-abs(v)*t) ua(i)=1;   end
         uplot(iout,i)=u(i);
        uaplot(iout,i)=ua(i);
      end
    end
%
% Next output
  end
%
% Plots for ncase = 1, 2
  figure(ncase);
  plot(z,uplot,'-o');
  if(ifd==1)axis([0 1 0 1]); end
  if(ifd==2)axis([0 1 0 1.5]); end
  if(ifd==3)axis([0 1 -0.5 1.5]); end
  if(ifd==4)axis([0 1 0 1]); end
  if(ifd==5)axis([0 1 0 1]); end
  if(ifd==6)axis([0 1 0 1]); end
  ylabel('u(z,t),ua(z,t)');xlabel('z');
  if(ncase==1)
    title('ncase = 1, v > 0; t = 0.25, 0.5, 0.75; num - o; anal - line');
  end
  if(ncase==2)
    title('ncase = 2, v < 0; t = 0.25, 0.5, 0.75; num - o; anal - line');
```

```
  end
  hold on
  plot(z,uaplot,'-');
%
% Next case
  end
```

Listing 1.9 Main program `pde_1_main` for the solution of eqs. (1.1) to (1.3) with six MOL approximations

We can note the following details about Listing 1.9.

- Earlier files are cleared. Then a set of comments summarizes the PDE problem, basically eqs. (1.1) to (1.3) for the Heaviside unit step function, $f(z)=0, g(t)=1$ of eqs. (1.2) and (1.3), respectively. These lines are not repeated here to conserve space, but note that the six MOL approximations of eqs. (1.1) to (1.3) are summarized for `ifd = 1` to `6` and will be discussed subsequently. Also, global variables are defined that can be shared with other routines. The first execution of `pde_1_main` is for `ifd = 1`, which is the two point approximation discussed previously (eqs. (1.4b) and (1.4f)).
- As before, a spatial grid of 51 points is defined for $0 \leq z \leq 1$.

```
%
% Grid (in z)
  zL=1; n=51; dz=0.02;
  z =[0:dz:zL];
```

- Two cases are again programmed for $v>0, v<0$,

```
%
% Step through cases
%
%   ncase = 1: v > 0
%
%   ncase = 2: v < 0
%
  for ncase=1:2
    if ncase==1 v= 1; end
    if ncase==2 v=-1; end
%
% Parameters for Euler integration
  nsteps=250;
  h=0.001;
```

  `euler` of Listing 1.2 is used for the integration in t. The `for` loop in `euler` takes 250 Euler steps of length 0.001 so that this loop covers an interval of 0.250 for each output (this interval is longer than before because spatial profiles are plotted for only three values of t).
- The IC of eq. (1.2) is specified for $f(z)=0$. The BC of eq. (1.3) is specified for $g(t)=1$ (at $z=0$ for $v>0$ and $z=z_L$ for $v<0$). t is initialized to zero.

```
%
% Initial condition
  if(ncase==1)
    for i=2:n
      u(i)=0;
    end
    u(1)=1;
  end
  if(ncase==2)
    for i=1:n-1
      u(i)=0;
    end
    u(n)=1;
  end
  t=0;
```

- A brief heading displays only `ncase, h, v`, and three outputs (passes through the `for` loop) corresponding to $t = 0.25, 0.5, 0.75$ (from the integrator parameters above). The counter for the ODE routine, `pde_1`, is initialized.

```
%
% Write ncase, h, v
  fprintf('\n\n ncase = %5d     h = %10.3e    v = %4.2f\n\n',ncase,h,v);
%
% nout output points
  nout=3;
  ncall=0;
  for iout=1:nout
```

- The integration is by `euler` of Listing 1.2. The solution vector u is returned at $t = 0.25, 0.5, 0.75$.

```
%
%   Euler integration
    u0=u; t0=t;
    [u,t]=euler(u0,t0,h,nsteps);
```

- The numerical and analytical solutions are stored for subsequent plotting. The analytical solution is from eq. (1.5) (the point of discontinuity $z = vt$ is given the value zero; this could just as well be 0.5 or 1 since the solution is not defined at the discontinuity).

```
%
%   Store solution for plotting at t = 0.25, 0.5, 0.75
    if(ncase==1)
      for i=1:n
        if(z(i)>= v*t) ua(i)=0;    end
        if(z(i)<  v*t) ua(i)=1;    end
         uplot(iout,i)=u(i);
        uaplot(iout,i)=ua(i);
      end
    end
    if(ncase==2)
      for i=1:n
```

```
        if(z(i)>=z(n)-abs(v)*t) ua(i)=0;    end
        if(z(i)< z(n)-abs(v)*t) ua(i)=1;    end
         uplot(iout,i)=u(i);
        uaplot(iout,i)=ua(i);
      end
    end
%
% Next output
  end
```

The end ends the `for` loop in `iout`.

- The plotting of the solutions for `ncase=1,2` requires a set of calls to the `axis` utility because the solutions vary considerably with `ifd`; an alternative would be to rely on the automatic axis scaling, but the resulting plots are not quite as well-formatted as with the specification of the axes through `axis`.

```
%
% Plots for ncase = 1, 2
  figure(ncase);
  plot(z,uplot,'-o');
  if(ifd==1)axis([0 1 0 1]); end
  if(ifd==2)axis([0 1 0 1.5]); end
  if(ifd==3)axis([0 1 -0.5 1.5]); end
  if(ifd==4)axis([0 1 0 1]); end
  if(ifd==5)axis([0 1 0 1]); end
  if(ifd==6)axis([0 1 0 1]); end
  ylabel('u(z,t),ua(z,t)');xlabel('z');
  if(ncase==1)
    title('ncase=1, v > 0; t=0.25, 0.5, 0.75; num - o; anal - line');
  end
  if(ncase==2)
    title('ncase=2, v < 0; t=0.25, 0.5, 0.75; num - o; anal - line');
  end
  hold on
  plot(z,uaplot,'-');
%
% Next case
  end
```

The end ends the `for` loop for `ncase`. Note that the abscissa (horizontal) variable is z, not t as in Figs. 1.1 and 1.2. The exact solution could be drawn with a vertical line at the point of discontinuity $z = vt$. In other words, `plot` does not require single-valued data, but rather, two different points could be plotted as $ua(z = vt, t) = 0$ and $ua(z = vt, t) = 1$. This alternative is not difficult to program but it does require a little elementary logic and two values of ua for the same value of z. Instead, we plot the solution with the analytical solution departing from a vertical line at the three points $z = vt$, $t = 0.25, 0.5, 0.75$ or $z = 0.25, 0.5, 0.75$ with $v = 1$ (owing to the interval `dz=0.02`).

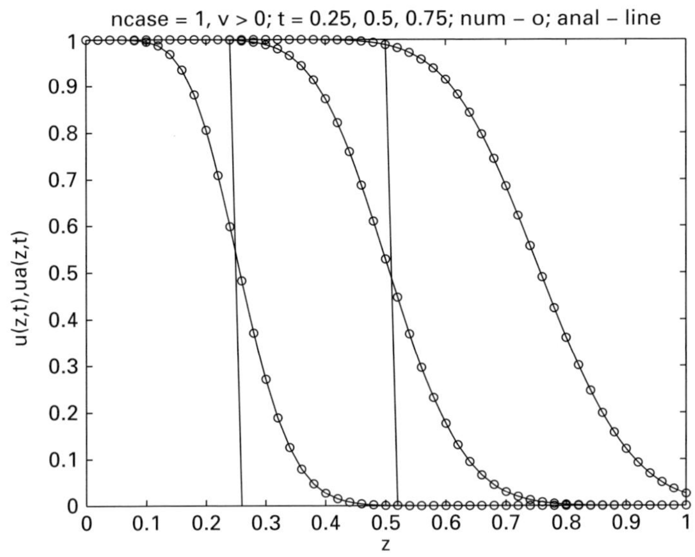

Figure 1.4 Spatial profiles of the MOL solution of eqs. (1.1) to (1.3) with two point upwinding

The tabular output is just

```
ncase =     1     h = 1.000e-003     v = 1.00

ncase =     2     h = 1.000e-003     v = -1.00
```

which provides an indication that the two cases, `ncase=1,2`, executed.

The plot for `ncase=1` is in Fig. 1.4.

We can arrive at the following conclusions about this plot.

- The numerical diffusion is again apparent (as in Figs. 1.1 and 1.2) as the solution moves left to right.
- Generally, any application for which an accurate resolution of a moving front is required probably should not be based on a two point upwind FD approximation of a convective derivative, in this case $(\partial u/\partial z)$ approximated by eq. (1.4a).

The plot for `ncase=2` is not presented since it is identical to Fig. 1.4 (but the front moves right to left).

The ODE routine `pde_1` called by `euler` is listed next.

```
  function ut=pde_1(u,t)
%
% Function pde_1 computes the t derivative vector of the u vector
%
  global z dz zL v ifd n ncase ncall
%
% Boundary condition
  if(ncase==1) u(1)=1; end
```

```
  if(ncase==2) u(n)=1; end
%
% uz; approximation selected by ifd
%
%   ifd = 1: Two point upwind finite difference (2pu)
    if(ifd==1) [uz]=dss012(0,zL,n,u,v); end
%
%   ifd = 2: Three point center finite difference (3pc)
    if(ifd==2) [uz]=dss002(0,zL,n,u); end
%
%   ifd = 3: Five point biased upwind approximation (5pbu)
    if(ifd==3) [uz]=dss020(0,zL,n,u,v); end
%
%   ifd = 4: van Leer flux limiter
    if(ifd==4) [uz]=vanl(0,zL,n,u,v); end
%
%   ifd = 5: Superbee flux limiter
    if(ifd==5) [uz]=super(0,zL,n,u,v); end
%
%   ifd = 6: Smart flux limiter
    if(ifd==6) [uz]=smart(0,zL,n,u,v); end
%
% ut (PDE)
  ut=-v*uz;
  if(ncase==1) ut(1)=0; end
  if(ncase==2) ut(n)=0; end
%
% Increment calls to pde_1
  ncall=ncall+1;
```

Listing 1.10 ODE routine pde_1 called by euler of Listing 1.2

We can note the following details about pde_1.

- The function is defined and selected variables are declared global so they can be shared with other routines.

```
  function ut=pde_1(u,t)
%
% Function pde_1 computes the t derivative vector of the u vector
%
  global z dz zL v ifd n ncase ncall
```

- BC (1.3) is specified as $g(t) = 1$ for the two cases $v > 0, v < 0$.

```
%
% Boundary condition
  if(ncase==1) u(1)=1; end
  if(ncase==2) u(n)=1; end
```

- The convective derivative $(\partial u/\partial z)$ in eq. (1.1) is approximated by one of six methods selected by ifd (discussed subsequently). In particular, dss012 implements the two point upwind approximation of eqs. (1.4b) and (1.4f) with `ifd = 1` set in `pde_1_main` of Listing 1.9.

```
%
% uz; approximation selected by ifd
%
%   ifd = 1: Two point upwind finite difference (2pu)
    if(ifd==1) [uz]=dss012(0,zL,n,u,v); end
%
%   ifd = 2: Three point center finite difference (3pc)
    if(ifd==2) [uz]=dss002(0,zL,n,u); end
%
%   ifd = 3: Five point biased upwind approximation (5pbu)
    if(ifd==3) [uz]=dss020(0,zL,n,u,v); end
%
%   ifd = 4: van Leer flux limiter
    if(ifd==4) [uz]=vanl(0,zL,n,u,v); end
%
%   ifd = 5: Superbee flux limiter
    if(ifd==5) [uz]=super(0,zL,n,u,v); end
%
%   ifd = 6: Smart flux limiter
    if(ifd==6) [uz]=smart(0,zL,n,u,v); end
```

- Equation (1.1) is programmed using the MATLAB vector facility; the derivative vector `ut` is returned as the LHS argument of `pde_1`.

```
%
% ut (PDE)
  ut=-v*uz;
  if(ncase==1) ut(1)=0; end
  if(ncase==2) ut(n)=0; end
%
% Increment calls to pde_1
  ncall=ncall+1;
```

Note again that the BCs at $z = 0$ (`ncase=1` and grid point `1` for $v > 0$) and $z = z_L = 1$ (`ncase=2` and grid point `n` for $v < 0$) are applied by zeroing the derivatives in t at the two boundary points. Finally, the number of calls to `pde_1` is incremented (and displayed in `pde_1_main` at the end of each solution).

`dss012` is listed next.

```
  function [uz]=dss012(zl,zu,n,u,v)
%
% Function dss012 is an application of first order directional
% differencing in the numerical method of lines.
%
% Compute the spatial increment, then select the finite difference
% approximation depending on the sign of v.
%
    dz=(zu-zl)/(n-1);
    if v > 0
```

```
%
%    (1)  Finite difference approximation for positive v
          uz(1)=(u(2)-u(1))/dz;
          for i=2:n
            uz(i)=(u(i)-u(i-1))/dz;
          end
     end
     if v < 0
%
%    (2)  Finite difference approximation for negative v
          for i=1:n-1
            uz(i)=(u(i+1)-u(i))/dz;
          end
          uz(n)=(u(n)-u(n-1))/dz;
     end
```

Listing 1.11 dss012 for the two point upwind FD approximation of a convective first derivative

We can note the following details about dss012.

- The function is defined with the input (RHS) and output (LHS) arguments.

  ```
  function [uz]=dss012(zl,zu,n,u,v)
  ```

  The arguments are

  Input:

  – zl: lower (left value) value of the spatial variable ($z = 0$).
  – zu: upper (right value) of the spatial variable ($z = z_L = 1$).
  – n: number of points in the spatial grid, counting both end points ($n = 51$).
  – u: dependent variable vector to be differentiated with respect to z.
  – v: velocity in the convective term $vu_z = v(\partial u/\partial z)$

  Output:

  – uz: derivative vector u_z.

- The grid spacing is computed. Then for $v > 0$, the for loop implements the two point FD approximation (used in eq. (1.4b)). Note that for the left end, a two point downwind approximation is used to provide a full set of n values of the derivative approximation in uz.

  ```
       dz=(zu-zl)/(n-1);
       if v > 0
  %
  %    (1)  Finite difference approximation for positive v
            uz(1)=(u(2)-u(1))/dz;
            for i=2:n
              uz(i)=(u(i)-u(i-1))/dz;
            end
       end
  ```

The downwind approximation is used at `i=1` in order to avoid going outside the grid in z (by referencing `u(0)`; also a zero subscript is not allowed in MATLAB). Note also that the `for` loop starts at `i=2`.

- For $v < 0$, the `for` loop implements the two point FD approximation (used in eq. (1.4f)). Again, for the right end, a two point downwind approximation is used to provide a full set of n values of the derivative approximation in `uz`.

```
      if v < 0
%
%     (2)  Finite difference approximation for negative v
           for i=1:n-1
             uz(i)=(u(i+1)-u(i))/dz;
           end
           uz(n)=(u(n)-u(n-1))/dz;
      end
```

The downwind approximation is used at `i=n` to avoid going outside the grid in z (by referencing `u(n+1)`). Note also that the `for` loop ends at `i=n-1`.

- v is not used in the calculations. Rather, the sign of v is used to determine the FD with the required upwinding.

In summary, `dss012` performs the same calculation of $(\partial u/\partial z)$ as used previously (in eqs. (1.4b) and (1.4f)). The plotted solution in Fig. 1.4 demonstrates the large numerical diffusion of this two point upwind approximation, and this diffusion is not reduced substantially by using more grid points in z.

This conclusion would suggest that the solution from the first order, two point FD approximation could be improved by using a higher order method. To investigate this idea, we now consider a three point FD approximation of the derivative $(\partial u/\partial z)$ implemented in `dss002` that is second order correct. This is accomplished by setting `ifd=2` in `pde_1_main` of Listing 1.9, which in turn calls `dss002` in `pde_1` of Listing 1.11.

Briefly, the FD approximation is

$$\frac{\partial u_i}{\partial z} \approx \frac{u_{i+1} - u_{i-1}}{2\Delta z} + O(\Delta z^2). \tag{1.14}$$

More details about the FD approximations will be considered when `dss002` is discussed.

The solution for `ifd=2` in `pde_1_main` of Listing 1.9 and `pde_1` of Listing 1.10 is in Fig. 1.5.

The numerical solution is clearly in error due to numerical oscillation (the second major form of numerical error, in addition to numerical diffusion). Also, the magnitude of the oscillations increases with t, suggesting that the solution would eventually become unstable for greater t (beyond $t = 0.75$). As a related point, these oscillations take the solution outside the interval $0 \le u(z,t) \le 1$, which is the reason for the rescaling of the vertical axis in `pde_1_main` of Listing 1.9 as `if(ifd==2)axis([0 1 0 1.5]); end`. Some additional analysis of the oscillations is given after the following discussion of `dss002` (Listing 1.12).

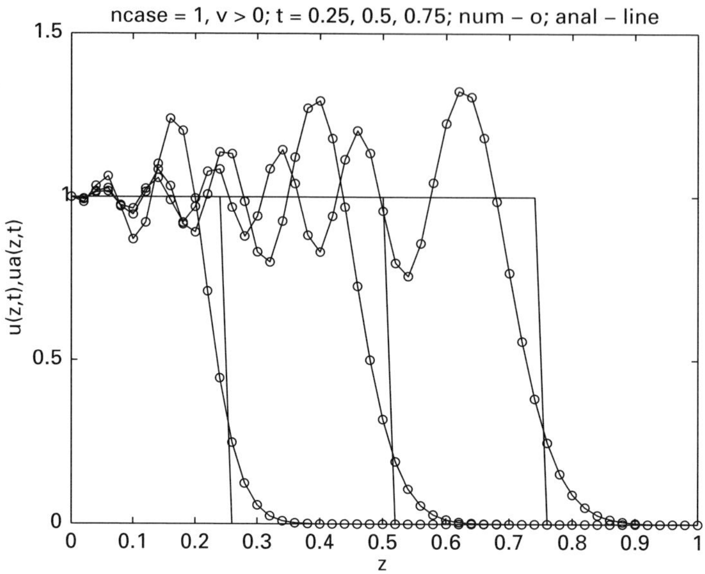

Figure 1.5 Spatial profiles of the MOL solution of eqs. (1.1) to (1.3) with three point centered FDs

```
  function [uz]=dss002(zl,zu,n,u)
%
% Function dss002 computes the first derivative uz of a variable
% u over the interval zl <= z <= zu
%
% The finite difference approximations for uz are based on the
% differentiation matrix
%
%            -3   4  -1
%
%      1/2  -1   0   1
%
%             1  -4   3
%
% Compute the spatial increment
  dz=(zu-zl)/(n-1);
  r2fdz=1./(2.*dz);
%
% Left end.  The following coding has been formatted so that the
% numerical weighting coefficients can be more easily associated
% with the differentiation matrix
    uz(1)=r2fdz*...
    (      -3.   *u(  1)      +4.   *u(  2)      -1.   *u(  3));
%
% Interior points
  for i=2:n-1
    uz(i)=r2fdz*...
    (      -1.   *u(i-1)      +0.   *u(  i)      +1.   *u(i+1));
```

```
  end
%
% Right end
    uz(n)=r2fdz*...
    (      1.    *u(n-2)     -4.    *u(n-1)      +3.    *u(  n));
```

Listing 1.12 dss002 for the three point centered FD approximation of a convective first derivative

We can note the following details about dss002.

- The function is defined with the input (RHS) and output (LHS) arguments.

```
  function [uz]=dss002(zl,zu,n,u)
%
% Function dss002 computes the first derivative uz of a variable
% u over the interval zl <= z <= zu
%
% The finite difference approximations for uz are based on the
% differentiation matrix
%
%            -3   4  -1
%
%      1/2  -1   0   1
%
%             1  -4   3
```

  The four arguments are the same as for dss012 in Listing 1.11. The fifth argument, v, of dss012 is not required for the FD approximations of dss002.

  The documentation comments briefly explain how the numerical derivative uz is computed with a 3×3 differentiation matrix. The download copy of dss002 has a more extensive set of comments that includes a derivation of the elements of the differentiation matrix (generally, from a Taylor series). Additional discussion of routines based on differentiation matrices is given in [10], Appendix 5. The calculation of the weighting coefficients can be accomplished with readily available library routines ([6], pp 201–234).
- The grid spacing is computed.

```
%
% Compute the spatial increment
  dz=(zu-zl)/(n-1);
  r2fdz=1./(2.*dz);
```

- The FD approximation of the left point derivative uz(1) = $(\partial u(z=0,t)/\partial z)$ is computed according to the first row of the differentiation matrix.

```
%
% Left end.  The following coding has been formatted so that the
% numerical weighting coefficients can be more easily associated
% with the differentiation matrix
    uz(1)=r2fdz*...
    (      -3.    *u(  1)      +4.    *u(  2)      -1.    *u(  3));
```

Note that the RHS consists of a weighted sum with the coefficients from the first row of the differentiation matrix applied to u at points $1, 2, 3$ (this is generally how the weighting coefficients of differentiation matrices discussed subsequently are used). An important point is that only values of u at the boundary (u(1)) and in the interior (u(2),u(3)) are used in the calculation of uz(1); approximations of this form are termed one-sided.

The division of this weighted sum by $2\Delta z$ (according to eq. (1.14)) is accomplished by multiplication by r2fdz. The components of this variable name are derived in the following way:

- r: reciprocal;
- 2f: two factorial, 2!;
- dz: grid spacing.

Thus r2fdz = $(1/2!\Delta z)$.

- The FD approximation of the interior point derivatives uz(i) = $(\partial u(z,t)/\partial z)$, i=2,3,...,n-1 or $z \neq 0, z \neq z_L$, are computed according to the second row of the differentiation matrix.

```
%
% Interior points
  for i=2:n-1
    uz(i)=r2fdz*...
    (      -1.    *u(i-1)      +0.    *u(  i)      +1.    *u(i+1));
  end
```

Note that the RHS consists of a weighted sum with the coefficients from the second row of the differentiation matrix applied to u at points $i-1, i, i+1$. Since the values of u are located symmetrically around point i, the approximation is termed a centered FD.

Also, the weighting coefficient for the center point i (zero) is included in the code even though multiplication by zero is a do-nothing operation in forming the weighted sum of uz(i). This was done to illustrate the correspondence with the second row of the differentiation matrix.

- The FD approximation of the right point derivative uz(n) = $(\partial u(z = z_u, t)/\partial z)$ is computed according to the third row of the differentiation matrix.

```
%
% Right end
    uz(n)=r2fdz*...
    (       1.    *u(n-2)      -4.    *u(n-1)      +3.    *u(  n));
```

Again, the RHS consists of a weighted sum with the coefficients from the third row of the differentiation matrix applied u at points $n-2, n-1, n$ so that only values of u at the boundary (u(n)) and in the interior (u(n-1),u(n-2)) are used in the calculation of uz(n); this is again a one-sided FD approximation.

- The final result of these calculations is the derivative n-vector uz that is returned as the output (LHS) argument of dss002.

- Two basic characteristics of the differentiation matrix in `dss002` can be noted.
  - The weighting coefficients in any row sum to zero. For example, in the first row, $-3+4-1=0$. This basic property is required for the differentiation of a constant to zero (consider, for example, if `u(1) = u(2) = u(3) = c` in the calculation of `uz(1)`).
  - If a diagonal is drawn through the central element of the matrix (through `0`), the coefficients along the diagonal are antisymmetric, that is, they change sign. This is a characteristic of differentiation matrices for odd order derivatives (such as first order).

  These two properties apply to differentiation matrices of any order (size); they are useful in checking a new matrix and the associated programming.

In summary, `dss002` performs the calculation of $(\partial u/\partial z)$ in eqs. (1.4b) and (1.4f). The plotted solution in Fig. 1.5 demonstrates the large numerical oscillation produced by the three point approximations in `dss002`. This oscillation increases substantially with more grid points in z (larger values of n). Also, increasing the order (size) of the differentiation matrix does not reduce the numerical oscillation. Thus, we come to the conclusion that centered FDs generally should not be used to approximate first order convective derivatives.

Since two point upwind FD approximations give excessive numerical diffusion, but no oscillation, possibly including upwinding in the higher order centered approximations could be used to reduce the oscillation of the latter. To test this idea, we next consider five point, biased upwind FD approximations (in `dss020`) by using `ifd=3` in `pde_1_main` and `pde_1` of Listings 1.9 and 1.10.

`dss020` is listed next.

```
  function [uz]=dss020(zl,zu,n,u,v)
%
% Function dss020 computes the first derivative, uz, of a vector u
% by five point, biased upwind approximations.
%
% Compute the common factor for each FD approximation.  Then select
% the FD approximation depending on the sign of v (fifth argument).
  dz=(zu-zl)/(n-1);
  r4fdz=1./(12.*dz);
%
% (1)  FD approximation for positive v
  if v > 0.
    uz(  1)=r4fdz*...
    ( -25.      *u(  1)...
      +48.      *u(  2)...
      -36.      *u(  3)...
      +16.      *u(  4)...
       -3.      *u(  5));
    uz(  2)=r4fdz*...
    (  -3.      *u(  1)...
      -10.      *u(  2)...
```

```
      +18.     *u(  3)...
       -6.     *u(  4)...
       +1.     *u(  5));
    uz(  3)=r4fdz*...
    (  +1.     *u(  1)...
       -8.     *u(  2)...
       +0.     *u(  3)...
       +8.     *u(  4)...
       -1.     *u(  5));
    for i=4:n-1
    uz(  i)=r4fdz*...
    (  -1.     *u(i-3)...
       +6.     *u(i-2)...
      -18.     *u(i-1)...
      +10.     *u(i  )...
       +3.     *u(i+1));
    end
    uz(  n)=r4fdz*...
    (  +3.     *u(n-4)...
      -16.     *u(n-3)...
      +36.     *u(n-2)...
      -48.     *u(n-1)...
      +25.     *u(n  ));
    end
%
% (2)  FD approximation for negative v
  if v < 0.
    uz(  1)=r4fdz*...
    ( -25.     *u(  1)...
      +48.     *u(  2)...
      -36.     *u(  3)...
      +16.     *u(  4)...
       -3.     *u(  5));
    nm3=n-3;
    for i=2:nm3
    uz(  i)=r4fdz*...
    (  -3.     *u(i-1)...
      -10.     *u(i  )...
      +18.     *u(i+1)...
       -6.     *u(i+2)...
       +1.     *u(i+3));
    end
    uz(n-2)=r4fdz*...
    (  +1.     *u(n-4)...
       -8.     *u(n-3)...
       +0.     *u(n-2)...
       +8.     *u(n-1)...
       -1.     *u(n  ));
    uz(n-1)=r4fdz*...
    (  -1.     *u(n-4)...
       +6.     *u(n-3)...
```

```
    -18.      *u(n-2)...
    +10.      *u(n-1)...
     +3.      *u(n  ));
  uz(  n)=r4fdz*...
  (  +3.      *u(n-4)...
    -16.      *u(n-3)...
    +36.      *u(n-2)...
    -48.      *u(n-1)...
    +25.      *u(n  ));
  end
```

Listing 1.13 dss020 for the five point biased upwind FD approximation of a convective first derivative

We can note the following details about dss020.

- The function is defined with the input (RHS) and output (LHS) arguments.

```
  function [uz]=dss020(zl,zu,n,u,v)
%
% Function dss020 computes the first derivative, uz, of a vector u
% by five point, biased upwind approximations.
```

  The arguments are the same as for dss012 in Listing 1.11.
- The grid spacing is computed.

```
%
% Compute the common factor for each FD approximation.  Then select
% the FD approximation depending on the sign of v (fifth argument).
  dz=(zu-zl)/(n-1);
  r4fdz=1./(12.*dz);
```

- The FD approximation of the left point derivative uz(1) = $(\partial u(z = z_l = 0,t)/\partial z)$ is computed.

```
%
% (1)  FD approximation for positive v
  if v > 0.
    uz(  1)=r4fdz*...
    ( -25.      *u(  1)...
      +48.      *u(  2)...
      -36.      *u(  3)...
      +16.      *u(  4)...
       -3.      *u(  5));
```

  This coding indicates that the first row of the 5×5 differentiation matrix is

$$-25 \quad 48 \quad -36 \quad 16 \quad -3.$$

  Only values of u at the boundary (u(1)) and in the interior (u(2),u(3),u(4),u(5)) are used in the calculation of uz(1); thus, this approximation is one-sided. Also, the coefficients sum to zero, as noted previously.
- The FD approximation one grid point inside the left boundary (at $z = z_l + \Delta z$) is

```
uz( 2)=r4fdz*...
( -3.     *u( 1)...
 -10.     *u( 2)...
 +18.     *u( 3)...
  -6.     *u( 4)...
  +1.     *u( 5));
```

This coding indicates that the second row of the 5×5 differentiation matrix is

$$-3 \quad -10 \quad 18 \quad -6 \quad 1.$$

Only values of u at the boundary (u(1)) and in the interior (u(2),u(3),u(4),u(5)) are used in the calculation of uz(2), so this approximation is one-sided. Also, the coefficients sum to zero as noted previously.

- The FD approximation two grid points inside the left boundary (at $z = z_l + 2\Delta z$) is

```
uz( 3)=r4fdz*...
( +1.     *u( 1)...
  -8.     *u( 2)...
  +0.     *u( 3)...
  +8.     *u( 4)...
  -1.     *u( 5));
```

This coding indicates that the second row of the 5×5 differentiation matrix is

$$1 \quad -8 \quad 0 \quad 8 \quad -1.$$

Values of u at the boundary (u(1)) and in the interior (u(2),u(3),u(4),u(5)) are used in the calculation of uz(3). However, this is a centered approximation (the derivative is calculated at $i = 3$, which is at the center of the points $i = 1,2,3,4,5$). Just to emphasize a basic point, although a centered approximation is used for uz(3), this approximation is used at only one point (i=3) and not throughout the interior of the z grid. This will be done with the next approximation. Also, the coefficients sum to zero and have the antisymmetric property (change in sign around the center point 0), as noted previously.

- The FD approximation of the interior point derivatives uz(i) = $(\partial u(z,t)/\partial z)$, i=4,5,...,n-3,n-2,n-1 are computed within a for loop.

```
for i=4:n-1
uz( i)=r4fdz*...
( -1.     *u(i-3)...
  +6.     *u(i-2)...
 -18.     *u(i-1)...
 +10.     *u(i  )...
  +3.     *u(i+1));
end
```

This coding indicates that the fourth row of the 5×5 differentiation matrix is

$$-1 \quad 6 \quad 18 \quad 10 \quad 3.$$

Note that the numerical derivative at point `i`, `uz(i))`, is computed using three upwind points `u(i-3),u(i-2),u(i-1)` and one downwind point `u(i+1)`. Thus the approximation weights the upwind direction more heavily and is therefore termed a biased upwind FD. Qualitatively, the idea is that by using some upwinding, the numerical oscillations of the centered FDs (see Fig. 1.5) would be reduced. While this does occur, the result is still not satisfactory, as demonstrated in Fig. 1.6.

- The FD approximation of the right point derivative `uz(n)` = $(\partial u(z = z_u = z_L, t)/\partial z)$ is computed.

```
uz(  n)=r4fdz*...
(  +3.      *u(n-4)...
  -16.      *u(n-3)...
  +36.      *u(n-2)...
  -48.      *u(n-1)...
  +25.      *u(n  ));
end
```

  This coding indicates that the fifth row of the 5×5 differentiation matrix is

$$3 \quad -16 \quad 36 \quad -48 \quad 25.$$

  Values of `u` at the boundary (`u(n)`) and in the interior (`u(n-4),u(n-3),u(n-2),u(n-1)`) are used in the calculation of `uz(n)`, so this approximation is one-sided. Also, the coefficients sum to zero, as noted previously.
- The final result of these calculations is the derivative n-vector `uz` that is returned as the output (LHS) argument of `dss020`.
- The usual basic characteristic of the differentiation matrix in `dss020` can be noted, that is, the weighting coefficients in any row sum to zero.
- Although the differentiation matrix of eq. (1.15) (below) is $O(\Delta z^4)$, this higher order does not assure an accurate numerical PDE solution.

The preceding sets of weighting coefficients can be combined into a 5×5 differentiation matrix.

$$\frac{2}{4!}\begin{bmatrix} -25 & 48 & -36 & 16 & -3 \\ -3 & -10 & 18 & -6 & 1 \\ 1 & -8 & 0 & 8 & -1 \\ -1 & 6 & 18 & 10 & 3 \\ 3 & -16 & 36 & -48 & 25 \end{bmatrix}. \tag{1.15}$$

A common factor of 2 has been placed outside the matrix so that $(2/4!) = (2/24) = (1/12)$ is the constant used in `r24fdz` of Listing 1.13. The antisymmetric property of the differentiation matrix of eq. (1.15) is clear. The coding for $v < 0$ involves a straightforward reversal of the weighting coefficients in the second half of `dss020` in Listing 1.13.

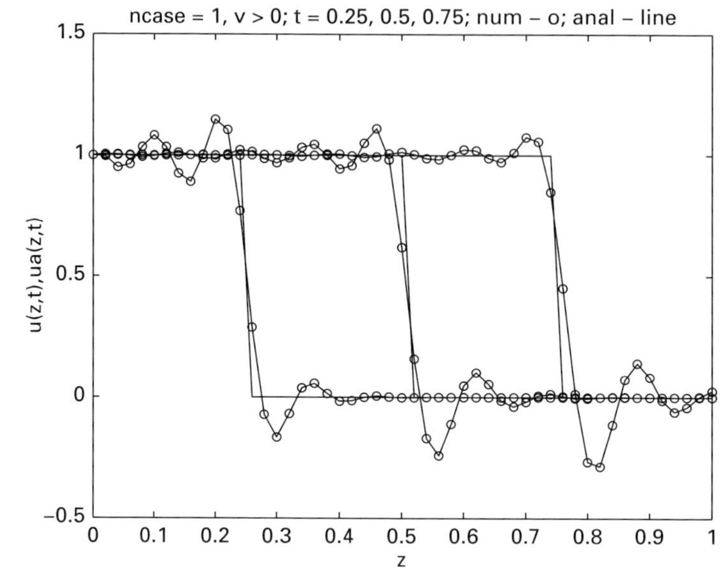

Figure 1.6 Spatial profiles of the MOL solution of eqs. (1.1) to (1.3) with five point biased upwind FDs

In summary, `dss020` performs the approximate calculation of $(\partial u/\partial z)$ in eqs. (1.4b) and (1.4f). The plotted solution in Fig. 1.6 demonstrates the large numerical diffusion and oscillation produced by the five point biased upwind approximations in `dss020` (which necessitated the scaling of the vertical axis according to `if(ifd==3)axis([0 1 -0.5 1.5]; end` in `pde_1` of Listing 1.9). The quality of the numerical solution does not improve substantially with more points in z (larger values of n). Also, increasing the order (size) of the differentiation matrix does not reduce the numerical distortions. Thus, we come to the conclusion that biased upwind FDs generally should not be used to resolve discontinuities and sharp moving fronts.

The oscillations of the numerical solutions in Figs. 1.5 and 1.6 illustrate the conclusion from the *Godunov barrier theorem*, which states that there is no linear approximation above first order for the Riemann problem that is nonoscillatory. The details of this theorem are explained next.

- Linear approximation: The FDs used in `dss012, dss002, dss020` are linear in the sense that the dependent variable `u` in the weighted sums at the various grid points in z is to the first power (linear).
- Above first order: The FD approximations in `dss002, dss020` are second and fourth order, respectively (above first order).
- Riemann problem: As explained previously, a Riemann problem has a discontinuous IC, in this case, the Heaviside unit step of eq. (1.5) with $t = 0$.
- Nonoscillatory: The second and fourth order FDs of `dss002` and `dss020` produced numerical solutions with oscillations (Figs. 1.5, 1.6).

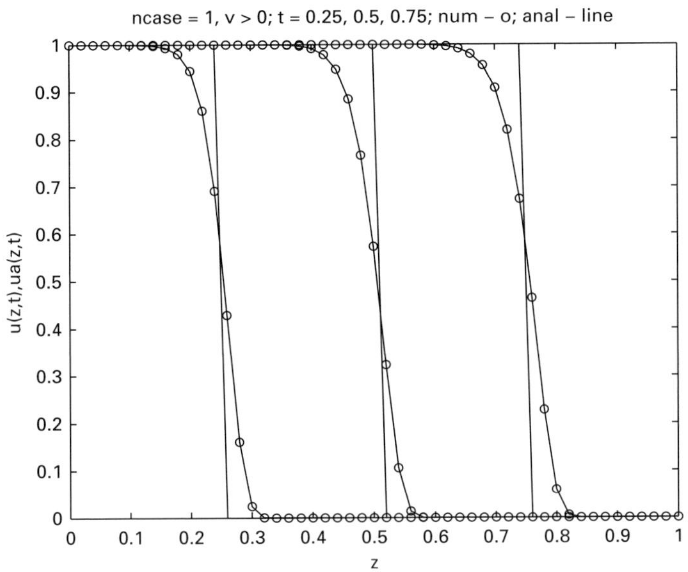

Figure 1.7 Spatial profiles of the MOL solution of eqs. (1.1) to (1.3) with the van Leer flux limiter

As a related point, the first order FD approximations in `dss012` produced a numerical solution that was nonoscillatory (Fig. 1.4).

Thus, we can infer that there is no approach to a numerical solution based on FDs that will give small numerical diffusion and oscillation (in the resolution of discontinuities and steep fronts for strongly convective or strongly hyperbolic PDEs such as eq. (1.1)). However, we note that the Godunov theorem applies to linear approximations such as FDs. This suggests the possibility that nonlinear approximations, e.g., for the Riemann problem, might give numerical solutions of acceptable accuracy (free of numerical distortions), and we next consider some nonlinear approximations that fulfill this requirement.

These nonlinear approximations are termed flux limiters. We will not go into the theory of flux limiters, but rather, demonstrate their use and effectiveness through the continued discussion of eqs. (1.1) to (1.3). Additional details of the theory are available in [6], Chapter 2. The first of these is the van Leer limiter implemented in a routine `vanl` and called by `pde_1` of Listing 1.10 with `ifd = 4` set in `pde_1_main` of Listing 1.9. To conserve space, we will not discuss the details of `vanl` here; this routine is included in the available downloads.

With `ifd = 4` (van Leer flux limiter), `pde_1_main` of Listing 1.9 gives the plotted output in Fig. 1.7 for $f(z) = 0, g(t) = 1$ in eqs. (1.2) and (1.3).
We can note the following details of Fig. 1.7.

- Numerical oscillation has been eliminated.
- Numerical diffusion is relatively small; also recall that this Riemann problem is essentially impossible numerically, at least within the MOL context, since $u(z,t)$ and its

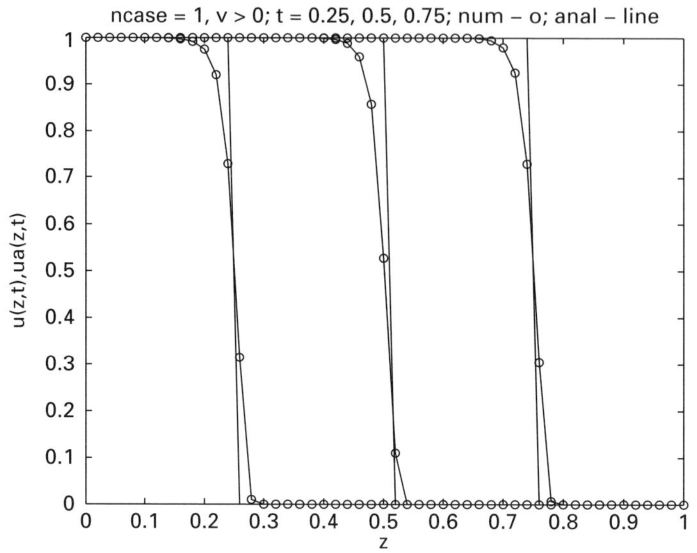

Figure 1.8 Spatial profiles of the MOL solution of eqs. (1.1) to (1.3) with the superbee flux limiter

derivative in z are undefined at $z = vt$; the numerical solution of Fig. 1.7 is a good approximation to the analytical solution, eq. (1.5), at least relative to the solutions from FDs (Figs. 1.4, 1.5, 1.6).

With `ifd = 5` (superbee flux limiter), `pde_1_main` of Listing 1.9 gives the plotted output in Fig. 1.8 (again, for $f(z) = 0, g(t) = 1$ in eqs. (1.2) and (1.3)). The numerical solution of Fig. 1.8 is slightly better than that of Fig. 1.7.

With `ifd = 6` (smart flux limiter), `pde_1_main` of Listing 1.9 gives the plotted output in Fig. 1.9 (again, for $f(z) = 0, g(t) = 1$ in eqs. (1.2) and (1.3)). The numerical solution of Fig. 1.9 is comparable to that of Fig. 1.8.

Note that near the point of discontinuity, $z = vt$, there are relatively few points for the numerical solution. This would suggest that increasing the number of points in z might improve the numerical solution. To test this idea, the coding in `pde_1_main` was changed to `zL=1,n=101,dz=0.01`, that is the number of grid points in z was doubled. The resulting plot for `ifd = 6` is in Fig. 1.10, which shows even less numerical diffusion than Fig. 1.9. Thus is in contrast to the use of FDs, which produced no improvement in the numerical solution with increasing points in z, and in fact, the oscillations such as in Fig. 1.5 became substantially larger.

In summary, the three flux limiters, van Leer, superbee, and smart, produced numerical solutions with no oscillations and substantially reduced diffusion relative to FDs. The calls to the flux limiters were the same as for the FDs, and the additional calculations did not appreciably slow the execution (the routines `vanl, super, smart` called by `pde_1` in Listing 1.10 are available in the downloads).

These results would suggest that flux limiters should always be used in place of FDs. However, this is not necessarily the case. The Godunov theorem pertains to a Riemann

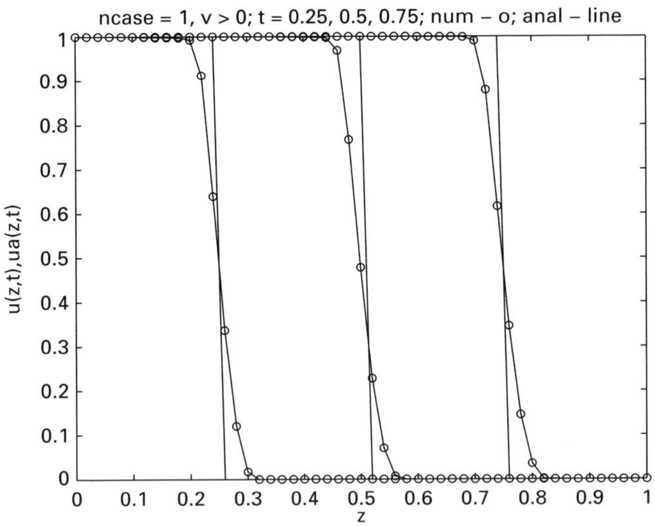

Figure 1.9 Spatial profiles of the MOL solution of eqs. (1.1) to (1.3) with the smart flux limiter

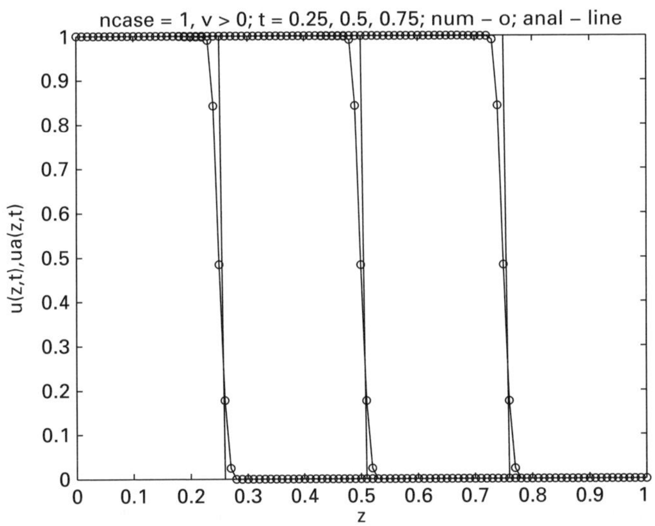

Figure 1.10 Spatial profiles of the MOL solution of eqs. (1.1) to (1.3) with the smart flux limiter, $n = 101$ points in z

problem with a discontinuous IC such as eq. (1.5) with $t = 0$. For smoother ICs, the FDs generally work well, with the exception of the two point FDs of `dss012`. To demonstrate this conclusion, we now consider the Gaussian function as an IC, that is continuous (and with continuous derivatives of all orders).

$$u(z, t = 0) = e^{-cz^2}. \tag{1.16}$$

$u(z,t=0)$ of eq. (1.16) is a pulse centered at $z=0$ where c is a constant to be specified.

The previous six numerical methods (`ifd=1,...,6`) are next applied to eqs. (1.1) to (1.3) with eq. (1.16) as an IC. Since there are several changes in the preceding `pde_1_main` and `pde_1`, new versions are listed next.

```
  clc
  clear all
%
%  Linear advection equation
%
%  The linear advection equation
%
%    ut + v*uz = 0                                        (1)
%
%  is integrated by the method of lines (MOL) subject to
%  the IC
%
%    u(z,t=0) = f(z)                                      (2)
%
%  BC
%
%    u(z=0,t) = g(t)                                      (3)
%
%  We consider in particular f(z) = e^(-c*z^2), g(t) = 0
%  corresponding to the Gaussian function; the solution to
%  eqs. (1) to (3) is
%
%    u(z,t)=f(t - z/v)                                    (4)
%
% which is used to evaluate the numerical (MOL) solution.
%
%  The numerical algorithms are:
%
%    z (spatial, boundary value) integration: Selected by ifd
%      (see comments below)
%
%    t (temporal, initial value) integration: Explicit Euler
%
  global z dz zL v ifd n ncase ncall
%
% Select an approximation for the convective derivative uz
%
%   ifd = 1: Two point upwind approximation
%
%   ifd = 2: Centered approximation
%
%   ifd = 3: Five point, biased upwind approximation
%
%   ifd = 4: van Leer flux limiter
%
```

```
%   ifd = 5: Superbee flux limiter
%
%   ifd = 6: Smart flux limiter
%
  ifd=1;
%
% Grid (in z)
  zL=1; n=101; dz=0.02;
  z=[-zL:dz:zL];
%
% Step through cases
%
%   ncase = 1: v > 0
%
%   ncase = 2: v < 0
%
  for ncase=1:2
    if ncase==1 v= 1; end
    if ncase==2 v=-1; end
%
% Parameters for Euler integration
  nsteps=250;
  h=0.001;
%
% Initial condition
  for i=1:n
    u(i)=exp(-40*z(i)^2);
  end
  t=0;
%
% Store solution for plotting at t = 0, 0.25, 0.5, 0.75
  for i=1:n
    ua(i)=exp(-40*z(i)^2);
     uplot(1,i)=u(i);
    uaplot(1,i)=ua(i);
  end
%
% Write ncase, h, v
  fprintf('\n\n ncase = %5d    h = %10.3e   v = %4.2f\n\n',
          ncase,h,v);
%
% nout output points
  nout=4;
  ncall=0;
  for iout=2:nout
%
%   Euler integration
    u0=u; t0=t;
    [u,t]=euler(u0,t0,h,nsteps);
%
%   Store solution for plotting at t = 0, 0.25, 0.5, 0.75
```

```
      for i=1:n
        ua(i)=exp(-40*(z(i)-v*t)^2);
         uplot(iout,i)=u(i);
        uaplot(iout,i)=ua(i);
      end
%
% Next output
    end
%
% Plots for ncase = 1, 2
    figure(ncase);
    plot(z,uplot,'-o');
    axis([-1 1 0 1.1]);
    ylabel('u(z,t),ua(z,t)');xlabel('z');
    if(ncase==1)
      title('ncase = 1, v > 0; t = 0, 0.25, 0.5, 0.75; num - o;
             anal - line');
    end
    if(ncase==2)
      title('ncase = 2, v < 0; t = 0, 0.25, 0.5, 0.75; num - o;
             anal - line');
    end
    hold on
    plot(z,uaplot,'-');
%
% Next case
    end
```

Listing 1.14 Main program pde_1_main for the solution of eqs. (1.1) to (1.3) with six MOL approximations, Gaussian IC of eq. (1.14)

We can note the following details about pde_1_main.

- Previous files are cleared and selected variables are declared global.

```
clc
clear all
global z dz zL v ifd n ncase ncall
```

  The documentation comments that define the problem are not repeated here to conserve space.

- The previous six MOL approximations are again explained and one is selected.

```
%
% Select an approximation for the convective derivative uz
%
%   ifd = 1: Two point upwind approximation
%
%   ifd = 2: Centered approximation
%
%   ifd = 3: Five point, biased upwind approximation
%
%   ifd = 4: van Leer flux limiter
```

```
%
%   ifd = 5: Superbee flux limiter
%
%   ifd = 6: Smart flux limiter
%
  ifd=1;
```

- A grid in z is defined as $-z_L \leq z \leq z_L$ with $z_L = 1$ and 101 points so that the grid spacing is $\Delta z = 0.02$.

```
%
% Grid (in z)
  zL=1; n=101; dz=0.02;
  z=[-zL:dz:zL];
```

This grid in z was selected (negative and positive z) since the initial Gaussian pulse from eq. (1.16) is centered at $z = 0$ and moves left to right for $v > 0$ (`ncase=1`) and right to left for $v < 0$ (`ncase=2`). These features of the solution will be clear when the graphical output is discussed.

- Two cases are again programmed and the parameters for the explicit Euler integration are the same as in Listing 1.9.

```
%
% Step through cases
%
%   ncase = 1: v > 0
%
%   ncase = 2: v < 0
%
  for ncase=1:2
    if ncase==1 v= 1; end
    if ncase==2 v=-1; end
%
% Parameters for Euler integration
  nsteps=250;
  h=0.001;
```

- The IC from eq. (1.16) is programmed with $c = 40$.

```
%
% Initial condition
  for i=1:n
    u(i)=exp(-40*z(i)^2);
  end
  t=0;
```

- The IC is stored for subsequent plotting. This was not done in the case of eq. (1.5) since the IC is a unit step that cannot be easily plotted using the grid in z, that is, whether the value of the IC at $z = 0$ should be zero or one. In the case of the Gaussian pulse of eq. (1.16), this is not a problem since $u(z = 0, t = 0) = e^0 = 1$.

```
%
% Store solution for plotting at t = 0, 0.25, 0.5, 0.75
```

```
for i=1:n
  ua(i)=exp(-40*z(i)^2);
   uplot(1,i)=u(i);
  uaplot(1,i)=ua(i);
end
```

- The parameters `ncase,h,v` are displayed and the solution at `t=0.25,0.5,0.75` is produced within the `for` loop. Note that this loop starts at `iout=2` since the solution at $t = 0$ is also now included in the graphical output. Thus, a total of `nout=4` outputs are subsequently plotted.

```
%
% Write ncase, h, v
  fprintf('\n\n ncase = %5d    h = %10.3e    v = %4.2f\n\n',ncase,h,v);
%
% nout output points
  nout=4;
  ncall=0;
  for iout=2:nout
```

- The numerical solution is again computed with `euler` of Listing 1.2. The numerical solution is then stored along with the analytical solution,

$$u(z,t) = \mathrm{e}^{-c(z-vt)^2}, \tag{1.17}$$

with $c = 40$.

```
%
%   Euler integration
    u0=u; t0=t;
    [u,t]=euler(u0,t0,h,nsteps);
%
%   Store solution for plotting at t = 0, 0.25, 0.5, 0.75
    for i=1:n
      ua(i)=exp(-40*(z(i)-v*t)^2);
       uplot(iout,i)=u(i);
      uaplot(iout,i)=ua(i);
    end
%
% Next output
  end
```

The `end` concludes the loop in `iout`. Equation (1.17) follows from the general analytical solution to eq. (1.1)

$$u(z,t) = f(z - vt),$$

that is, the Gaussian pulse of eq. (1.16) displaced in z by vt. Equation (1.5) is another example of this general solution (a unit step displaced in z by vt).

- The plotting of the solution for the two cases $v > 0, v < 0$ is the same as before (Listing 1.9).

```
%
% Plots for ncase = 1, 2
  figure(ncase);
  plot(z,uplot,'-o');
  axis([-1 1 0 1.1]);
  ylabel('u(z,t),ua(z,t)');xlabel('z');
  if(ncase==1)
    title('ncase = 1, v > 0; t = 0, 0.25, 0.5, 0.75; num - o;
           anal - line');
  end
  if(ncase==2)
    title('ncase = 2, v < 0; t = 0, 0.25, 0.5, 0.75; num - o;
           anal - line');
  end
  hold on
  plot(z,uaplot,'-');
%
% Next case
  end
```

The end concludes the loop in ncase.

Execution of pde_1_main for ifd=1 produces Fig. 1.11. We see that again, even for the IC of eq. (1.16), the two point upwind approximations of dss012 produce excessive numerical diffusion. This implies that these FD approximations in general are not a good choice for strongly convective (hyperbolic) problems (since in the present case they did not produce an acceptable numerical solution for the IC of either eq. (1.5) with $t = 0$ (discontinuous) or eq. (1.16) (smooth)).

We can note a detail about the numerical solution in Fig. 1.11. The numerical solution for $t = 0.75$ has a distortion near $z = 1$ due to the imposed homogeneous (zero) BC in pde_1. Therefore, the z domain was extended to $-1.5 \leq z \leq 1.5$ with the following code in pde_1_main in Listing 1.14.

```
%
% Grid (in z)
  zL=1.5; n=151; dz=0.02;
  z=[-zL:dz:zL];
```

and

```
axis([-1.5 1.5 0 1.1]);
```

Everything else remained the same in the programming. The result of this change is indicated in Fig. 1.12. Note that the effect of the boundary condition at $z = 1$ (set in pde_1) is to keep the solution at zero. But otherwise, the results of Figs. 1.11 and 1.12 are essentially the same.

This analysis does indicate, however, that when a PDE solution approaches the spatial boundaries, the BCs may affect the solution. An alternative approach would be to

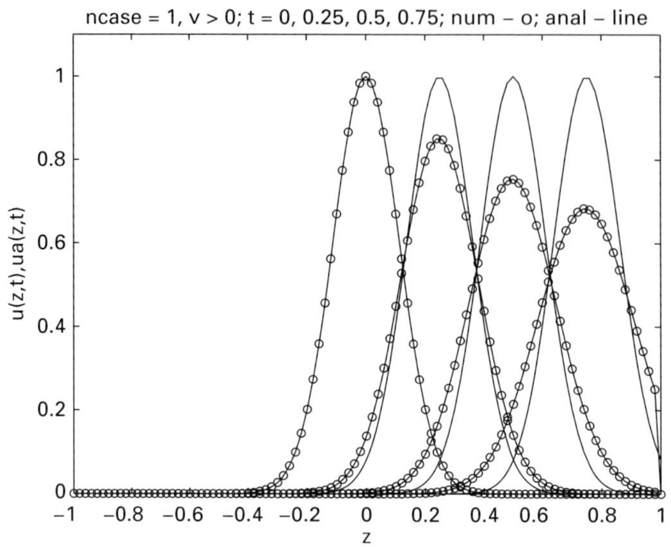

Figure 1.11 Spatial profiles of the MOL solution of eqs. (1.1) to (1.3) with two point upwind FDs, Gaussian IC; $t = 0, 0.25, 0.5, 0.75$ (left to right)

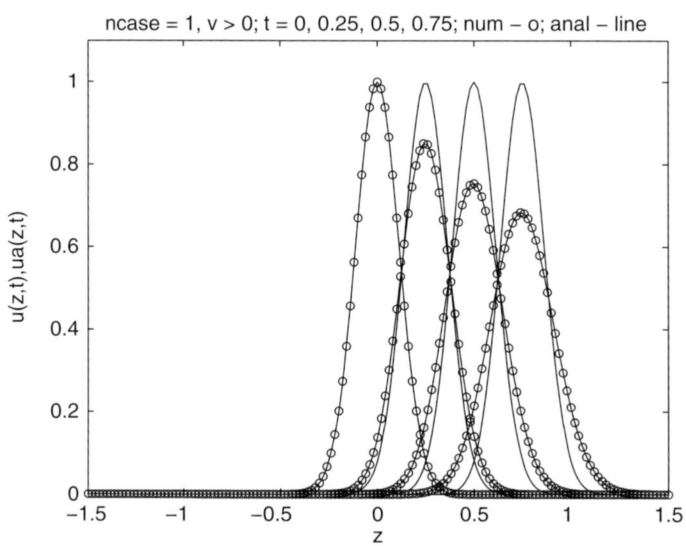

Figure 1.12 Spatial profiles of the MOL solution of eqs. (1.1) to (1.3) $-1.5 \leq z \leq 1.5$

apply the analytical solution, in this case eq. (1.17), at the boundaries. Of course, this will not be possible if an analytical solution is not available (which is generally the case).

If `pde_1_main` is executed with `ifd=2`, the plotted solution is as in Fig. 1.13.

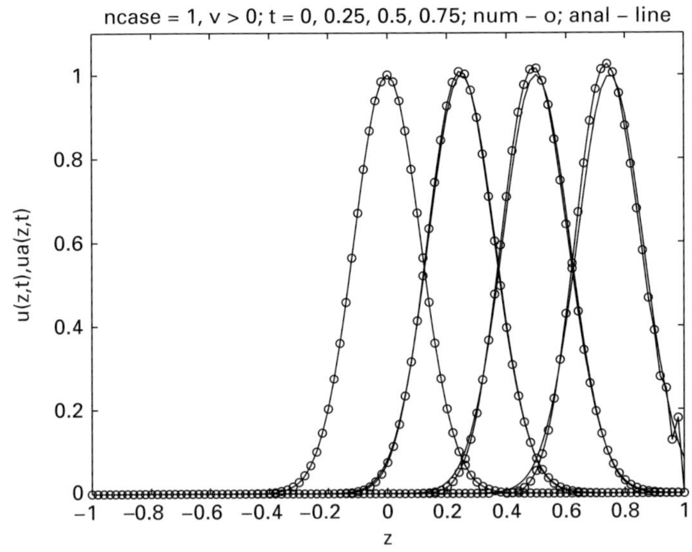

Figure 1.13 Spatial profiles of the MOL solution of eqs. (1.1) to (1.3) with three point centered FDs, Gaussian IC; $t = 0, 0.25, 0.5, 0.75$ (left to right)

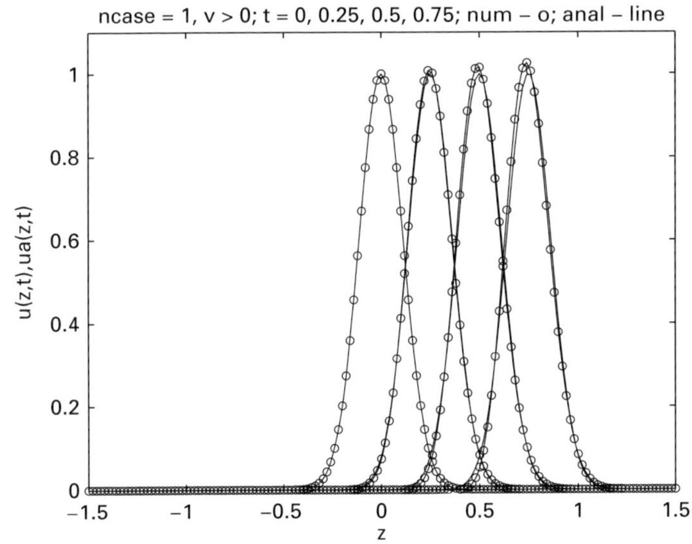

Figure 1.14 Spatial profiles of the MOL solution of eqs. (1.1) to (1.3) with three point centered FDs, Gaussian IC; $t = 0, 0.25, 0.5, 0.75$ (left to right); $-1.5 \leq z \leq 1.5$

We can note again the boundary effect on the solution at $t = 0.75$. Therefore, in the remaining solutions, the extended grid $-1.5 \leq z \leq 1.5$ is used, starting again with the solution for `ifd=2`, shown in Fig. 1.14.

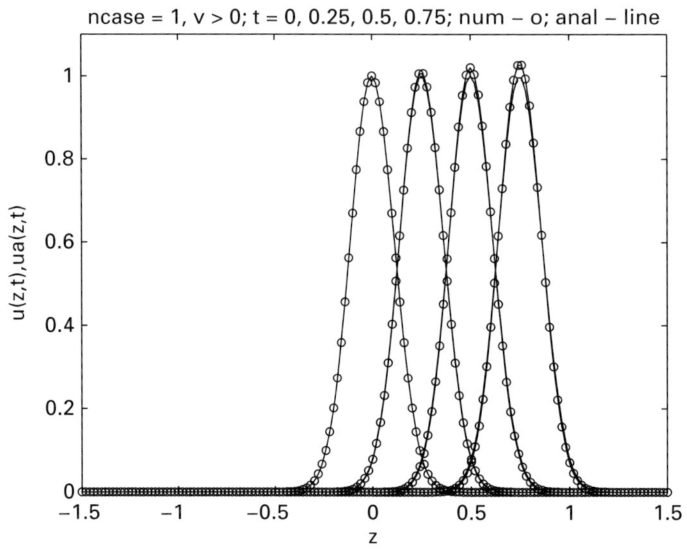

Figure 1.15 Spatial profiles of the MOL solution of eqs. (1.1) to (1.3) with five point biased upwind FDs, Gaussian IC; $t = 0, 0.25, 0.5, 0.75$ (left to right)

We can note that there is no numerical oscillation as in Fig. 1.5, although there is a small increase in the peak height with increasing t (it should remain at one). But clearly the smooth IC of eq. (1.16) results in a much better numerical solution than the discontinuous IC of eq. (1.5) (with $t = 0$).

For `pde_1_main` with `ifd=3`, the plotted solution is in Fig. 1.15.

Again, there is no numerical oscillation as in Fig. 1.6, although there is a small increase in the peak height with increasing t (it should remain at one). But clearly the smooth IC of eq. (1.16) results in a much better numerical solution than the discontinuous IC of eq. (1.5) (with $t = 0$).

For `pde_1_main` with `ifd=4`, the plotted solution is in Fig. 1.16.

Again, there is good agreement between the numerical and analytical solutions, although there is a small decrease in the peak height with increasing t (it should remain at one).

For `pde_1_main` with `ifd=5`, the plotted solution is in Fig. 1.17.

Again, there is good agreement between the numerical and analytical solutions, although there is a small decrease in the peak height with increasing t and a slight rounding of the peak.

For `pde_1_main` with `ifd=6`, the plotted solution is in Fig. 1.18.

Again, there is good agreement between the numerical and analytical solutions, although there is a small decrease in the peak height with increasing t.

Of the six cases (`ifd=1,...,6`), `ifd=6` gives about the best agreement between the numerical and analytical solutions. But generally, the agreement between the two solutions is satisfactory except for `ifd=1`. This is in contrast with the case of the discontinuous

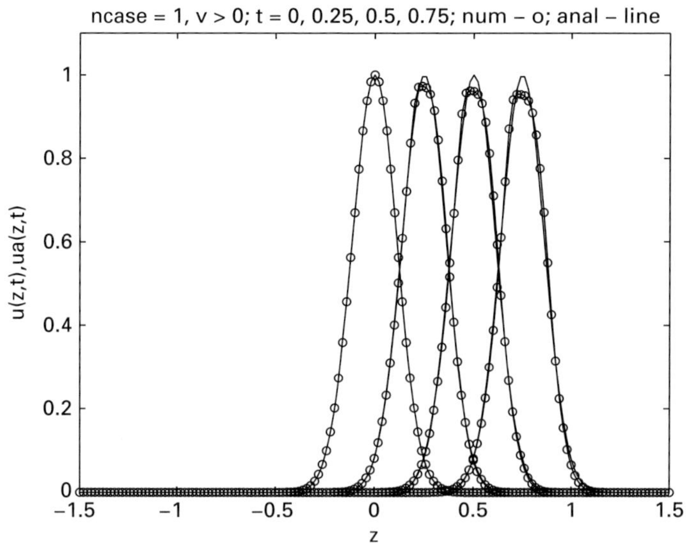

Figure 1.16 Spatial profiles of the MOL solution of eqs. (1.1) to (1.3) with the van Leer flux limiter, Gaussian IC; $t = 0, 0.25, 0.5, 0.75$ (left to right)

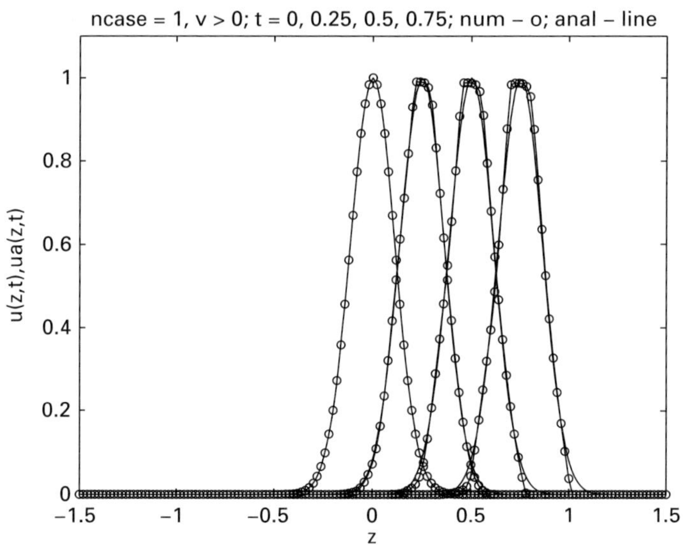

Figure 1.17 Spatial profiles of the MOL solution of eqs. (1.1) to (1.3) with the superbee flux limiter, Gaussian IC; $t = 0, 0.25, 0.5, 0.75$ (left to right)

IC of eq. (1.5) with $t = 0$ (the Riemann problem) for which, with `ifd=1,2,3`, the numerical solution was unacceptable owing to numerical diffusion and oscillation. Generally, then, the smoothness of the problem for strongly convective systems is an important consideration in the selection of a MOL approximation.

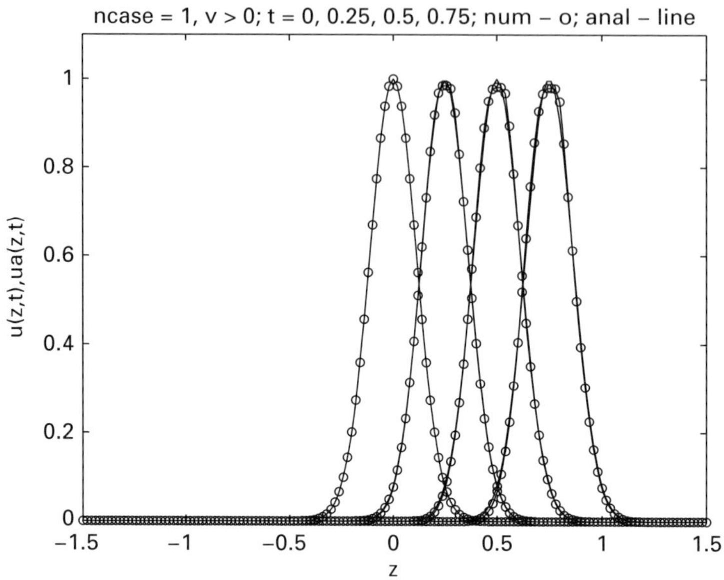

Figure 1.18 Spatial profiles of the MOL solution of eqs. (1.1) to (1.3) with the smart flux limiter, Gaussian IC; $t = 0, 0.25, 0.5, 0.75$ (left to right)

As an overall conclusion, hyperbolic PDEs can present a particularly challenging requirement for an accurate numerical solution, particularly when the solution exhibits a discontinuity or steep moving front. Generally, linear FDs will not give satisfactory solutions for a nonsmooth case and some special nonlinear approximation, such as a flux limiter, is required.

We now go on to a much easier problem, a parabolic PDE. Generally, such a problem is first order in t (as in eq. (1.1)), but second order in z (in contrast with the first order derivative in z of eq. (1.1)). We first illustrate the parabolic case with the classical Fourier's second law (also termed Fick's second law or the diffusion equation), which is derived in Appendix 1 based on conservation of mass or energy.

1.3 Parabolic PDEs

Fourier's second law in 1D is

$$\frac{\partial u}{\partial t} = D\frac{\partial^2 u}{\partial z^2}, \tag{1.18}$$

where D is a diffusivity.

Since eq. (1.18) is first order in t and second order in z, it requires one IC and two BCs.

$$u(z,t=0) = f(z). \tag{1.19}$$

The BCs can be of several types:

$$u(z = z_l, t) = g_{d,1}(t), \ u(z = z_u, t) = g_{d,2}(t); \tag{1.20a,b}$$

$$\frac{u(z = z_l, t)}{\partial z} = g_{n,1}(t), \ \frac{u(z = z_u, t)}{\partial z} = g_{n,2}(t); \tag{1.20c,d}$$

$$\frac{u(z = z_l, t)}{\partial z} + c_1 u(z = z_l, t) = g_{t,1}(t), \ \frac{u(z = z_u, t)}{\partial z} + c_2 u(z = z_u, t) = g_{t,2}(t). \tag{1.20e,f}$$

$$g_{b,1}(z, t, u(z = z_l, t), \frac{u(z = z_l, t)}{\partial z}) = 0, \ g_{b,2}(z, t, u(z = z_u, t), \frac{u(z = z_u, t)}{\partial z}) = 0. \tag{1.20g,h}$$

$D, f, g_{d,1}, g_{d,2}, g_{n,1}, g_{n,2}, g_{t,1}, g_{t,2}, g_{b,1}, g_{b,2}, c_1, c_2, z_l, z_u$ are functions and constants to be specified as part of the PDE problem. Equations (1.20a) and (1.20b) are termed Dirichlet; they specify the dependent variable $u(z,t)$ at the boundaries $z = z_l, z_u$. Equations (1.20c) and (1.20d) are termed Neumann; they specify the derivative of the solution, $(\partial u(z,t)/\partial z)$, at the boundaries. Boundary conditions (1.20e) and (1.20f) are a combination of Dirichlet and Neumann and are termed third type or Robin. Boundary conditions (1.20g) and (1.20h) are general boundary conditions that include eqs. (1.20a) to (1.20f), and can be nonlinear (if $g_{b,1}, g_{b,2}$ are nonlinear). Any combination of two of these BCs will satisfy the BC requirements of eq. (1.18), such as, for example, eqs. (1.20a) and (1.20d). Generally the BCs have an important physical interpretation as will be illustrated in the applications discussed in subsequent chapters. As an example, BC (1.3) at $z = 0$ for $v > 0$ is the inflow or entering value of $u(z = 0, t)$.

1.3.1 Dirichlet BCs

To illustrate the MOL solution of eq. (1.18), we select the IC and BCs

$$u(z, t = 0) = f(z) = \sin(\pi * z/z_L); \quad 0 \le z \le z_L \tag{1.21a}$$

$$u(z = 0, t) = 0 \tag{1.21b}$$

$$u(z = z_L, t) = 0 \tag{1.21c}$$

The corresponding analytical solution that is used to evaluate the numerical solution is

$$u(z, t) = e^{-D(\pi/z_L)^2 t} \sin(\pi * z/z_L). \tag{1.22}$$

Equation (1.21a) is a special case of IC (1.19) with $f(z) = \sin(\pi z/z_L)$. Equations (1.21b) and (1.21c) are special cases of Dirichlet BCs (1.20a) and (1.20b) with $g_{d,1}(t) = g_{d,2}(t) = 0$.

A main program for eqs. (1.18) to (1.22), `pde_1_main`, parallels the main programs in Section (1.2).

```
  clc
  clear all
%
%   One dimensional diffusion
```

```
%
%   The PDE that models the diffusion mass transfer is
%
%      ut = D*uzz                                              (1)
%
%   with the initial and Dirichlet boundary conditions
%
%      u(z,0) = u0(z), u(0,t) = 0, u(zL,t) = 0           (2)(3)(4)
%
%   where
%
%      u      dependent variable, e.g., concentration
%
%      t      time
%
%      z      position
%
%      D      diffusivity
%
%      u0(z) initial u
%
%      zL     length
%
%   Of particular interest is the concentration, u(z=zL/2,t).
%
%   The method of lines (MOL) solution of eq. (1) is coded below.
%   The resulting system of ODEs in t, defined on a 21 point grid in z,
%   is then integrated by the classical fourth order Runge Kutta method.
%
%   The analytical solution to eqs. (1) to (4) is also programmed
%   for comparison with the numerical solution.
%
%   The following code is run for the six special cases:
%
%      Case 1: uzz by three point finite differences (3pc)
%              and stagewise differentiation
%
%      Case 2: uzz by five point finite differences  (5pc)
%              and stagewise differentiation
%
%      Case 3: uzz by seven point finite differences (7pc)
%              and stagewise differentiation
%
%      Case 4: uzz by three point finite differences (3pc)
%              and direct second order differentiation
%
%      Case 5: uzz by five point finite differences  (5pc)
%              and direct second order differentiation
%
%      Case 6: uzz by seven point finite differences (7pc)
%              and direct second order differentiation
```

```
%
  global zL D ncase n ncall
%
% Model parameters (defined in the comments above)
  D=1; zL=1; n=21; n2=11;
%
% Step through cases
  for ncase=1:6
%
% Level of output
%
%   Detailed output - ip = 1
%
%   Brief (IC) output - ip = 2
%
  ip=1;
%
% Parameters for fourth order Runge Kutta integration (Note: for
% nsteps = 10, h = 0.002, the numerical solution is unstable for
% ncase = 4,5,6)
  nsteps=20;
  h=0.001;
%
% Initial condition
  for i=1:n
    z(i)=(i-1)/(n-1)*zL;
    u(i)=sin(pi*z(i)/zL);
  end
  t=0;
%
% Write ncase, h
  fprintf('\n\n ncase = %1d    h = %10.3e\n\n',ncase,h);
%
% Write heading
  fprintf('   t      u(zL/2,t)   ua(zL/2,t)      diff\n');
%
% Display numerical, analytical solutions at t = 0, z = zL/2
  ua=sin(pi*z(n2)/zL);
  diff=u(n2)-ua;
  fprintf('%5.2f%12.5f%12.5f%15.4e\n',t,u(n2),ua,diff);
%
% Store solution for plotting
   uplot(ncase,1)=u(n2);
  uaplot(ncase,1)=ua;
   tplot(1)=t;
%
% nout output points
  nout=51;
  ncall=0;
  for iout=2:nout
%
```

```
%   Fourth order Runge Kutta integration
    u0=u; t0=t;
    [u,t]=rk4(u0,t0,h,nsteps);
%
%   Numerical, analytical solutions
    ua=exp(-(pi/zL)^2*t)*sin(pi*z(n2)/zL);
    diff=u(n2)-ua;
    if(ip==1)
      fprintf('%5.2f%12.5f%12.5f%15.4e\n',t,u(n2),ua,diff);
    end
%
%   Store solution for plotting
     uplot(ncase,iout)=u(n2);
    uaplot(ncase,iout)=ua;
     tplot(iout)=t;
%
% Next output
  end
%
% Plots for ncase = 1 to 6
  figure(ncase);
  plot(tplot,uplot(1,:),'-o');
  axis([0 1 0 1]);
  ylabel('u(z=zL/2,t),ua(z=zL/2,t)');xlabel('t');
  if(ncase==1)title('ncase = 1; num - o; anal - line');end
  if(ncase==2)title('ncase = 2; num - o; anal - line');end
  if(ncase==3)title('ncase = 3; num - o; anal - line');end
  if(ncase==4)title('ncase = 4; num - o; anal - line');end
  if(ncase==5)title('ncase = 5; num - o; anal - line');end
  if(ncase==6)title('ncase = 6; num - o; anal - line');end
  hold on
  plot(tplot,uaplot(1,:),'-');
%
% Next case
  end
```

Listing 1.15 Main program pde_1_main for the solution of eqs. (1.18) to (1.22) with a series of FD approximations in pde_1 of Listing 1.16

We can note the following details about pde_1_main.

- Previous files are cleared and selected variables are declared global. The documentation comments pertaining to eqs. (1.18) to (1.22) are not repeated here to conserve space; the comments pertaining to the calculation of the derivative $(\partial^2 u/\partial z^2)$ (= uzz) in eq. (1.18) indicate the FD approximations for six cases.

```
    clc
    clear all
%
%   The following code is run for the six special cases:
%
%      Case 1: uzz by three point finite differences (3pc)
```

```
%              and stagewise differentiation
%
%       Case 2: uzz by five point finite differences  (5pc)
%              and stagewise differentiation
%
%       Case 3: uzz by seven point finite differences (7pc)
%              and stagewise differentiation
%
%       Case 4: uzz by three point finite differences (3pc)
%              and direct second order differentiation
%
%       Case 5: uzz by five point finite differences  (5pc)
%              and direct second order differentiation
%
%       Case 6: uzz by seven point finite differences (7pc)
%              and direct second order differentiation
%
  global zL D ncase n ncall
```

- The diffusivity in eq. (1.18) is defined. The grid in z is $0 \leq z \leq 1$ with 21 points; the midpoint is also specified (at `zL = 0.5`) with `n2=11`) for use later in the output.

```
%
% Model parameters (defined in the comments above)
  D=1; zL=1; n=21; n2=11;
```

- The `for` loop in `ncase` steps through the six cases, with the selection of detailed or brief output.

```
%
% Step through cases
  for ncase=1:6
%
% Level of output
%
%   Detailed output - ip = 1
%
%   Brief (IC) output - ip = 2
%
  ip=1;
```

- The parameters for the integration in t are specified (the integrator is `rk4` in Listing 1.5). Also, an incidental note indicates that if the integration step is doubled (from `0.001` to `0.002`), the solution becomes unstable; this reflects the limited stability of explicit methods as discussed previously (just after eq. (1.10e) for `rk4`); this occurs only for `ncase=4,5,6` which also indicates that the FD approximation in z affects the t integration.

```
%
% Parameters for fourth order Runge Kutta integration (Note: for
% nsteps = 10, h = 0.002, the numerical solution is unstable for
```

```
% ncase = 4,5,6)
  nsteps=20;
  h=0.001;
```

- The grid in z and the IC of eq. (1.21a) is programmed (this sets the ICs of the 21 ODEs for the MOL solution of eq. (1.18)).

```
%
% Initial condition
  for i=1:n
    z(i)=(i-1)/(n-1)*zL;
    u(i)=sin(pi*z(i)/zL);
  end
  t=0;
```

- Two headings for the tabulated numerical solution, and the IC for the numerical and analytical solutions at $z = z_L/2$ (midpoint in z) are displayed.

```
%
% Write ncase, h
  fprintf('\n\n ncase = %1d    h = %10.3e\n\n',ncase,h);
%
% Write heading
  fprintf('   t      u(zL/2,t)   ua(zL/2,t)       diff\n');
%
% Display numerical, analytical solutions at t = 0, z = zL/2
  ua=sin(pi*z(n2)/zL);
  diff=u(n2)-ua;
  fprintf('%5.2f%12.5f%12.5f%15.4e\n',t,u(n2),ua,diff);
```

- The ICs for the numerical and analytical solutions are stored for subsequent plotting. Note the use of the subscript 1 for the first point ($t = 0$) in the plots.

```
%
% Store solution for plotting
   uplot(ncase,1)=u(n2);
  uaplot(ncase,1)=ua;
   tplot(1)=t;
```

- The parameters are set for the t integration with 51 outputs (including $t = 0$) over the interval $0 \le t \le 1$ in steps of $(20)(0.001) = 0.02$ (from the preceding programming of `nsteps=20` and `h=0.001`). Also, the number of calls to the ODE routine, `pde_1`, is initialized.

```
%
% nout output points
  nout=51;
  ncall=0;
  for iout=2:nout
```

The integration in t then proceeds with a `for` loop. Note the starting index of `2` to include the previous IC.

- rk4 of Listing 1.5 is called for the integration of the 21 ODEs (programmed in pde_1, considered subsequently).

```
%
%   Fourth order Runge Kutta integration
    u0=u; t0=t;
    [u,t]=rk4(u0,t0,h,nsteps);
```

  Each call to rk4 advances the solution $20(0.001) = 0.02$ in t. $51 - 1$ steps, each of length 0.02, produce the complete solution over the interval $0 \leq t \leq 1$.
- The analytical solution of eq. (1.22) is evaluated and the difference between the numerical and analytical solutions is computed at the 51 output points. These results are then displayed in tabular format and stored for graphical format.

```
%
%   Numerical, analytical solutions
    ua=exp(-(pi/zL)^2*t)*sin(pi*z(n2)/zL);
    diff=u(n2)-ua;
    if(ip==1)
      fprintf('%5.2f%12.5f%12.5f%15.4e\n',t,u(n2),ua,diff);
    end
%
%   Store solution for plotting
     uplot(ncase,iout)=u(n2);
    uaplot(ncase,iout)=ua;
     tplot(iout)=t;
%
% Next output
  end
```

  The end concludes the for loop in iout.
- At $t = 1$, the numerical and analytical solutions are plotted.

```
%
% Plots for ncase = 1 to 6
  figure(ncase);
  plot(tplot,uplot(1,:),'-o');
  axis([0 1 0 1]);
  ylabel('u(z=zL/2,t),ua(z=zL/2,t)');xlabel('t');
  if(ncase==1)title('ncase = 1; num - o; anal - line');end
  if(ncase==2)title('ncase = 2; num - o; anal - line');end
  if(ncase==3)title('ncase = 3; num - o; anal - line');end
  if(ncase==4)title('ncase = 4; num - o; anal - line');end
  if(ncase==5)title('ncase = 5; num - o; anal - line');end
  if(ncase==6)title('ncase = 6; num - o; anal - line');end
  hold on
  plot(tplot,uaplot(1,:),'-');
%
% Next case
  end
```

  The end concludes the outer for loop for the six values of ncase.

The routine for the 21 ODEs is in Listing 1.16.

```
  function ut=pde_1(u,t)
%
% Function pde_1 computes the t derivative vector of the u vector
%
  global zL D ifd n ncase ncall
%
% Boundary conditions at z = 0, z=zL
  u(1)=0; u(n)=0;
%
% Second order spatial derivative
  if(ncase==1)
     [uz]=dss002(0,zL,n,u);
    [uzz]=dss002(0,zL,n,uz);
  end
  if(ncase==2)
     [uz]=dss004(0,zL,n,u);
    [uzz]=dss004(0,zL,n,uz);
  end
  if(ncase==3)
     [uz]=dss006(0,zL,n,u);
    [uzz]=dss006(0,zL,n,uz);
  end
  if(ncase==4)
    nl=1; nu=1; uz(1)=0;
    [uzz]=dss042(0,zL,n,u,uz,nl,nu);
  end
  if(ncase==5)
    nl=1; nu=1; uz(1)=0;
    [uzz]=dss044(0,zL,n,u,uz,nl,nu);
  end
  if(ncase==6)
    nl=1; nu=1; uz(1)=0;
    [uzz]=dss046(0,zL,n,u,uz,nl,nu);
  end
%
% Temporal derivative
  ut(1)=0.0; ut(n)=0;
  for i=2:n-1
    ut(i)=D*uzz(i);
  end
%
% Increment calls to pde_1
  ncall=ncall+1;
```

Listing 1.16 pde_1 for the solution of eqs. (1.18) to (1.22) with a series of FD approximations

We can note the following details about Listing 1.16.

- The function is defined and selected variables are declared global.

```
  function ut=pde_1(u,t)
%
% Function pde_1 computes the t derivative vector of the u vector
%
  global zL D ifd n ncase ncall
```

  The arguments of pde_1 were discussed previously, after Listing 1.3.
- Homogeneous (zero) Dirichlet BCs (1.21b) and (1.21c) are programmed at grid points 1 ($z = 0$) and n ($z = z_L$).

```
%
% Boundary conditions at z = 0, z=zL
  u(1)=0; u(n)=0;
```

- Six cases are then programmed for the calculation of $(\partial^2 u/\partial z^2)$ in eq. (1.18). The programming for ncase=1 is

```
%
% Second order spatial derivative
  if(ncase==1)
     [uz]=dss002(0,zL,n,u);
    [uzz]=dss002(0,zL,n,uz);
  end
```

  The first derivative uz is calculated by a call to dss002 in Listing 1.12. Then a second call to dss002 calculates the second derivative, uzz, by differentiation of the first derivative. This procedure of successive differentiations is termed stagewise differentiation.
- This procedure of successive differentiation is also used for ncase=2,3 for which dss004 and dss006 are called, respectively. These two routines implement five and seven point FDs, respectively, which are fourth and sixth order correct. We can make a brief comparison of the various FDs by looking at just the central row in the differentiation matrix of each routine. Also, we look at just one line of output from each routine, with a more complete discussion of the output from pde_1_main discussed subsequently.

dss002 (i=2,...,n-1)

```
uz(i)=r2fdz*...
(      -1.    *u(i-1)      +0.    *u(  i)      +1.    *u(i+1));
```

dss004 (i=3,...,n-2)

```
uz(  i)=r4fdz*...
(  +1.*u(i-2)   -8.*u(i-1)   +0.*u(  i)   +8.*u(i+1)   -1.*u(i+2));
```

dss006 (i=4,...,n-3)

```
uz(  i)=r6fdz*...
(    -12.*u(i-3)    +108.*u(i-2)    -540.*u(i-1)      +0.*u(  i)...
    +540.*u(i+1)    -108.*u(i+2)     +12.*u(i+3));
```

Listing 1.17 Calculation of the derivative uz(i) by the FDs of dss002, dss004, dss006 of FD approximations

Table 1.6. Output from pde_1_main of Listing 1.15 for $t = 0.1$, ncase = 1,2,3

```
dss002 (ncase = 1)
   t       u(zL/2,t)    ua(zL/2,t)        diff
 0.10       0.37574      0.37271     3.0277e-003

dss004 (ncase = 2)
   t       u(zL/2,t)    ua(zL/2,t)        diff
 0.10       0.37272      0.37271     1.2245e-005

dss006 (ncase = 3)
   t       u(zL/2,t)    ua(zL/2,t)        diff
 0.10       0.37271      0.37271     5.9622e-008
```

We can note the following points about Listing 1.17 and Table 1.6.

- The FDs for uz(i) in Listing 1.17 are based on three, five and seven weighting coefficients, respectively. These coefficients constitute the center row of a differentiation matrix, which is 3×3, 5×5, and 7×7; for example, the three weighting coefficients for ncase=1 appear in dss002 of Listing 1.12, and are discussed just after this listing.
- The calculation of uz for the points identified by the values of the index i are for interior points. For example, uz(i) is calculated for i=2,...,n-1 for ncase=1. For the boundary points, i=1,n, one-sided FDs are used as indicated in Listing 1.12. Thus, for ncase=2, points near the boundaries, that is, for i=1,2,n-1,n, require one-sided FDs.
- The weighting coefficients of Listing 1.17 have the antisymmetric property discussed previously, that is, they change sign around the central point with a weighting coefficient of zero. This is a property of FD approximations of odd order derivatives such as the first derivative uz. For even order derivatives, the weighting coefficients are symmetric (do not change sign).
- The effectiveness of using additional weighting coefficients (higher order FDs) is demonstrated in Table 1.6, where the error in the numerical solution decreases approximately two to three orders of magnitude with the use of two additional weighting coefficients. In other words, the additional computational effort in using more weighting coefficients is very worthwhile.
- This conclusion might suggest that higher order FDs should always be used. This would be true if we were differentiating polynomials (on which the order conditions such as second, fourth, and sixth order are based). However, PDE solutions are generally not polynomials (see, for example, eq. (1.22)), so the conclusion that higher

order is always better is not necessarily true. In fact, as higher order FDs are used, the numerical solutions tend to oscillate unrealistically (a numerical effect from the underlying polynomials of the FDs). Practical experience has indicated that the five point, fourth order FDs are a good compromise to achieve improved accuracy while avoiding unwanted numerical effects; admittedly, this is a rather vague statement, and some experimentation as we have done with `ncase=1,2,3` is usually worthwhile. This is an example of p refinement since we are varying the order of the approximations, and the order is generally designated with p, that is, $O(h^p)$ where h is the grid spacing in z; for `ncase=1,2,3`, $p = 2,4,6$, respectively.

- As a related point, two additional routines, `dss008` and `dss010`, are also available with FDs for which $p = 8,10$.
- Some additional tabular output from `pde_1_main` of Listing 1.15 is given in Table 1.7 for `ncase=1,...,6`. Also the first of six plots (for `ncase=1`) is given in Fig. 1.19. We defer discussion of this numerical and graphical output until after the discussion of `ncase=4,5,6` in `pde_1` of Listing 1.16.

For `ncase=1,2,3`, stagewise differentiation was used to compute uz from u, then uzz from uz. While this seems mathematically to be logical, it does not always work computationally and experience has indicated that the success of stagewise differentiation is dependent on the particular PDE problem (as well as how the grid in z is implemented). However, stagewise differentiation, when it performs as expected, offers some important advantages. To illustrate this point, consider the nonlinear extension of eq. (1.18).

$$\frac{\partial u}{\partial t} = \frac{\partial\left(D(u)\dfrac{\partial u}{\partial z}\right)}{\partial z}. \tag{1.23}$$

In eq. (1.23) we have generalized the diffusivity D so that it is now a function of u. This is an important extension in applications, where, for example, the diffusivity might be a quadratic function of u, such as $D = a_0 + a_1u + a_2u^2$, or an exponential function, such as $D = b_0e^{b_1u}$, where a_0, a_1, a_2, b_0, b_1 are constants determined from experimental data.

The RHS of eq. (1.23) could be implemented in `pde_1` with the following code, which is based on the idea of stagewise differentiation.

```
%
% Generalized second order spatial derivative
  if(ncase==1)
     [uz]=dss002(0,zL,n,u);
     for i=1:n
       uz(i)=D(i)*uz(i);
     end
    [uzz]=dss002(0,zL,n,uz);
  end
```

Note that `uz(i)` is multiplied by `D(i)` before a second call to `dss002` to compute the RHS of eq. (1.23). `D(i)` is a function that defines $D(u)$ in eq. (1.23). Or `D(i)` could be computed directly as, for example, in the case of an exponential function

Table 1.7. Selected output from `pde_1_main` of Listing 1.15

```
ncase = 1     h = 1.000e-003

   t      u(zL/2,t)   ua(zL/2,t)       diff
 0.00      1.00000      1.00000     0.0000e+000
 0.02      0.82220      0.82087     1.3294e-003
 0.04      0.67601      0.67383     2.1842e-003
 0.06      0.55581      0.55312     2.6916e-003
 0.08      0.45699      0.45404     2.9484e-003
 0.10      0.37574      0.37271     3.0277e-003
              .            .
              .            .
              .            .
 0.90      0.00015      0.00014     1.0482e-005
 0.92      0.00012      0.00011     8.8030e-006
 0.94      0.00010      0.00009     7.3893e-006
 0.96      0.00008      0.00008     6.1997e-006
 0.98      0.00007      0.00006     5.1995e-006
 1.00      0.00006      0.00005     4.3588e-006

ncase = 2     h = 1.000e-003

   t      u(zL/2,t)   ua(zL/2,t)       diff
 0.00      1.00000      1.00000     0.0000e+000
 0.02      0.82087      0.82087     5.5833e-006
 0.04      0.67383      0.67383     8.5987e-006
 0.06      0.55313      0.55312     1.0564e-005
 0.08      0.45405      0.45404     1.1731e-005
 0.10      0.37272      0.37271     1.2245e-005
              .            .
              .            .
              .            .
 0.90      0.00014      0.00014     4.6031e-008
 0.92      0.00011      0.00011     3.8639e-008
 0.94      0.00009      0.00009     3.2418e-008
 0.96      0.00008      0.00008     2.7186e-008
 0.98      0.00006      0.00006     2.2788e-008
 1.00      0.00005      0.00005     1.9093e-008


ncase = 3     h = 1.000e-003

   t      u(zL/2,t)   ua(zL/2,t)       diff
 0.00      1.00000      1.00000     0.0000e+000
 0.02      0.82087      0.82087     3.9933e-008
 0.04      0.67383      0.67383     5.7230e-008
```

```
0.06      0.55312      0.55312     6.2306e-008
0.08      0.45404      0.45404     6.2166e-008
0.10      0.37271      0.37271     5.9622e-008
             .            .
             .            .
             .            .
0.90      0.00014      0.00014     1.4684e-010
0.92      0.00011      0.00011     1.2309e-010
0.94      0.00009      0.00009     1.0314e-010
0.96      0.00008      0.00008     8.6390e-011
0.98      0.00006      0.00006     7.2329e-011
1.00      0.00005      0.00005     6.0534e-011


ncase = 4     h = 1.000e-003

  t      u(zL/2,t)   ua(zL/2,t)       diff
0.00      1.00000      1.00000     0.0000e+000
0.02      0.82120      0.82087     3.3296e-004
0.04      0.67437      0.67383     5.4674e-004
0.06      0.55380      0.55312     6.7335e-004
0.08      0.45478      0.45404     7.3712e-004
0.10      0.37346      0.37271     7.5650e-004
             .            .
             .            .
             .            .
0.90      0.00014      0.00014     2.5558e-006
0.92      0.00012      0.00011     2.1450e-006
0.94      0.00010      0.00009     1.7994e-006
0.96      0.00008      0.00008     1.5088e-006
0.98      0.00006      0.00006     1.2646e-006
1.00      0.00005      0.00005     1.0595e-006


ncase = 5     h = 1.000e-003

  t      u(zL/2,t)   ua(zL/2,t)       diff
0.00      1.00000      1.00000     0.0000e+000
0.02      0.82087      0.82087     1.0807e-006
0.04      0.67383      0.67383     1.7233e-006
0.06      0.55312      0.55312     2.0842e-006
0.08      0.45404      0.45404     2.2576e-006
0.10      0.37271      0.37271     2.3015e-006
             .            .
             .            .
             .            .
0.90      0.00014      0.00014     7.5324e-009
0.92      0.00011      0.00011     6.3201e-009
```

```
0.94      0.00009      0.00009      5.3004e-009
0.96      0.00008      0.00008      4.4433e-009
0.98      0.00006      0.00006      3.7231e-009
1.00      0.00005      0.00005      3.1184e-009


ncase = 6     h = 1.000e-003

  t       u(zL/2,t)    ua(zL/2,t)       diff
0.00      1.00000      1.00000      0.0000e+000
0.02      0.82087      0.82087      4.5830e-009
0.04      0.67383      0.67383      8.6263e-009
0.06      0.55312      0.55312      1.1457e-008
0.08      0.45404      0.45404      1.3063e-008
0.10      0.37271      0.37271      1.3738e-008
             .            .
             .            .
             .            .
0.90      0.00014      0.00014      5.0064e-011
0.92      0.00011      0.00011      4.2018e-011
0.94      0.00009      0.00009      3.5249e-011
0.96      0.00008      0.00008      2.9556e-011
0.98      0.00006      0.00006      2.4772e-011
1.00      0.00005      0.00005      2.0753e-011
```

```
%
% Generalized second order spatial derivative
  if(ncase==1)
     [uz]=dss002(0,zL,n,u);
     for i=1:n
       uz(i)=b0*exp(b1*u(i))*uz(i);
     end
    [uzz]=dss002(0,zL,n,uz);
  end
```

Here we assume that b0 and b1 are constants set numerically, perhaps in the main program and passed as global variables to pde_1. Note that the programming of eq. (1.23) is straightforward; the variation of D with u almost certainly precludes an analytical solution.

Also, FD routines are available for the direct calculation of a second derivative (rather than through stagewise differentiation), such as the second derivative in eq. (1.18). Three of these routines, dss042, dss044, dss046, are called in pde_1 of Listing 1.16. Their use is now discussed, starting with the code from Listing 1.16.

```
  if(ncase==4)
    nl=1; nu=1; uz(1)=0;
    [uzz]=dss042(0,zL,n,u,uz,nl,nu);
```

```
end
if(ncase==5)
  nl=1; nu=1; uz(1)=0;
  [uzz]=dss044(0,zL,n,u,uz,nl,nu);
end
if(ncase==6)
  nl=1; nu=1; uz(1)=0;
  [uzz]=dss046(0,zL,n,u,uz,nl,nu);
end
```

We can note the following details about this code (for `ncase=4`, which also applies to `ncase=5,6`).

- The first four input arguments, `0,zl,n,u`, are the same as for `dss002`. The additional three arguments are:
  - `uz`: The first derivative, which is set at the boundaries for Neumann and third type BCs (see eqs. (1.20b), (1.20c), (1.20d), (1.20e)). In the present case, we are considering Dirichlet BCs (eqs. (1.21b),(1.21c)) so `uz` is not used in the calculations within `dss042`, but the value `uz(1)=0` is used as an input to meet the general requirement that all input arguments to a MATLAB routine must be defined numerically).
  - `nl`: The type of BC at $z = 0$ (the first argument). `nl=1` specifies a Dirichlet BC (eq. (1.21b)). `nl=2` specifies a Neumann (and also third type) BC at $z = 0$.
  - `nu`: The type of BC at $z = z_L$ (the second argument). `nu=1` specifies a Dirichlet BC (eq. (1.21c)). `nu=2` specifies a Neumann (and also third type) BC at $z = z_L$.

- In other words, `dss042` computes the second derivative, `uzz`, of `u`, including the BCs at the first and second argument values of z (a few details for how this is done are considered subsequently).
- To reiterate, `dss042` returns as the output (LHS) argument the vector of `n` second derivatives, `uzz`.

We now consider some abbreviated tabular output (Table 1.7) for all six cases, and the plot for `ncase = 1` (Fig. 1.19).

We can note the following details about this output.

- The solution decays with t as expected according to the exponential $e^{-D(\pi/z_L)^2 t}$ of eq. (1.22), starting from the IC of eq. (1.21a) ($u(z = z_L/2, t = 0) = \sin(\pi/2) = 1$).
- The comparison of the numerical and analytical solutions of Table 1.6 can be extended to `ncase=4,5,6` (Table 1.8).
  We again note two orders of magnitude reduction in the error of the numerical solution for `ncase=4,5,6` (FDs of order $p = 2, 4, 6$).
- The three routines for `uzz` are in Listing 1.18; an extensive set of comments in each routine detail the derivation of the FD approximations; these have been deleted to conserve space, but are in the download versions.

Table 1.8. Output from pde_1_main of Listing 1.15 for $z = z_L/2 = 0.5, t = 0.1$, ncase = 1,...,6

```
dss002 (ncase = 1)
   t      u(zL/2,t)    ua(zL/2,t)        diff
 0.10      0.37574      0.37271    3.0277e-003

dss004 (ncase = 2)
   t      u(zL/2,t)    ua(zL/2,t)        diff
 0.10      0.37272      0.37271    1.2245e-005

dss006 (ncase = 3)
   t      u(zL/2,t)    ua(zL/2,t)        diff
 0.10      0.37271      0.37271    5.9622e-008

dss042 (ncase = 4)
   t      u(zL/2,t)    ua(zL/2,t)        diff
 0.10      0.37346      0.37271    7.5650e-004

dss044 (ncase = 5)
   t      u(zL/2,t)    ua(zL/2,t)        diff
 0.10      0.37271      0.37271    2.3015e-006

dss046 (ncase = 6)
   t      u(zL/2,t)    ua(zL/2,t)        diff
 0.10      0.37271      0.37271    1.3738e-008
```

```
-------------------------------dss042______________________________

   function [uzz]=dss042(zl,zu,n,u,uz,nl,nu)
%
% Function dss042 computes a second order approximation of a
% second order derivative, with or without the normal derivative
% at the boundary.
%
% Grid spacing
   dz=(zu-zl)/(n-1);
%
% uzz at the left boundary, without uz
   if nl==1
     uzz(1)=(( 2.)*u(  1)...
            +(-5.)*u(  2)...
            +( 4.)*u(  3)...
            +(-1.)*u(  4))/(dz^2);
%
% uzz at the left boundary, including uz
   elseif nl==2
     uzz(1)=((-7.)*u(  1)...
            +( 8.)*u(  2)...
```

```
            +(-1.)*u(  3))/(2.*dz^2)...
            +(-6.)*uz( 1) /(2.*dz);
      end
%
%  uzz at the right boundary, without uz
   if nu==1
     uzz(n)=(( 2.)*u(n  )...
            +(-5.)*u(n-1)...
            +( 4.)*u(n-2)...
            +(-1.)*u(n-3))/(dz^2);
%
%  uzz at the right boundary, including uz
   elseif nu==2
     uzz(n)=((-7.)*u(n  )...
            +( 8.)*u(n-1)...
            +(-1.)*u(n-2))/(2.*dz^2)...
            +( 6.)*uz(n ) /(2.*dz);
   end
%
%  uzz at the interior grid points
   for i=2:n-1
     uzz(i)=(u(i+1)-2.*u(i)+u(i-1))/dz^2;
   end
```

```
-------------------------------dss044------------------------------

   function [uzz]=dss044(zl,zu,n,u,uz,nl,nu)
%
%  Function dss044 computes a fourth order approximation of a
%  second order derivative, with or without the normal derivative
%  at the boundary.
%
%  Grid spacing
   dz=(zu-zl)/(n-1);
%
%  1/(12*dz**2) for subsequent use
   r12dzs=1./(12.0*dz^2);
%
%  uzz at the left boundary
%
%     Without uz
      if nl==1
        uzz(1)=r12dzs*...
                         (      45.0*u(1)...
                              -154.0*u(2)...
                              +214.0*u(3)...
                              -156.0*u(4)...
                               +61.0*u(5)...
                               -10.0*u(6));
%
%     With uz
```

```
      elseif nl==2
        uzz(1)=r12dzs*...
                      (-415.0/6.0*u(1)...
                              +96.0*u(2)...
                              -36.0*u(3)...
                         +32.0/3.0*u(4)...
                          -3.0/2.0*u(5)...
                                 -50.0*uz(1)*dz);
         end
%
%  uzz at the right boundary
%
%     Without uz
      if nu==1
        uzz(n)=r12dzs*...
                      (      45.0*u(n  )...
                           -154.0*u(n-1)...
                           +214.0*u(n-2)...
                           -156.0*u(n-3)...
                            +61.0*u(n-4)...
                            -10.0*u(n-5));
%
%     With uz
      elseif nu==2
        uzz(n)=r12dzs*...
                      (-415.0/6.0*u(n  )...
                              +96.0*u(n-1)...
                              -36.0*u(n-2)...
                         +32.0/3.0*u(n-3)...
                          -3.0/2.0*u(n-4)...
                             +50.0*uz(n  )*dz);
      end
%
%  uzz at the interior grid points
%
%     i = 2
         uzz(2)=r12dzs*...
                       (     10.0*u(1)...
                            -15.0*u(2)...
                             -4.0*u(3)...
                            +14.0*u(4)...
                             -6.0*u(5)...
                             +1.0*u(6));
%
%     i = n-1
         uzz(n-1)=r12dzs*...
                        (   10.0*u(n  )...
                           -15.0*u(n-1)...
                            -4.0*u(n-2)...
                           +14.0*u(n-3)...
                            -6.0*u(n-4)...
```

```
                              +1.0*u(n-5));
%
%     i = 3, 4,..., n-2
         for i=3:n-2
         uzz(i)=r12dzs*...
                       (     -1.0*u(i-2)...
                            +16.0*u(i-1)...
                            -30.0*u(i  )...
                            +16.0*u(i+1)...
                             -1.0*u(i+2));
         end
```

_______________________________dss046______________________________

```
   function [uxx]=dss046(xl,xu,n,u,ux,nl,nu)
%
%  Function dss046 computes a sixth order approximation of a
%  second order derivative, with or without the normal derivative
%  at the boundary.
%
%  Grid spacing
   dx=(xu-xl)/(n-1);
   rdxs=1.0/dx^2;
%
%  uxx at the left boundary
%
%     Without ux
         if nl==1
         uxx(1)=rdxs*...
               (  5.211111111111110*u(1)...
                -22.300000000000000*u(2)...
                +43.950000000000000*u(3)...
                -52.722222222222200*u(4)...
                +41.000000000000000*u(5)...
                -20.100000000000000*u(6)...
                 +5.661111111111110*u(7)...
                 -0.700000000000000*u(8));
%
%     With ux
         elseif nl==2
         uxx(1)=rdxs*...
               ( -7.493888888888860*u(1)...
                +12.000000000000000*u(2)...
                 -7.499999999999940*u(3)...
                 +4.444444444444570*u(4)...
                 -1.874999999999960*u(5)...
                 +0.479999999999979*u(6)...
                 -0.055555555555568*u(7)...
                 -4.900000000000000*ux(1)*dx);
         end
%
```

```
%  uxx at the right boundary
%
%     Without ux
         if nu==1
         uxx(n)=rdxs*...
                (  5.211111111111110*u(n  )...
                 -22.300000000000000*u(n-1)...
                 +43.950000000000000*u(n-2)...
                 -52.722222222222200*u(n-3)...
                 +41.000000000000000*u(n-4)...
                 -20.100000000000000*u(n-5)...
                  +5.661111111111110*u(n-6)...
                  -0.700000000000000*u(n-7));
%
%     With ux
         elseif nu==2
         uxx(n)=rdxs*...
                ( -7.493888888888860*u(n  )...
                 +12.000000000000000*u(n-1)...
                  -7.499999999999940*u(n-2)...
                  +4.444444444444570*u(n-3)...
                  -1.874999999999960*u(n-4)...
                  +0.479999999999979*u(n-5)...
                  -0.055555555555568*u(n-6)...
                  +4.900000000000000*ux(n)*dx);
         end
%
%  uxx at the interior grid points
%
%     i = 2
         uxx(2)=rdxs*...
                (  0.700000000000000*u(1)...
                  -0.388888888888889*u(2)...
                  -2.700000000000000*u(3)...
                  +4.750000000000000*u(4)...
                  -3.722222222222220*u(5)...
                  +1.800000000000000*u(6)...
                  -0.500000000000000*u(7)...
                  +0.061111111111111*u(8));
%
%     i = 3
          uxx(3)=rdxs*...
                ( -0.061111111111111*u(1)...
                  +1.188888888888890*u(2)...
                  -2.100000000000000*u(3)...
                  +0.722222222222223*u(4)...
                  +0.472222222222222*u(5)...
                  -0.300000000000000*u(6)...
                  +0.088888888888889*u(7)...
                  -0.011111111111111*u(8));
%
```

```
%     i = n-1
        uxx(n-1)=rdxs*...
                ( 0.700000000000000*u(n)...
                 -0.388888888888889*u(n-1)...
                 -2.700000000000000*u(n-2)...
                 +4.750000000000000*u(n-3)...
                 -3.722222222222220*u(n-4)...
                 +1.800000000000000*u(n-5)...
                 -0.500000000000000*u(n-6)...
                 +0.061111111111111*u(n-7));
%
%     i = n-2
        uxx(n-2)=rdxs*...
                ( -0.061111111111111*u(n  )...
                  +1.188888888888890*u(n-1)...
                  -2.100000000000000*u(n-2)...
                  +0.722222222222223*u(n-3)...
                  +0.472222222222222*u(n-4)...
                  -0.300000000000000*u(n-5)...
                  +0.088888888888889*u(n-6)...
                  -0.011111111111111*u(n-7));
%
%     i = 4, 5, ..., n-3
        for i=4:n-3
        uxx(i)=rdxs*...
                ( 0.011111111111111*u(i-3)...
                 -0.150000000000000*u(i-2)...
                 +1.500000000000000*u(i-1)...
                 -2.722222222222220*u(i  )...
                 +1.500000000000000*u(i+1)...
                 -0.150000000000000*u(i+2)...
                 +0.011111111111111*u(i+3));
        end
```

Listing 1.18 Calculation of the derivative uzz by dss042, dss044, dss046

We can note the following points about these routines.

- dss042
  - After the definition of the function, the grid spacing in z (= dz) is calculated.

```
  function [uzz]=dss042(zl,zu,n,u,uz,nl,nu)
%
% Function dss042 computes a second order approximation of a
% second order derivative, with or without the normal derivative
% at the boundary.
%
% Grid spacing
  dz=(zu-zl)/(n-1);
```

– uzz(1) (second derivative at the left boundary, $z = 0$) is computed by a one-sided FD approximation, that is based on four points, i=1,2,3,4. Note the use of nl=1 for a Dirichlet BC.

```
%
%  uzz at the left boundary, without uz
   if nl==1
     uzz(1)=(( 2.)*u(  1)...
            +(-5.)*u(  2)...
            +( 4.)*u(  3)...
            +(-1.)*u(  4))/(dz^2);
```

– uzz(1) is computed by a one-sided FD approximation that is based on three points, i=1,2,3,, but also includes the derivative at the left boundary, uz(1), which is available as the fifth input argument. Note the use of nl=2 for a Neumann BC.

```
%
%  uzz at the left boundary, including uz
   elseif nl==2
     uzz(1)=((-7.)*u(  1)...
            +( 8.)*u(  2)...
            +(-1.)*u(  3))/(2.*dz^2)...
            +(-6.)*uz( 1) /(2.*dz);
    end
```

– uzz(n) (second derivative at the right boundary, $z = z_L$) is computed by a one-sided FD approximation, which is based on four points, i=n,n-1,n-2,n-3. Note the use of nu=1 for a Dirichlet BC.

```
%
%  uzz at the right boundary, without uz
   if nu==1
     uzz(n)=(( 2.)*u(n  )...
            +(-5.)*u(n-1)...
            +( 4.)*u(n-2)...
            +(-1.)*u(n-3))/(dz^2);
```

This FD can be obtained from the left boundary (i=1) counterpart by permutation of the subscripts (e.g., 1 replaced by n to 4 replaced by n-3) and reversal of the sign of dz, which actually has no effect in this case since dz is squared).

– uzz(n) is computed by a one-sided FD approximation that is based on three points, i=n, n-1,n-2, but again also includes the derivative at the right boundary, uz(n), which is available as the fifth input argument. Note the use of nu=2 for a Neumann BC.

```
%
%  uzz at the right boundary, including uz
   elseif nu==2
     uzz(n)=((-7.)*u(n  )...
            +( 8.)*u(n-1)...
            +(-1.)*u(n-2))/(2.*dz^2)...
            +( 6.)*uz(n ) /(2.*dz);
   end
```

Note the sign reversal of the uz(n) term due to the change in sign of dz of the previous uz(1) term.

- For the interior points (i=2,...,n-1), a centered approximations is used.

```
%
%  uzz at the interior grid points
   for i=2:n-1
     uzz(i)=(u(i+1)-2.*u(i)+u(i-1))/dz^2;
   end
```

- dss044
  - The coding of dss044 parallels that of dss042. Note the use of additional points (values of u) to achieve $O(h^4)$ compared with $O(h^2)$ of dss042. Also, two FD approximations are programmed for uzz(1) and uzz(n) that include the first derivatives uz(1) and uz(n) for Neumann BCs (with nl=2, nu=2, respectively).
  - One additional feature of dss044 is the separate programming for uzz(2) (for one point to the right of the left boundary at $z=0$) and for uzz(n-1) (for one point to the left of the right boundary at $z=z_L$). Again, the derivation of all of the FDs is given in a set of documentation comments in the download version of dss044.
- dss046
  - The coding of dss046 parallels that of dss044. Note the use of additional points (values of u) to achieve $O(h^6)$ compared with $O(h^4)$ of dss044. Also, two FD approximations are programmed for uzz(1) and uzz(n) that include the first derivatives uz(1) and uz(n) for Neumann BCs (with nl=2, nu=2, respectively).
  - One additional feature of dss046 is the separate programming for uzz(2) and uzz(3) (for one and two points to the right of the left boundary at $z=0$), and for uzz(n-1) and uzz(n-2) (for one and two points to the left of the right boundary at $z=z_L$). Again, the derivation of all of the FDs is given in a set of documentation comments in the download version of dss046.
  - The format of the weighting coefficients with 16 figures, e.g., 5.211111111111110, resulted from the use of a routine based on the algorithm by Fornberg [3, 4]. As a related point, two additional routines for second derivatives, dss048 and dss050, are also available with FDs for which $p=8,10$.
- One additional detail concerning the FD approximations can be noted. For first derivatives, the weighting coefficients have a length in the denominator that results from $1/\Delta z$; this is expected for the multiplication of u(i) by the weighting coefficients to give uz(i). Similarly, for second derivatives, the weighting coefficients have a squared length in the denominator that results from $1/\Delta z^2$; this is expected for the multiplication of u(i) by the weighting coefficients to give uzz(i).

Figure 1.19 confirms the close agreement between the numerical and analytical solutions, as reflected in the output of Table 1.7. The other five plots for ncase=2,...,6 are identical to Fig. 1.19 and are therefore not presented here. This agreement is to be expected since the problem of eqs. (1.18) to (1.21) is smooth in the sense that the solution and its derivatives of all orders are smooth according to eq. (1.22). In particular, the IC

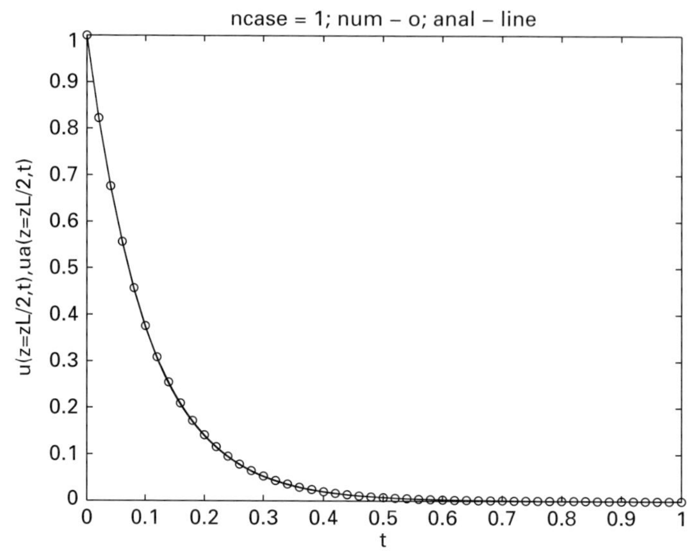

Figure 1.19 $u(zL/2,t)$ from `pde_1_main` of Listing 1.15 for `ncase = 1`

(1.21a), and BCs (1.21b) and (1.21c) are consistent (they agree). If the IC and BCs were inconsistent, perhaps by having boundary values other than zero, a discontinuity would be introduced that could possibly cause computational problems (consider the effect of a discontinuity in the case of the hyperbolic problem of eqs. (1.1) to (1.3), as reflected, for example in eq. (1.5)). However, for eq. (1.18), a discontinuity between the IC and BCs would probably not cause a computational problem because eq. (1.18) is parabolic and thus tends to smooth discontinuities; physically, this is to be expected since eq. (1.18) models diffusion, which is a smoothing process. In other words, parabolic PDEs are generally much easier to handle numerically than hyperbolic PDEs.

We conclude this discussion of parabolic PDEs with a few remaining ideas.

- The routines that calculate `uzz` directly from `u`, that is `dss042`, `dss044`, `dss046`, cannot accommodate a PDE like eq. (1.23) and stagewise differentiation is the obvious choice of a method for eq. (1.23).
- However, the second derivative routines can be applied to higher order PDEs through stagewise differentiation. For example, the fourth order PDE

$$\frac{\partial^2 u}{\partial t^2} + c^2 \frac{\partial^4 u}{\partial z^4} = 0 \tag{1.24}$$

could be investigated numerically by applying the second derivative routines twice to compute the fourth derivative. The required four BCs can be included through various combinations of Dirichlet and Neumann BCs (defined with arguments `nl,nu` as the second derivative routines are applied).

- Third type BCs such as eqs. (1.20e) and (1.20f) can also be accommodated with the second derivative routines by programming them as Neumann BCs. This case will be demonstrated subsequently by an example.

1.3.2 Neumann BCs

We now consider eqs. (1.18) to (1.22) with the Dirichlet BCs replaced by Neumann BCs. The IC is

$$u(z,t=0) = f(z) = \cos(\pi z/z_L); \quad 0 \le z \le z_L, \tag{1.25a}$$

and BCs (1.21b) and (1.21c) are replaced by the Neumann BCs

$$\frac{\partial u(z=0,t)}{\partial z} = 0, \tag{1.25b}$$

$$\frac{\partial u(z=z_L,t)}{\partial z} = 0. \tag{1.25c}$$

Equations (1.25b) and (1.25c) are special cases of eqs. (1.20c) and (1.20d) with $g_{n,1}(t) = g_{n,2}(t) = 0$. The analytical solution of eq. (1.22) becomes

$$u(z,t) = e^{-D(\pi/z_L)^2 t}\cos(\pi z/z_L). \tag{1.26}$$

The problem then is stated as eqs. (1.18) and (1.25) with analytical solution (1.26) to evaluate the numerical solution.

A main program for eqs. (1.18) and (1.25) is listed next.

```
  clc
  clear all
%
%   One dimensional diffusion
%
%   The PDE that models the diffusion mass transfer is
%
%      ut = D*uzz                                          (1)
%
%   with the initial and Neumann boundary conditions
%
%      u(z,0) = u0(z), uz(0,t) = 0, uz(zL,t) = 0     (2)(3)(4)
%
%   where
%
%      u      dependent variable, e.g., concentration
%
%      t      time
%
%      z      position
%
%      D      diffusivity
%
```

```
%      u0(z) initial u
%
%      zL    length
%
%   The profiles of u(z,t) in z are plotted for selected t.
%
%   The method of lines (MOL) solution of eq. (1) is coded below.
%   The resulting system of ODEs in t, defined on a 21 point grid in z,
%   is then integrated by the classical fourth order Runge Kutta method.
%
%   The analytical solution to eqs. (1) to (4) is also programmed
%   for comparison with the numerical solution.
%
%   The following code is run for the six special cases:
%
%      Case 1: uzz by three point finite differences (3pc)
%              and stagewise differentiation
%
%      Case 2: uzz by five point finite differences  (5pc)
%              and stagewise differentiation
%
%      Case 3: uzz by seven point finite differences (7pc)
%              and stagewise differentiation
%
%      Case 4: uzz by three point finite differences (3pc)
%              and direct second order differentiation
%
%      Case 5: uzz by five point finite differences  (5pc)
%              and direct second order differentiation
%
%      Case 6: uzz by seven point finite differences (7pc)
%              and direct second order differentiation
%
  global zL D ncase n ncall
%
% Model parameters (defined in the comments above)
  D=1; zL=1; n=21;
%
% Step through cases
  for ncase=1:6
%
% Parameters for fourth order Runge Kutta integration
  nsteps=100;
  h=0.0005;
%
% Initial condition
  for i=1:n
    z(i)=(i-1)/(n-1)*zL;
    u(i)=cos(pi*z(i)/zL);
  end
  t=0;
```

```
%
% Write ncase, h
  fprintf('\n\n ncase = %1d    h = %10.3e\n\n',ncase,h);
%
% Analytical solution at t = 0
  for i=1:n
    ua(i)=cos(pi*z(i)/zL);
%
%   Store solutions for plotting at t = 0
     uplot(1,i)=u(i);
    uaplot(1,i)=ua(i);
     zplot(i)=z(i);
  end
%
% nout output points
  nout=7;
  ncall=0;
  for iout=2:nout
%
%   Fourth order Runge Kutta integration
    u0=u; t0=t;
    [u,t]=rk4(u0,t0,h,nsteps);
%
%   Analytical solution
    for i=1:n
      ua(i)=exp(-(pi/zL)^2*t)*cos(pi*z(i)/zL);
%
%     Store solutions for plotting
       uplot(iout,i)=u(i);
      uaplot(iout,i)=ua(i);
%
%   Next point in z
    end
%
% Next output
  end
%
% Plot z profiles of solution
  figure(ncase);
  plot(zplot,uplot(1,:),'-o',zplot,uaplot(1,:),'-');
  axis([0 1 -1 1]);
  ylabel('u(z,t),ua(z,t)');xlabel('t');
  if(ncase==1)title('ncase = 1; t = 0, 0.05,..., 0.3;
    num - o; anal - line');end
  if(ncase==2)title('ncase = 2; t = 0, 0.05,..., 0.3;
    num - o; anal - line');end
  if(ncase==3)title('ncase = 3; t = 0, 0.05,..., 0.3;
    num - o; anal - line');end
  if(ncase==4)title('ncase = 4; t = 0, 0.05,..., 0.3;
    num - o; anal - line');end
  if(ncase==5)title('ncase = 5; t = 0, 0.05,..., 0.3;
```

```
     num - o; anal - line');end
   if(ncase==6)title('ncase = 6; t = 0, 0.05,..., 0.3;
     num - o; anal - line');end
   hold on
   for iout=2:nout
     plot(zplot,uplot(iout,:),'-o',zplot,uaplot(iout,:),'-');
     hold on
   end
%
% Next case
   end
```

Listing 1.19 Main program pde_1_main for the solution of eqs. (1.18) and (1.25) with a series of FD approximations in pde_1 of Listing 1.20

We can note the following details about pde_1_main.

- Previous files are cleared and selected variables are declared global. The documentation comments pertaining to eqs. (1.18) to (1.25) and the calculation of uzz are not repeated here to conserve space.

```
  clc
  clear all
%
%   One dimensional diffusion
%
%
  global zL D ncase n ncall
```

- The diffusivity in eq. (1.18) is defined. The grid in z is $0 \leq z \leq 1$ with 21 points.

```
%
% Model parameters (defined in the comments above)
  D=1; zL=1; n=21;
```

- The for loop in ncase steps through the six cases.

```
%
% Step through cases
  for ncase=1:6
```

- The parameters for the integration in t are specified (the integrator is rk4 in Listing 1.5).

```
%
% Parameters for fourth order Runge Kutta integration
  nsteps=100;
  h=0.0005;
```

- The grid in z and the IC of eq. (1.25a) are programmed (this sets the ICs of the 21 ODEs for the MOL solution of eq. (1.18)).

```
%
% Initial condition
```

```
  for i=1:n
    z(i)=(i-1)/(n-1)*zL;
    u(i)=cos(pi*z(i)/zL);
  end
  t=0;
```

- A line for each case is displayed.

```
%
% Write ncase, h
  fprintf('\n\n ncase = %1d    h = %10.3e\n\n',ncase,h);
```

- The IC for the analytical solution is computed, and the ICs for the numerical and analytical solutions are stored for subsequent plotting. Note the use of the subscript 1 for the first point ($t = 0$) in the plots.

```
%
% Analytical solution at t = 0
  for i=1:n
    ua(i)=cos(pi*z(i)/zL);
%
%   Store solutions for plotting at t = 0
     uplot(1,i)=u(i);
    uaplot(1,i)=ua(i);
     zplot(i)=z(i);
  end
```

- The parameters are set for the t integration with seven outputs (including $t = 0$) over the interval $0 \leq t \leq 0.3$ in steps of $(100)(0.0005) = 0.05$ (from the preceding programming of `nsteps=100` and `h=0.0005`). Also, the number of calls to the ODE routine, `pde_1`, is initialized.

```
%
% nout output points
  nout=7;
  ncall=0;
  for iout=2:nout
```

The integration in t then proceeds with a `for` loop. Note the starting index of `iout=2` (to include the previous IC with `iout=1`).

- `rk4` of Listing 1.5 is called for the integration of the 21 ODEs (programmed in `pde_1`, considered subsequently).

```
%
%   Fourth order Runge Kutta integration
    u0=u; t0=t;
    [u,t]=rk4(u0,t0,h,nsteps);
```

Each call to `rk4` advances the solution $100(0.0005) = 0.05$ in t. $7 - 1$ steps, each of length 0.05, produce the complete solution over the interval $0 \leq t \leq 0.3$.

- The analytical solution of eq. (1.26) is evaluated and the numerical and analytical solutions are stored for plotting.

```
%
%   Analytical solution
    for i=1:n
      ua(i)=exp(-(pi/zL)^2*t)*cos(pi*z(i)/zL);
%
%     Store solutions for plotting
       uplot(iout,i)=u(i);
      uaplot(iout,i)=ua(i);
%
%   Next point in z
    end
%
% Next output
  end
```

The second end concludes the for loop in iout.

- The profiles in z are plotted for $t = 0, 0.05, \cdots, 0.3$ for ncase = 1,...,6.

```
%
% Plot z profiles of solution
  figure(ncase);
  plot(zplot,uplot(1,:),'-o',zplot,uaplot(1,:),'-');
  axis([0 1 -1 1]);
  ylabel('u(z,t),ua(z,t)');xlabel('t');
  if(ncase==1)title('ncase = 1; t = 0, 0.05,..., 0.3;
    num - o; anal - line');end
  if(ncase==2)title('ncase = 2; t = 0, 0.05,..., 0.3;
    num - o; anal - line');end
  if(ncase==3)title('ncase = 3; t = 0, 0.05,..., 0.3;
    num - o; anal - line');end
  if(ncase==4)title('ncase = 4; t = 0, 0.05,..., 0.3;
    num - o; anal - line');end
  if(ncase==5)title('ncase = 5; t = 0, 0.05,..., 0.3;
    num - o; anal - line');end
  if(ncase==6)title('ncase = 6; t = 0, 0.05,..., 0.3;
    num - o; anal - line');end
  hold on
  for iout=2:nout
    plot(zplot,uplot(iout,:),'-o',zplot,uaplot(iout,:),'-');
    hold on
  end
%
% Next case
  end
```

The end concludes the outer for loop for the six values of ncase.

The graphical output for ncase=1 is in Fig. 1.20. The plotted output for ncase=2,...,6 is identical to Fig. 1.20 and is not repeated here.

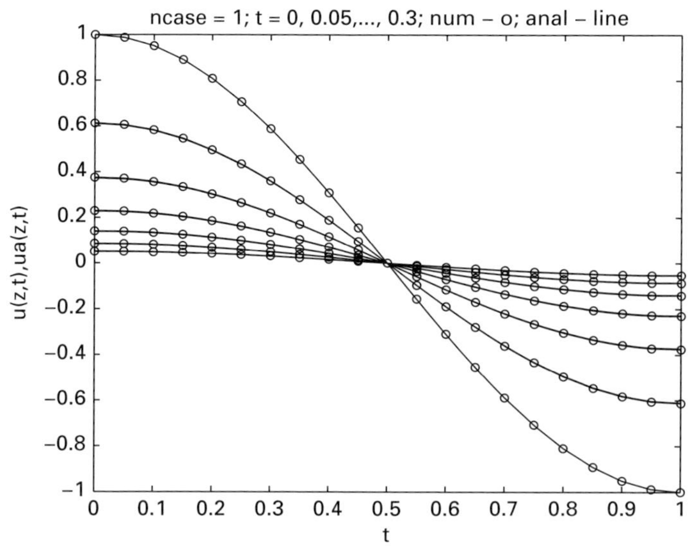

Figure 1.20 $u(z,t)$ from `pde_1_main` of Listing 1.19 for `ncase = 1`

We can note the following details about Fig. 1.20.

- The numerical and analytical solutions are in close agreement so that the two solutions are indistinguishable.
- The homogeneous (zero) Neumann BCs of eqs. (1.25b) and (1.25c) are evident (zero slope at $z = 0, 1$).
- The solutions approach the limiting value $u(z,t=\infty) = 0$ as indicated by eq. (1.26).

The ODE routine `pde_1` called by `pde_1_main` of Listing 1.19 is listed next.

```
  function ut=pde_1(u,t)
%
% Function pde_1 computes the t derivative vector of the u vector
%
  global zL D ifd n ncase ncall
%
% Second order spatial derivative
  if(ncase==1)
     [uz]=dss002(0,zL,n,u);
     uz(1)=0; uz(n)=0;
    [uzz]=dss002(0,zL,n,uz);
  end
  if(ncase==2)
     [uz]=dss004(0,zL,n,u);
     uz(1)=0; uz(n)=0;
    [uzz]=dss004(0,zL,n,uz);
  end
  if(ncase==3)
     [uz]=dss006(0,zL,n,u);
```

```
      uz(1)=0; uz(n)=0;
     [uzz]=dss006(0,zL,n,uz);
  end
  if(ncase==4)
    nl=2; nu=2; uz(1)=0; uz(n)=0;
    [uzz]=dss042(0,zL,n,u,uz,nl,nu);
  end
  if(ncase==5)
    nl=2; nu=2; uz(1)=0; uz(n)=0;
    [uzz]=dss044(0,zL,n,u,uz,nl,nu);
  end
  if(ncase==6)
    nl=2; nu=2; uz(1)=0; uz(n)=0;
    [uzz]=dss046(0,zL,n,u,uz,nl,nu);
  end
%
% Temporal derivative
  for i=1:n
    ut(i)=D*uzz(i);
  end
%
% Increment calls to pde_1
  ncall=ncall+1;
```

Listing 1.20 pde_1 for the solution of eqs. (1.18) and (1.25) with a series of FD approximations

We can note the following details about pde_1.

- The function is defined and selected variables are declared as global.

```
  function ut=pde_1(u,t)
%
% Function pde_1 computes the t derivative vector of the u vector
%
  global zL D ifd n ncase ncall
```

- For ncase=1, dss002 is called to compute the second derivative in eq. (1.18) by stagewise differentiation.

```
%
% Second order spatial derivative
  if(ncase==1)
      [uz]=dss002(0,zL,n,u);
      uz(1)=0; uz(n)=0;
     [uzz]=dss002(0,zL,n,uz);
  end
```

After the first call to dss002 to compute the first derivative, uz, the homogeneous (zero) Neumann BCs of eqs. (1.25b) and (1.25c) are used to reset uz(1) and uz(n) (the first derivatives at the boundaries $z = 0, 1$). Then a second call to dss002 gives the second derivative uzz. Thus, in this way the two BCs for eq. (1.18) are included in the numerical solution.

- The same procedure is used to calculate uzz with dss004 (ncase=2) and dss006 (ncase=3).
- A second approach is to use the routines that calculate the second derivative directly. For ncase=4, dss042 is called.

```
if(ncase==4)
  nl=2; nu=2; uz(1)=0; uz(n)=0;
  [uzz]=dss042(0,zL,n,u,uz,nl,nu);
end
```

  Neumann BCs are declared with nl=2; nu=2; before dss042 is called, the two homogeneous BCs of eqs. (1.25b) and (1.25c) are specified as uz(1)=0; uz(n)=0;. Then dss042 is called to calculate the second derivative uzz.
- The same procedure is used to calculate uzz with dss044 (ncase=5) and dss046 (ncase=6).
- Equation (1.18) is programmed as the approximating 21 ODEs in a for loop.

```
%
% Temporal derivative
  for i=1:n
    ut(i)=D*uzz(i);
  end
%
% Increment calls to pde_1
  ncall=ncall+1;
```

  This could also have been done with a single statement ut=D*uzz; using the MATLAB vector facility. The counter for the calls to pde_1 is incremented at the end of pde_1. This final step provides the derivative vector ut returned as the output (LHS) argument of pde_1.

As in the case of Dirichlet BCs (see Tables 1.7 and 1.8), the accuracy of the numerical solutions improves through the use of higher order FDs. The numbers to demonstrate this are not presented here to conserve space.

1.3.3 Third type BCs

We conclude the discussion of BCs with an example of third type (Robin) BCs. The approach is a straightforward extension of the methods used in Section 1.3.2 for Neumann BCs. The problem is again based on eq. (1.18) with the following BCs, which are a special case of eqs. (1.20e) and (1.20f) with $c_1 = -1, c_2 = 1, g_{t,1}(t) = g_{t,2}(t) = 0$:

$$\frac{u(z=0,t)}{\partial z} - u(z=0,t) = 0, \tag{1.27a}$$

$$\frac{u(z=z_L,t)}{\partial z} + u(z=z_L,t) = 0. \tag{1.27b}$$

Although an analytical solution might be available for this problem, it would be relatively complicated and we will therefore not attempt to develop and use it. Instead, we can infer the validity of the numerical solution by h and p refinement, a more realistic situation for most applications; that is, we generally do not have available an analytical solution to evaluate the numerical solution.

To complete the specification of the problem, we will consider two cases for $f(z)$ in IC (1.19). The details of the two cases will be considered as the computer code is discussed. The main program is listed next.

```
  clc
  clear all
%
%   One dimensional diffusion
%
%   The PDE that models the diffusion mass transfer is
%
%      ut = D*uzz                                             (1)
%
%   with the initial and third type boundary conditions
%
%      u(z,0) = u0(z)                                         (2)
%
%      uz(0,t) - u(0,t) = 0, uz(zL,t) + u(zL,t) = 0        (3)(4)
%
%   where
%
%      u      dependent variable, e.g., concentration
%
%      t      time
%
%      z      position
%
%      D      diffusivity
%
%      u0(z) initial u
%
%      zL     length
%
%   The profiles of u(z,t) in z are plotted for selected t.
%
%   The method of lines (MOL) solution of eq. (1) is coded below.
%   The resulting system of ODEs in t, defined on a 21 point grid in z,
%   is then integrated by the classical fourth order Runge Kutta method.
%
%   The following code is run for the six special cases:
%
%      Case 1: uzz by three point finite differences (3pc)
%              and stagewise differentiation
%
%      Case 2: uzz by five point finite differences  (5pc)
%              and stagewise differentiation
%
%      Case 3: uzz by seven point finite differences (7pc)
```

```
%                and stagewise differentiation
%
%        Case 4: uzz by three point finite differences (3pc)
%                and direct second order differentiation
%
%        Case 5: uzz by five point finite differences  (5pc)
%                and direct second order differentiation
%
%        Case 6: uzz by seven point finite differences (7pc)
%                and direct second order differentiation
%
  global zL D ncase n ncall
%
% Model parameters (defined in the comments above)
  D=1; zL=1; n=21;
%
% Step through cases
  for ncase=1:6
%
% Parameters for fourth order Runge Kutta integration
  nsteps=200;
  h=0.0005;
%
% Initial condition
  for i=1:n
    z(i)=(i-1)/(n-1)*zL;
    if(i<=11)
      u(i)=1;
    else
%
%   Smooth
    u(i)=1;
%
%   Nonsmooth
%   u(i)=0;
    end
  end
  t=0;
%
% Write ncase, h
  fprintf('\n\n ncase = %1d    h = %10.3e\n\n',ncase,h);
%
% Store solution for plotting at t = 0
  uplot(1,:)=u(:);
  zplot=z;
%
% nout output points
  nout=11;
  ncall=0;
  for iout=2:nout
%
```

```
%   Fourth order Runge Kutta integration
    u0=u; t0=t;
    [u,t]=rk4(u0,t0,h,nsteps);
%
%    Store solution for plotting
     uplot(iout,:)=u(:);
%
% Next output
  end
%
% Plot z profiles of solution
  figure(ncase);
  plot(zplot,uplot(1,:),'-');
  axis([0 1 0 1]);
  ylabel('u(z,t),ua(z,t)');xlabel('t');
  if(ncase==1)title('ncase = 1; t = 0, 0.1,..., 1');end
  if(ncase==2)title('ncase = 2; t = 0, 0.1,..., 1');end
  if(ncase==3)title('ncase = 3; t = 0, 0.1,..., 1');end
  if(ncase==4)title('ncase = 4; t = 0, 0.1,..., 1');end
  if(ncase==5)title('ncase = 5; t = 0, 0.1,..., 1');end
  if(ncase==6)title('ncase = 6; t = 0, 0.1,..., 1');end
  hold on
  for iout=2:nout
    plot(zplot,uplot(iout,:),'-');
    hold on
  end
%
% Next case
  end
```

Listing 1.21 Main program pde_1_main for the solution of eqs. (1.18) and (1.27) with a series of FD approximations in pde_1 of Listing 1.22

We can note the following details about pde_1_main.

- Previous files are cleared and selected variables are declared global. The documentation comments pertaining to eqs. (1.18) to (1.27) and the calculation of uzz are not repeated here to conserve space.

```
  clc
  clear all
%
%   One dimensional diffusion
%
  global zL D ncase n ncall
```

- The diffusivity in eq. (1.18) is defined. The grid in z is $0 \leq z \leq 1$ with 21 points.

```
%
% Model parameters (defined in the comments above)
  D=1; zL=1; n=21;
```

- The for loop in ncase steps through the six cases.

```
%
% Step through cases
  for ncase=1:6
```

- The parameters for the integration in t are specified (the integrator is `rk4` in Listing 1.5).

```
%
% Parameters for fourth order Runge Kutta integration
  nsteps=200;
  h=0.0005;
```

- The grid in z is defined over $0 \le z \le z_L$ with $z_L = 1$ defined previously. The IC of eq. (1.19) is defined for two cases selected by uncommenting a line. To start, the smooth case is selected with `u(i)=1;` (for `i>11`). After this case is completed (the output is discussed), the nonsmooth case is selected by uncommenting `u(i)=0;` (for `i>11`).

```
%
% Initial condition
  for i=1:n
    z(i)=(i-1)/(n-1)*zL;
    if(i<=11)
      u(i)=1;
    else
%
%   Smooth
    u(i)=1;
%
%   Nonsmooth
%   u(i)=0;
    end
  end
  t=0;
```

For the smooth case, the IC is 1 throughout $0 \le z \le 1$. For the nonsmooth case, the IC is one for the left half of the interval $0 \le z \le 1$ ($i \le 11$) and is zero for the right half of this interval ($i > 11$).

- A line for each case is displayed. Then the solution at $t = 0$ and the grid in z are stored for subsequent plotting. Note the use of the subscript 1 for the first point ($t = 0$) in the plots.

```
%
% Write ncase, h
  fprintf('\n\n ncase = %1d    h = %10.3e\n\n',ncase,h);
%
% Store solution for plotting at t = 0
  uplot(1,:)=u(:);
  zplot=z;
```

- The parameters are set for the t integration with 11 outputs (including $t = 0$) over the interval $0 \le t \le 1$ in steps of $(200)(0.0005) = 0.1$ (from the preceding programming of nsteps=200 and h=0.0005). Also, the number of calls to the ODE routine, pde_1, is initialized.

```
%
% nout output points
  nout=11;
  ncall=0;
  for iout=2:nout
```

The integration in t then proceeds with a for loop. Note the starting index of 2 to include the previous IC (iout=1).

- rk4 of Listing 1.5 is called for the integration of the 21 ODEs (programmed in pde_1 considered subsequently).

```
%
%   Fourth order Runge Kutta integration
    u0=u; t0=t;
    [u,t]=rk4(u0,t0,h,nsteps);
```

Each call to rk4 advances the solution $200(0.0005) = 0.1$ in t. $11 - 1$ steps, each of length 0.1, produce the complete solution over the interval $0 \leq t \leq 1$.

- The numerical solution of eq. (1.18) is stored for plotting.

```
%
%     Store solution for plotting
      uplot(iout,:)=u(:);
%
% Next output
  end
```

The end concludes the for loop in iout.

- The profiles in z are plotted for $t = 0, 0.1, \cdots, 1$ for ncase=1,...,6.

```
%
% Plot z profiles of solution
  figure(ncase);
  plot(zplot,uplot(1,:),'-');
  axis([0 1 0 1]);
  ylabel('u(z,t),ua(z,t)');xlabel('t');
  if(ncase==1)title('ncase = 1; t = 0, 0.1,..., 1');end
  if(ncase==2)title('ncase = 2; t = 0, 0.1,..., 1');end
  if(ncase==3)title('ncase = 3; t = 0, 0.1,..., 1');end
  if(ncase==4)title('ncase = 4; t = 0, 0.1,..., 1');end
  if(ncase==5)title('ncase = 5; t = 0, 0.1,..., 1');end
  if(ncase==6)title('ncase = 6; t = 0, 0.1,..., 1');end
  hold on
  for iout=2:nout
    plot(zplot,uplot(iout,:),'-');
    hold on
  end
%
% Next case
  end
```

The end concludes the outer for loop for the six values of ncase.

The ODE routine pde_1 called by pde_1_main of Listing 1.21 is listed next.

```
  function ut=pde_1(u,t)
%
% Function pde_1 computes the t derivative vector of the u vector
%
  global zL D ifd n ncase ncall
%
% Second order spatial derivative
  if(ncase==1)
     [uz]=dss002(0,zL,n,u);
     uz(1)=u(1); uz(n)=-u(n);
    [uzz]=dss002(0,zL,n,uz);
  end
  if(ncase==2)
     [uz]=dss004(0,zL,n,u);
     uz(1)=u(1); uz(n)=-u(n);
    [uzz]=dss004(0,zL,n,uz);
  end
  if(ncase==3)
     [uz]=dss006(0,zL,n,u);
     uz(1)=u(1); uz(n)=-u(n);
    [uzz]=dss006(0,zL,n,uz);
  end
  if(ncase==4)
    nl=2; nu=2; uz(1)=u(1); uz(n)=-u(n);
    [uzz]=dss042(0,zL,n,u,uz,nl,nu);
  end
  if(ncase==5)
    nl=2; nu=2; uz(1)=u(1); uz(n)=-u(n);
    [uzz]=dss044(0,zL,n,u,uz,nl,nu);
  end
  if(ncase==6)
    nl=2; nu=2; uz(1)=u(1); uz(n)=-u(n);
    [uzz]=dss046(0,zL,n,u,uz,nl,nu);
  end
%
% Temporal derivative
  ut=D*uzz;
% for i=1:n
%   ut(i)=D*uzz(i);
% end
%
% Increment calls to pde_1
  ncall=ncall+1;
```

Listing 1.22 pde_1 for the solution of eqs. (1.18) and (1.27) with a series of FD approximations

We can note the following details about Listing 1.22.

- The function is defined and selected variables are declared as global.

```
  function ut=pde_1(u,t)
%
% Function pde_1 computes the t derivative vector of the u vector
%
  global zL D ifd n ncase ncall
```

- For ncase=1, dss002 is called to compute the second derivative in eq. (1.18) by stagewise differentiation.

```
%
% Second order spatial derivative
  if(ncase==1)
      [uz]=dss002(0,zL,n,u);
      uz(1)=u(1); uz(n)=-u(n);
    [uzz]=dss002(0,zL,n,uz);
  end
```

After the first call to dss002 to compute the first derivative, uz, the third type BCs of eqs. (1.27a) and (1.27b) are used to reset uz(1) and uz(n) (the first derivatives at the boundaries $z = 0, 1$). Then a second call to dss002 gives the second derivative uzz. Thus, in this way the two BCs for eq. (1.18) are included in the numerical solution.

- The same procedure is used to calculate uzz with dss004 (ncase=2) and dss006 (ncase=3).
- A second approach is to use the routines that calculate the second derivative directly. For ncase=4, dss042 is called.

```
  if(ncase==4)
    nl=2; nu=2; uz(1)=u(1); uz(n)=-u(n);
    [uzz]=dss042(0,zL,n,u,uz,nl,nu);
  end
```

Third type BCs are declared with nl=2, nu=2 before dss042 is called, and the two BCs of eqs. (1.27a) and (1.27b) are specified as uz(1)=u(1); uz(n)=-u(n);. Then dss042 is called to calculate the second derivative uzz.

- The same procedure is used to calculate uzz with dss044 (ncase=5) and dss046 (ncase=6).
- Equation (1.18) is programmed with a single statement ut=D*uzz; using the MATLAB vector facility.

```
%
% Temporal derivative
  ut=D*uzz;
% for i=1:n
%   ut(i)=D*uzz(i);
% end
%
% Increment calls to pde_1
  ncall=ncall+1;
```

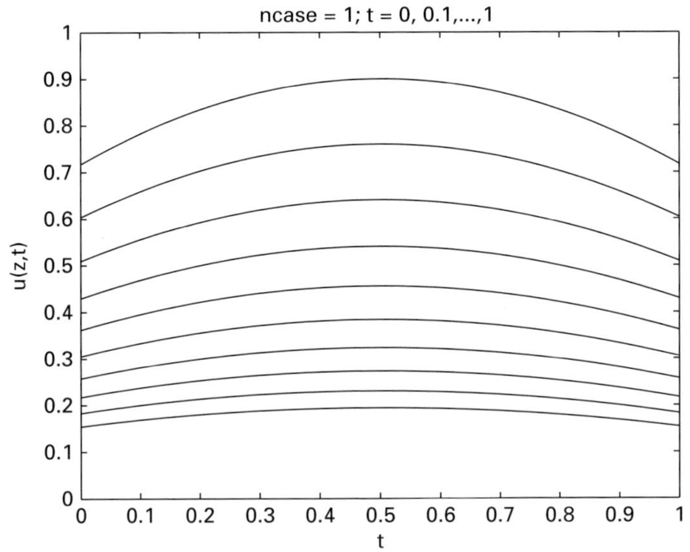

Figure 1.21 $u(z,t)$ from `pde_1_main` of Listing 1.21 for `ncase = 1`

A second approach is to use a `for` loop (commented) for the `n=21` ODEs. The counter for the calls to `pde_1` is incremented at the end of `pde_1`. This final step provides the derivative vector `ut` returned as the output (LHS) argument of `pde_1`.

The graphical output for `ncase=1` is in Fig. 1.21. The plotted output for `ncase=2,...,6` is identical to Fig. 1.21 and is not repeated here.

We can note the following details about Fig. 1.21.

- The solution is symmetrical about $z = 0.5$, as expected, since BCs (1.27a) and (1.27b) are symmetrical with respect to z.
- The solution appears to be approaching the limiting value $u(z, t = \infty) = 0$, which follows from BCs (1.27a) and (1.27b); one physical interpretation of these BCs is that the surrounding medium at the boundaries $z = 0, 1$ is at zero concentration and diffusion into these surroundings will continue until the concentration $u(z,t)$ is uniform and zero.

This concludes the discussion of eq. (1.18) for Dirichlet, Neumann, and third type BCs. In summary, eq. (1.1) is hyperbolic and eq. (1.18) is parabolic. A brief geometric classification of PDEs (hyperbolic, parabolic, elliptic) is given in Table 1.9. A more detailed classification of PDEs is given in [9].

We now consider the case for which two basic types of PDEs, first order hyperbolic and parabolic, are combined into a hyperbolic-parabolic PDE, or physically, a convective-diffusive PDE. This combination is an important mathematical description for physical and chemical systems, and will be used in applications in subsequent chapters.

Table 1.9. Brief geometric classification of PDEs; t – initial value variable; y, z – boundary value variables

Type	General characteristics	Example
First order Hyperbolic	First order in t First order in z	$(\partial u/\partial t) + v(\partial u/\partial z) = 0$ Linear advection eq. (1.1)
Second order Hyperbolic	Second order in t Second order in z	$(\partial^2 u/\partial t^2) = c^2(\partial^2 u/\partial z^2)$ Wave equation – can be expressed as two first order hyperbolic PDEs
Parabolic	First order in t Second order in z	$(\partial u/\partial t) = D(\partial^2 u/\partial z^2)$ Diffusion eq. (1.18)
Elliptic	Zeroth order in t Second order in y and z	$(\partial^2 u/\partial y^2) + (\partial^2 u/\partial z^2) = 0$ Laplace's equation

1.4 Hyperbolic-parabolic PDEs

The hyperbolic-parabolic PDE to be analyzed in several ways is

$$\frac{\partial u}{\partial t} = -v\frac{\partial u}{\partial z} + D\frac{\partial^2 u}{\partial z^2} + k_r u. \tag{1.28}$$

Note that in eq. (1.28) a reaction term, $k_r u$, has been included; k_r is a reaction rate constant with typical units of s^{-1}, as suggested by the LHS derivative in t. Thus, eq. (1.28) is a convection-diffusion-reaction (CDR) PDE. A derivation of eq. (1.28) is given in Appendix 1.

Since eq. (1.28) is first order in t and second order in z, it requires one IC and two BCs. For the IC, we will use eq. (1.2). For the BCs we will use

$$vu(z=0,t) = vu_e - D\frac{\partial u(z=0,t)}{\partial z} \tag{1.29a}$$

$$\frac{\partial u(z=z_L,t)}{\partial z} = 0 \tag{1.29b}$$

or

$$\frac{\partial u(z=z_L,t)}{\partial t} + v\frac{\partial u(z=z_L,t)}{\partial z} = 0. \tag{1.29c}$$

Boundary condition (1.29b) is frequently specified, but as we shall observe, it causes computational problems and unrealistic numerical solutions; BC (1.29c) circumvents these problems.

Boundary condition (1.29a) equates the convective flux $vu(z=0,t)$ to the sum of the entering flux vu_e and the diffusive flux $-D(\partial u(z=0,t)/\partial z)$, where u_e is the entering concentration. For the case of no diffusion, $D=0$, eq. (1.29a) reduces to $u(z=0,t)=u_e$, as expected. The minus in the diffusive flux follows from Fick's first law

$$N = -D\frac{\partial u}{\partial z}, \tag{1.29d}$$

where N is a diffusion flux (a vector with a sign indicating direction in z).

The analytical solution to eqs. (1.28) and (1.29) is available, but it is relatively complicated, so we will discuss only the numerical solution. As another detail concerning eqs. (1.28) and (1.29), the relative degree of convection to diffusion is usually expressed as the dimensionless Peclet number, $\text{Pe} = ((z_\text{L})(v)/D)$ where z_L, v, D appear in eqs. (1.28) and (1.29). Thus, for large Pe, the PDE system is strongly convective. For example, in the routines that follow, $z_\text{L} = v = 1, D = 0.0001$, so that $\text{Pe} = ((1)(1)/0.0001) = 10^4$, which corresponds to a strongly convective (or strongly hyperbolic) system; the consequence of this is that the solutions to eqs. (1.28) and (1.29) can display step moving fronts (as did eq. (1.1), for which Pe is infinite).

A main program, pde_1_main for eqs. (1.28) and (1.29) (with IC (1.2)) follows.

```
  clc
  clear all
%
%  One dimensional convection diffusion reaction (CDR) equation
%
%  The PDE is
%
%     ut = D*uzz - v*uz - kr*u                              (1)
%
%  with the initial condition
%
%     u(z,t=0) = f(z)                                       (2)
%
%  and boundary conditions
%
%     v*u(z=0,t) = v*ue - D*uz(z=0,t);                      (3)
%
%     ut(z=zl,t) + v*uz(z=zl,t) = 0                         (4)
%
%  where
%
%     u     dependent variable, e.g., concentration
%
%     t     time
%
%     z     position
%
%     D     diffusivity (dispersion coefficient)
%
%     v     velocity
%
%     kr    reaction rate constant
%
```

```
%       f(z)  initial condition function
%
%       ue    entering u
%
%       zl    length
%
%    The following code is run for five special cases:
%
%       Case 1: uz by two point upwind (2pu), uzz by three point
%               centered finite differences (3pc) and direct second
%               order differentiation
%
%       Case 2: uz and uzz by three point centered finite differences
%               (3pc) and direct second order differentiation
%
%       Case 3: uz by van Leer flux limiter (vanl), uzz by three
%               point centered finite differences (3pc) and direct
%               second order differentiation
%
%       Case 4: uz by superbee flux limiter (super), uzz by five
%               point centered finite differences (5pc) and direct
%               second order differentiation
%
%       Case 5: uz by smart flux limiter (smart), uzz by seven
%               point centered finite differences (7pc) and direct
%               second order differentiation
%
  global a b D v ue kr zl ncase n ncall
%
% Model parameters (defined in the comments above)
  kr=0; v=1; ue=1; zl=1; n=51; D=0.0001;
%
% Step through cases
  for ncase=1:5
%
% Level of output
%
%   Detailed output - ip = 1
%
%   Brief (IC) output - ip = 2
%
  ip=2;
%
% Parameters for fourth order Runge Kutta integration
  nsteps=200;
  h=0.001;
%
% Initial condition
  for i=1:n
    z(i)=(i-1)/(n-1)*zl;
    u(i)=0;
```

```
  end
  u(1)=ue;
  t=0;
%
% Write ncase, h
  fprintf('\n\n ncase = %1d   h = %10.3e\n\n',ncase,h);
%
% nout output points
  nout=6;
  ncall=0;
  for iout=1:nout
%
%   Fourth order Runge Kutta integration
    u0=u; t0=t;
    [u,t]=rk4(u0,t0,h,nsteps);
%
%   Numerical solution
    fprintf('\n t = %5.2f\n',t);
    for i=1:n
      uplot(iout,i)=u(i);
      if(ip==1)
        fprintf('%7.2f%12.3f\n',z(i),u(i));
      end
    end
%
% Next output
  end
%
% Plots for ncase = 1 to 5
  figure(ncase);
  plot(z,uplot,'-o');
  axis([0 1 0 1.2]);
  ylabel('u(z,t)'); xlabel('z');
  if(ncase==1)title('ncase = 1, u(z,t), t = 0.2, 0.4, ..., 1.2,');end
  if(ncase==2)title('ncase = 2, u(z,t), t = 0.2, 0.4, ..., 1.2,');
                                                 axis([0 1 0 1.4]);end
  if(ncase==3)title('ncase = 3, u(z,t), t = 0.2, 0.4, ..., 1.2,');end
  if(ncase==4)title('ncase = 4, u(z,t), t = 0.2, 0.4, ..., 1.2,');end
  if(ncase==5)title('ncase = 5, u(z,t), t = 0.2, 0.4, ..., 1.2,');end
%
% Next case
  end
```

Listing 1.23 Main program pde_1_main for the solution of eqs. (1.28) and (1.29) with a series of FD approximations in pde_1 of Listing 1.24

We can note the following details about pde_1_main.

- Previous files are cleared and selected variables are declared global. The documentation comments pertaining to eqs. (1.28) and (1.29) and the calculation of uzz are not repeated here to conserve space.

```
  clc
  clear all
%
%  One dimensional convection diffusion reaction (CDR) equation
%
  global a b D v ue kr zl ncase n ncall
```

- The parameters of eqs. (1.28), (1.29) are defined numerically. The grid in z is $0 \leq z \leq 1$ with 51 points.

```
%
% Model parameters (defined in the comments above)
  kr=0; v=1; ue=1; zl=1; n=51; D=0.0001;
```

  The Peclet number $\mathrm{Pe} = ((z_L)(v)/D)$ is simply $1/D$ with $z_L = v = 1$.
- The `for` loop in `ncase` steps through the five cases.

```
%
% Step through cases
  for ncase=1:5
%
% Level of output
%
%   Detailed output - ip = 1
%
%   Brief (IC) output - ip = 2
%
  ip=2;
```

  The level of the numerical output is specified with `ip`.
- The parameters for the integration in t are specified (the integrator is `rk4` in Listing 1.5).

```
%
% Parameters for fourth order Runge Kutta integration
  nsteps=200;
  h=0.001;
```

- The grid in z is defined over $0 \leq z \leq z_L$ with $z_L = 1$ defined previously. The IC of eq. (1.2) is a unit step at $z = 0$ (with ue=1).

```
%
% Initial condition
  for i=1:n
    z(i)=(i-1)/(n-1)*zl;
    u(i)=0;
  end
  u(1)=ue;
  t=0;
```

- A line for each case is displayed.

```
%
% Write ncase, h
  fprintf('\n\n ncase = %1d   h = %10.3e\n\n',ncase,h);
```

- The parameters are set for the t integration with six outputs in steps of $(200)(0.001) = 0.2$ from the preceding programming of nsteps=200 and h=0.001; that is, the output is at $t = 0.2, 0.4, \cdots, 1.2$. Also, the number of calls to the ODE routine, pde_1, is initialized.

```
%
% nout output points
  nout=6;
  ncall=0;
  for iout=1:nout
```

The integration in t then proceeds with a for loop.

- rk4 of Listing 1.5 is called for the integration of the 21 ODEs (programmed in pde_1 considered subsequently).

```
  for iout=1:nout
%
%   Fourth order Runge Kutta integration
    u0=u; t0=t;
    [u,t]=rk4(u0,t0,h,nsteps);
```

Each call to rk4 advances the solution $200(0.001) = 0.2$ in t. $6-1$ steps, each of length 0.2, produce the complete solution.

- The numerical solution of eq. (1.28) is stored for plotting with detailed numerical output for ip=1.

```
%
%   Numerical solution
    fprintf('\n t = %5.2f\n',t);
    for i=1:n
      uplot(iout,i)=u(i);
      if(ip==1)
        fprintf('%7.2f%12.3f\n',z(i),u(i));
      end
    end
```

The end concludes the for loop in iout.

- The profiles in z are plotted for $t = 0.2, 0.4, \cdots, 1.2$ for ncase=1, . . . ,5.

```
%
% Plots for ncase = 1 to 5
  figure(ncase);
  plot(z,uplot,'-o');
  axis([0 1 0 1.2]);
  ylabel('u(z,t)'); xlabel('z');
  if(ncase==1)title('ncase = 1, u(z,t), t = 0.2, 0.4,  ..., 1.2,');end
  if(ncase==2)title('ncase = 2, u(z,t), t = 0.2, 0.4,  ..., 1.2,');
                                              axis([0 1 0 1.4]);end
  if(ncase==3)title('ncase = 3, u(z,t), t = 0.2, 0.4,  ..., 1.2,');end
  if(ncase==4)title('ncase = 4, u(z,t), t = 0.2, 0.4,  ..., 1.2,');end
  if(ncase==5)title('ncase = 5, u(z,t), t = 0.2, 0.4,  ..., 1.2,');end
%
% Next case
  end
```

The vertical scale for ncase=2 is expanded to accommodate the oscillations in the numerical solution. The end concludes the outer for loop for the five values of ncase.

The ODE routine, pde_1, called by rk4 in pde_1_main is listed next.

```
  function ut=pde_1(u,t)
%
% Function pde_1 computes the t derivative vector of the u vector
%
  global a b D v ue kr zl n ncase ncall
%
% First, second order spatial derivatives
  nl=1; nu=2;
  if(ncase==1)
     [uz]=dss012(0,zl,n,u,v);
     u(1)=ue-D*uz(1);
     [uzz]=dss042(0,zl,n,u,uz,nl,nu);
  end
  if(ncase==2)
     [uz]=dss002(0,zl,n,u);
     u(1)=ue-D*uz(1);
     [uzz]=dss042(0,zl,n,u,uz,nl,nu);
  end
  if(ncase==3)
     [uz]=vanl(0,zl,n,u,v);
     u(1)=ue-D*uz(1);
     [uzz]=dss042(0,zl,n,u,uz,nl,nu);
  end
  if(ncase==4)
     [uz]=super(0,zl,n,u,v);
     u(1)=ue-D*uz(1);
     [uzz]=dss044(0,zl,n,u,uz,nl,nu);
  end
  if(ncase==5)
     [uz]=smart(0,zl,n,u,v);
     u(1)=ue-D*uz(1);
     [uzz]=dss046(0,zl,n,u,uz,nl,nu);
  end
%
% Temporal derivative
  for i=2:n-1
    ut(i)=D*uzz(i)-v*uz(i)-kr*u(i);
  end
  ut(1)=0; ut(n)=-v*uz(n);
%
% Increment calls to pde_1
  ncall=ncall+1;
```

Listing 1.24 pde_1 for the solution of eqs. (1.28) and (1.29)

We can note the following details about Listing 1.24.

- The function is defined and selected variables are declared as global.

```
  function ut=pde_1(u,t)
%
% Function pde_1 computes the t derivative vector of the u vector
%
  global a b D v ue kr zl n ncase ncall
```

- For ncase=1, the coding is

```
%
% First, second order spatial derivatives
  nl=1; nu=2;
  if(ncase==1)
     [uz]=dss012(0,zl,n,u,v);
     u(1)=ue-D*uz(1);
     [uzz]=dss042(0,zl,n,u,uz,nl,nu);
  end
```

  We can note the following details about this coding.

  - A Dirichlet BC is specified at $z = 0$ (nl=1) and a Neumann BC is specified at $z = z_L$ (nu=2).

    ```
    nl=1; nu=2;
    ```

  - The derivative $(\partial u/\partial z)$ in eq. (1.28) is computed by the two point upwind approximations in dss012 (in Listing 1.11).

    ```
    [uz]=dss012(0,zl,n,u,v);
    ```

  - With uz available, BC (1.29a) is implemented as

    ```
    u(1)=ue-D*uz(1);
    ```

    Note the use of the subscript 1 at $z = 0$. Calculating u(1) is one possible approach to the BC at $z = 0$; since the dependent variable is computed, it is a Dirichlet BC (and thus, nl=1). A second approach would be to calculate uz(1); since the derivative is computed, this would be a Neumann BC (and thus, nl=2). This second approach was not used because it would require a division by D which causes a problem for small D (the strongly convective or hyperbolic case with the limiting condition $D \rightarrow 0$).
  - The derivative $(\partial^2 u/\partial z^2)$ in eq. (1.28) is computed directly by the three point FDs in dss042 of Listing 1.18.

    ```
    [uzz]=dss042(0,zl,n,u,uz,nl,nu);
    ```

  - Thus, at this point the two derivatives in z of eq. (1.28) have been computed, and the MOL approximation of eq. (1.28) can then be completed (toward the end of pde_1).

- Similar programming is used for ncase=2 except that the derivative $(\partial u/\partial z)$ is computed by the three point centered FDs of dss002 (in Listing 1.12).

```
if(ncase==2)
   [uz]=dss002(0,zl,n,u);
   u(1)=ue-D*uz(1);
   [uzz]=dss042(0,zl,n,u,uz,nl,nu);
end
```

- For ncase=3, the van Leer flux limiter is used to calculate $(\partial u/\partial z)$.

```
if(ncase==3)
   [uz]=vanl(0,zl,n,u,v);
   u(1)=ue-D*uz(1);
   [uzz]=dss042(0,zl,n,u,uz,nl,nu);
end
```

- For ncase=4, the superbee flux limiter is used to calculate $(\partial u/\partial z)$ and the five point centered FDs of dss044 (in Listing 1.18) are used to calculate $(\partial^2 u/\partial z^2)$.

```
if(ncase==4)
   [uz]=super(0,zl,n,u,v);
   u(1)=ue-D*uz(1);
   [uzz]=dss044(0,zl,n,u,uz,nl,nu);
end
```

- For ncase=5, the smart flux limiter is used to calculate $(\partial u/\partial z)$ and the seven point centered FDs of dss046 (in Listing 1.18) are used to calculate $(\partial^2 u/\partial z^2)$.

```
if(ncase==5)
   [uz]=smart(0,zl,n,u,v);
   u(1)=ue-D*uz(1);
   [uzz]=dss046(0,zl,n,u,uz,nl,nu);
end
```

- Eq. (1.28) is programmed.

```
%
% Temporal derivative
  for i=2:n-1
    ut(i)=D*uzz(i)-v*uz(i)-kr*u(i);
  end
  ut(1)=0; ut(n)=-v*uz(n);
%
% Increment calls to pde_1
  ncall=ncall+1;
```

  Note that the index of the for loop starts at 2 because of the Dirichlet BC at $z = 0$; also, ut(1) is set to zero, so this BC is not changed. Boundary condition (1.29c) is programmed as ut(n)=-v*uz(n). Finally, the counter for the calls to pde_1 is incremented.

- The final result from pde_1 is the derivative vector ut that is returned as the LHS argument of pde_1. This completes the MOL programming of eq. (1.28).

We now consider the graphical output from the execution of pde_1_main of Listing 1.23. For ncase=1, the plot is in Fig. 1.22.

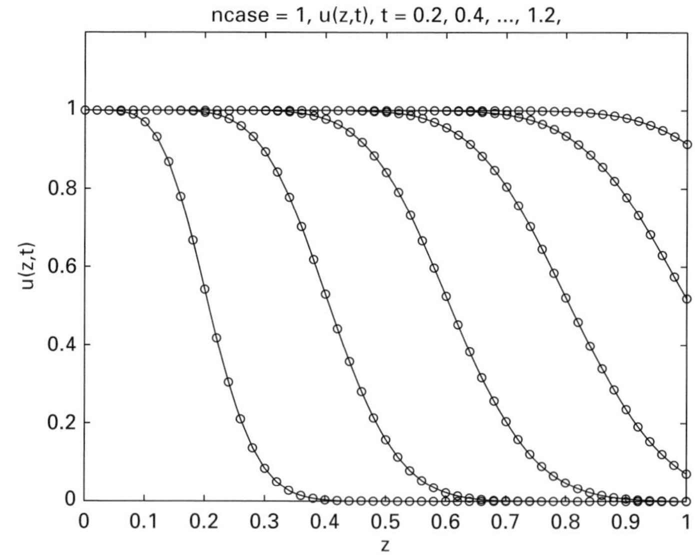

Figure 1.22 $u(z,t)$ from `pde_1_main` of Listing 1.23 for `ncase = 1`; $t = 0.2, 0.4, \cdots, 1.2$ (left to right)

Figure 1.22 superficially appears to be an acceptable solution. However, as we consider subsequent cases, it will be clear that the solution of Fig. 1.22 has excessive numerical diffusion, as might be expected from the two point upwind approximations of $(\partial u/\partial z)$ in eq. (1.28).

For `ncase=2`, the plot is in Fig. 1.23.

Figure 1.23 again indicates that centered FD approximations for strongly convective systems produce numerical oscillations, as discussed previously for Fig. 1.5.

For `ncase=3`, the plot is in Fig. 1.24.

Figure 1.24 indicates good front resolution with $(\partial u/\partial z)$ calculated by the van Leer flux limiter. Note in particular that the front moves past the boundary at $z = 1$ with no apparent distortion.

For `ncase=4`, the plot is in Fig. 1.25.

Figure 1.25 indicates good front resolution with $(\partial u/\partial z)$ calculated by the superbee flux limiter. Again in particular, the front moves past the boundary at $z = 1$ with no apparent distortion. Also, a visual comparison indicates good agreement between the solutions of Figs. 1.24 and 1.25 (of course, the numerical output for `ncase=3,4` could be compared by using `ip=1` in `pde_1_main`).

For `ncase=5`, the plot is in Fig. 1.26.

Figure 1.26 indicates good front resolution with $(\partial u/\partial z)$ calculated by the smart flux limiter. Again in particular, the front moves past the boundary at $z = 1$ with no apparent distortion. Also, a visual comparison indicates good agreement between the solutions of Figs. 1.24, 1.25, and 1.26 (and the numerical output for `ncase=3,4,5` could be compared by using `ip=1` in `pde_1_main`); generally, the van Leer, superbee, and smart flux limiters give solutions free of oscillation with little numerical diffusion.

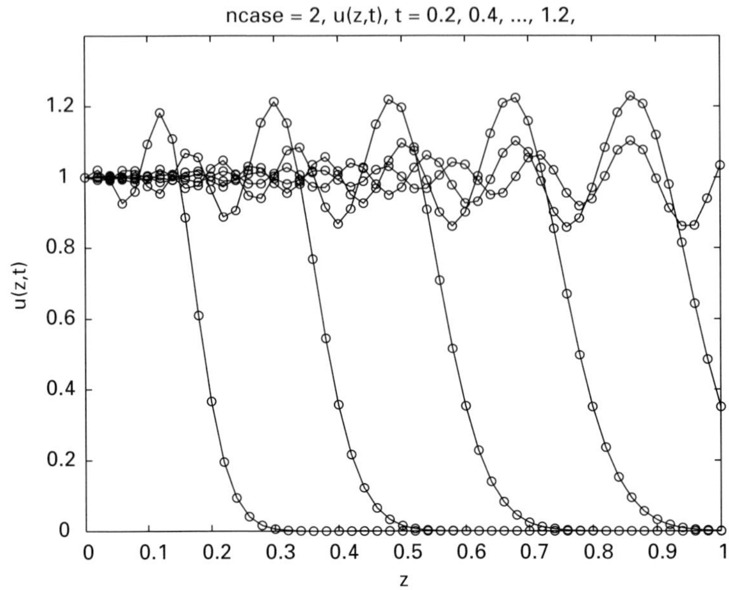

Figure 1.23 $u(z,t)$ from `pde_1_main` of Listing 1.23 for `ncase = 2`; $t = 0.2, 0.4, \cdots, 1.2$ (left to right)

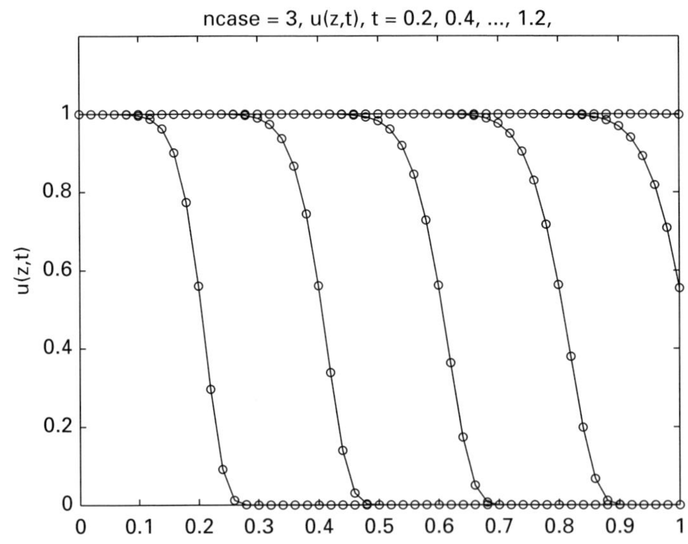

Figure 1.24 $u(z,t)$ from `pde_1_main` of Listing 1.23 for `ncase = 3`; $t = 0.2, 0.4, \cdots, 1.2$ (left to right)

To conclude this discussion of hyperbolic-parabolic PDEs, we again consider the execution of `pde_1_main` of Listing 1.23 but with BC (1.29b) implemented in `pde_1`. This is done because BC (1.29b) is frequently used in the solution of hyperbolic-parabolic

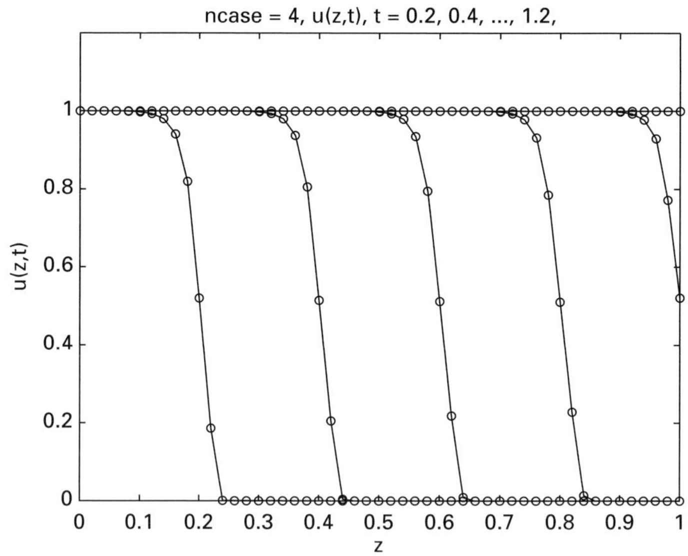

Figure 1.25 $u(z,t)$ from pde_1_main of Listing 1.23 for ncase = 4; $t = 0.2, 0.4, \cdots, 1.2$ (left to right)

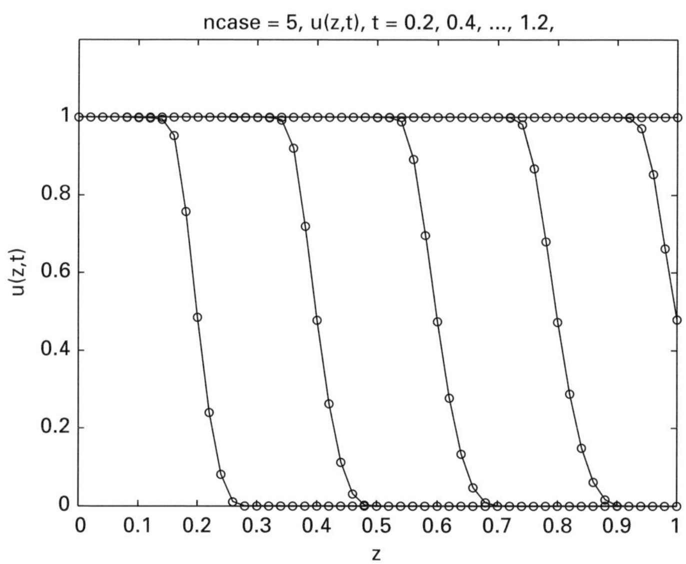

Figure 1.26 $u(z,t)$ from pde_1_main of Listing 1.23 for ncase = 5; $t = 0.2, 0.4, \cdots, 1.2$ (left to right)

PDEs that are second order in z and therefore require an outflow or exit BC (e.g., at $z = z_L = 1$).

```
  function ut=pde_1(u,t)
%
% Function pde_1 computes the t derivative vector of the u vector
```

```
%
  global a b D v ue kr zl n ncase ncall
%
% First, second order spatial derivatives
  nl=1; nu=2;
  if(ncase==1)
     [uz]=dss012(0,zl,n,u,v);
     u(1)=ue-D*uz(1); uz(n)=0;
     [uzz]=dss042(0,zl,n,u,uz,nl,nu);
  end
  if(ncase==2)
     [uz]=dss002(0,zl,n,u);
     u(1)=ue-D*uz(1); uz(n)=0;
     [uzz]=dss042(0,zl,n,u,uz,nl,nu);
  end
  if(ncase==3)
     [uz]=vanl(0,zl,n,u,v);
     u(1)=ue-D*uz(1); uz(n)=0;
     [uzz]=dss042(0,zl,n,u,uz,nl,nu);
  end
  if(ncase==4)
     [uz]=super(0,zl,n,u,v);
     u(1)=ue-D*uz(1); uz(n)=0;
     [uzz]=dss044(0,zl,n,u,uz,nl,nu);
  end
  if(ncase==5)
     [uz]=smart(0,zl,n,u,v);
     u(1)=ue-D*uz(1); uz(n)=0;
     [uzz]=dss046(0,zl,n,u,uz,nl,nu);
  end
%
% Temporal derivative
  for i=2:n
    ut(i)=D*uzz(i)-v*uz(i)-kr*u(i);
  end
  ut(1)=0;
%
% Increment calls to pde_1
  ncall=ncall+1;
```

Listing 1.25 pde_1 for the solution of eqs. (1.28) with BC (1.29b) in place of BC (1.29c)

We can note the following details about Listing 1.25 (which is similar to Listing 1.24).

- The function is defined and selected variables are declared as global.

```
  function ut=pde_1(u,t)
%
% Function pde_1 computes the t derivative vector of the u vector
%
  global a b D v ue kr zl n ncase ncall
```

- For ncase=1, the coding is

```
%
% First, second order spatial derivatives
  nl=1; nu=2;
  if(ncase==1)
     [uz]=dss012(0,zl,n,u,v);
     u(1)=ue-D*uz(1); uz(n)=0;
     [uzz]=dss042(0,zl,n,u,uz,nl,nu);
  end
```

We can note the following details about this coding.

  - A Dirichlet BC is specified at $z=0$ (nl=1) and a Neumann BC is specified at $z=z_L$ (nu=2).

```
nl=1; nu=2;
```

  - The derivative $(\partial u/\partial z)$ in eq. (1.28) is computed by the two point upwind approximations in dss012 (in Listing 1.11).

```
[uz]=dss012(0,zl,n,u,v);
```

  - With uz available, BC (1.29a) is implemented as

```
u(1)=ue-D*uz(1); uz(n)=0;
```

    Note the use of the subscript 1 at $z=0$. uz(n) is calculated from BC (1.29b).
  - The derivative $(\partial^2 u/\partial z^2)$ in eq. (1.28) is computed directly by the three point FDs in dss042 of Listing 1.18.

```
[uzz]=dss042(0,zl,n,u,uz,nl,nu);
```

  - At this point the two derivatives in z of eq. (1.28) have been computed, and the MOL approximation of eq. (1.28) can then be completed (toward the end of pde_1).

- Similar programming is used for ncase=2 except the derivative $(\partial u/\partial z)$ is computed by the three point centered FDs of dss002 (in Listing 1.12).

```
  if(ncase==2)
     [uz]=dss002(0,zl,n,u);
     u(1)=ue-D*uz(1); uz(n)=0;
     [uzz]=dss042(0,zl,n,u,uz,nl,nu);
  end
```

- For ncase=3, the van Leer flux limiter is used to calculate $(\partial u/\partial z)$.

```
  if(ncase==3)
     [uz]=vanl(0,zl,n,u,v);
     u(1)=ue-D*uz(1); uz(n)=0;
     [uzz]=dss042(0,zl,n,u,uz,nl,nu);
  end
```

- For ncase=4,5, the solutions are similar to that of ncase=3 and therefore will not be discussed subsequently.
- Eq. (1.28) is programmed.

```
%
% Temporal derivative
  for i=2:n
    ut(i)=D*uzz(i)-v*uz(i)-kr*u(i);
  end
  ut(1)=0;
%
% Increment calls to pde_1
  ncall=ncall+1;
```

Note that the index of the `for` loop starts at 2 because of the Dirichlet BC at $z = 0$; also, `ut(1)` is set to zero so this BC is not changed. The upper limit of the `for` loop is `n` (rather than `n-1` of Listing 1.24) so that eq. (1.28) is used at $z = 1$ (rather than using BC (1.29c) as in Listing 1.24). Finally, the counter for the calls to `pde_1` is incremented.

- The final result from `pde_1` is the derivative vector `ut` that is returned as the LHS argument of `pde_1`. This completes the MOL programming of eq. (1.28).

We now consider the graphical output from the execution of `pde_1_main` of Listing 1.23. For `ncase=1`, the plot is in Fig. 1.27.

Note that an unrealistic distortion occurs at $z = 1$ due to BC (1.29b) (in contrast to Fig. 1.22 based on BC (1.29c)). This result is not surprising; since BC (1.29b) requires that the moving front leave the system at $z = 1$ with zero slope, which cannot be achieved.

For `ncase=2`, the plot is in Fig. 1.28.

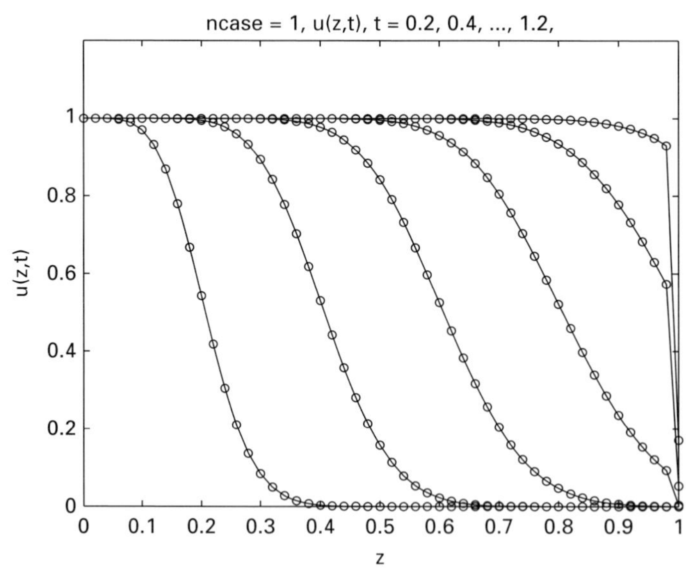

Figure 1.27 $u(z,t)$ from `pde_1_main` of Listing 1.23 for `ncase = 1`; $t = 0.2, 0.4, \cdots, 1.2$ (left to right)

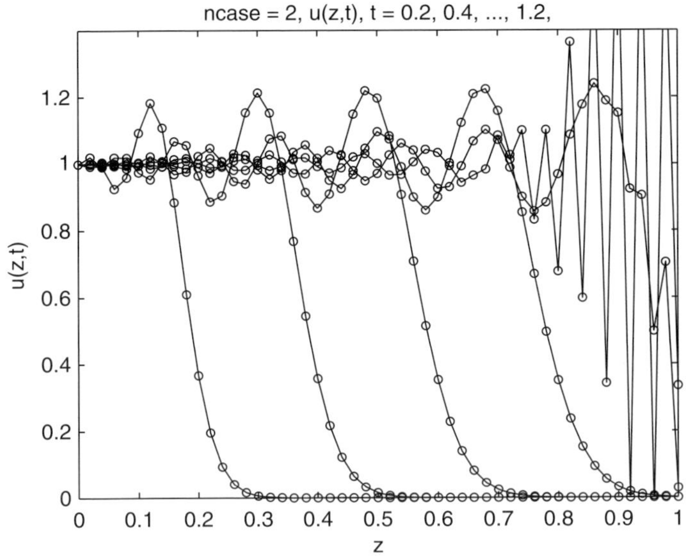

Figure 1.28 $u(z,t)$ from `pde_1_main` of Listing 1.23 for `ncase = 2`; $t = 0.2, 0.4, \cdots, 1.2$ (left to right)

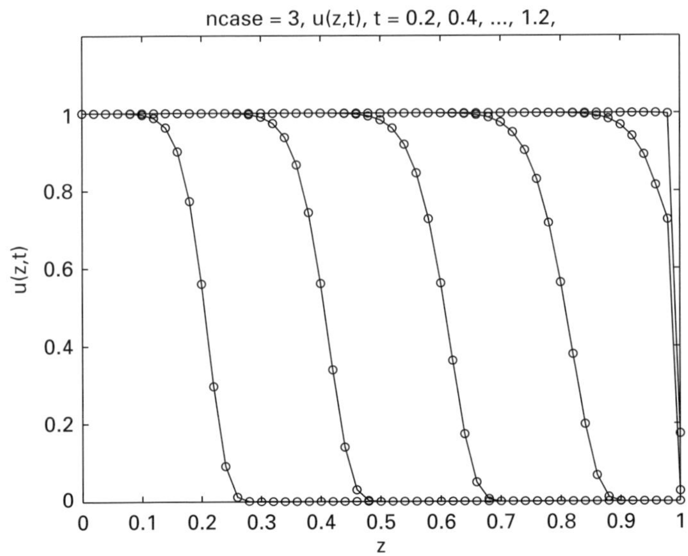

Figure 1.29 $u(z,t)$ from `pde_1_main` of Listing 1.23 for `ncase = 3`; $t = 0.2, 0.4, \cdots, 1.2$ (left to right)

Figure 1.28 indicates that the numerical solution is unacceptable due to numerical oscillations (which are more severe than in Fig. 1.23). Again, BC (1.29b) requires that the moving front leave the system at $z = 1$ with zero slope, which cannot be achieved.

For `ncase=3`, the plot is in Fig. 1.29.

Figure 1.29 indicates that the solution has an unrealistic distortion at $z = 1$, even though the van Leer flux limiter is used (compare this with Fig. 1.24); clearly the effect of BC (1.29b) is generally to produce unrealistic results at $z = 1$. This is also true for `ncase=4,5`, so the plots are not presented here.

As one minor variation of the programming of eq. (1.28) in `pde_1` of Listing 1.25, we can consider using eq. (1.28) at point `n` ($z = 1$) and setting the derivative $(\partial u/\partial z)$ to zero (according to BC (1.29b)).

```
%
% Temporal derivative
  for i=2:n-1
    ut(i)=D*uzz(i)-v*uz(i)-kr*u(i);
  end
  ut(1)=0; ut(n)=D*uzz(n)-kr*u(n);
```

It turns out the net result of this change (for `ncase=1,2,...,5`) is that the same distortions appeared at $z = 1$ as from the programming in Listing 1.25 (Figs. 1.27, 1.28, 1.29). In other words, using eq. (1.28) at $z = 1$ with BC (1.29b) included (rather than using just eq. (1.28) at $z = 1$ as in Listing 1.25) has essentially no effect in eliminating the distortions at $z = 1$.

This completes this introductory discussion of the MOL solution of hyperbolic-parabolic PDEs. The methods discussed can then be applied to the applications in subsequent chapters pertaining to the use of convection-diffusion-reaction PDEs. We now move on to PDE applications in biomedical engineering.

References

[1] Butcher, J. W. (2003), *Numerical Methods for Ordinary Differential Equations*, Hoboken, NJ: John Wiley and Sons, Inc

[2] Butcher, J. W. (2007), Runge-Kutta methods, *Scholarpedia*, **2** (9), 3147; www.scholarpedia.org/article/Runge-Kutta_methods

[3] Fornberg, B. (1992), Fast generation of weights in finite difference formulas, in *Recent Developments in Numerical Methods and Software for ODEs/DAEs/PDEs*, G. Byrne and W. E. Schiesser (eds.), River Edge, NJ: World Scientific

[4] Fornberg, B. (1998), Calculation of weights in finite difference formulas, *SIAM Rev.*, **40** (3), September, 685–691

[5] Gear, C. W. (1971), *Numerical Initial Value Problems in Ordinary Differential Equations*, Englewood Cliffs, NJ: Prentice-Hall

[6] Griffiths, G. W. and Schiesser, W. E. (2011), *Traveling Wave Analysis of Partial Differential Equations*, Burlington, MA: Academic Press/Elsevier

[7] Hindmarsh, A. C., Gresho, P. M., and Griffiths, D. F. (1984), The stability of explicit Euler method for certain finite difference approximations of the multi-dimensional advection-diffusion equation, *Int. J. Num. Meth. Fluids*, **4**, 853–897

[8] Lee, H. J. and Schiesser, W. E. (2004), *Ordinary and Partial Differential Equation Routines in C, C++, Fortran, Java, Maple, and MATLAB*, Appendix C, Boca Raton, FL: Chapman & Hall/CRC

[9] Polyanin, A. D., Schiesser, W. E, and Zhurov, A. I. (2008), Partial differenti
Scholarpedia, **3** (10), 4605 www.scholarpedia.org/article/partial_differential_e
[10] Schiesser, W. E. and Griffiths, G. W. (2009), *A Compendium of Partial Differe*
Models, Cambridge, UK: Cambridge University Press
[11] Shampine, L. F. and Thompson, S. (2007), Stiff systems, *Scholarpedia*,
www.scholarpedia.org/article/Stiff_systems
[12] Shampine, L. F. and Thompson, S. (2007), Initial value problems, *Scholarpe*
www.scholarpedia.org/article/Initial_value_problems
[13] Shampine, L. F. and Reichelt, M. W. (1997), The MATLAB ODE suite, *SIAM*
18, 1–22

2 ibody binding kinetics

ısider an example application consisting of an ordinary differential equation led with a PDE. The ODE/PDE model, taken originally from [7], pertains ıort and binding kinetics of an analyte, e.g., an antigen, on an antibody iber-optic biosensor. The model presented here[1] is a simplification of the l, which is intended to demonstrate the method of lines (MOL) approach E system. This simplified model could easily be extended to include the led in [7]. The overall intention of this discussion is to demonstrate the OL analysis in accommodating ODE/PDE systems.

2.1 el equations

the analyte concentration $c(z,t)$ is the classical one dimensional (1D) Fourier's second law for heat conduction (or Fick's second law for Cartesian coordinates (eq. (1.18) restated here with c as the dependent

$$\frac{\partial c}{\partial t} = D\frac{\partial^2 c}{\partial z^2}. \tag{2.1}$$

A .1) based on the mass conservation principle is given in Appendix 1. (B second order in z and therefore requires two boundary conditions n as

$$\frac{\partial c(z=0,t)}{\partial z} = k_f c(z=0,t)(c_{b,sat} - c_b) - k_r c_b, \tag{2.2}$$

$$c(z=h,t) = c_{bulk}. \tag{2.3}$$

Equa to $z =$ the binding of an analyte at the antibody surface corresponding The l ig. 2.1 (a detailed discussion of biofilm models is given in [2]). analyt of eq. (2.2), $D(\partial c(z=0,t)/\partial z)$, is the rate of diffusion of the or Fic face at $z=0$ according to Fourier's first law for heat conduction ss diffusion. The right-hand side (RHS) of eq. (2.2), $k_f c(z=$

[1] The O Kanpu g numerical values for the parameters, was provided by Dr. D. Rath, IIT,

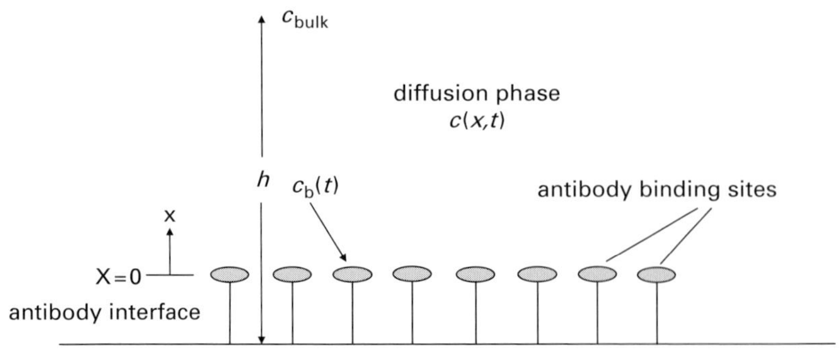

Figure 2.1 Schematic of diffusion-binding system

$0,t)(c_{b,sat} - c_b) - k_r c_b$, is the difference between the forward rate of adsorption (or binding) of the analyte, $k_f c(z=0,t)(c_{b,sat} - c_b)$, and the rate of desorption (or unbinding), $k_r c_b$. c_b is the concentration of the analyte bound to the antibody; k_f and k_r are mass transfer constants (or rate constants) for the forward and reverse binding, respectively. Note that the forward rate goes to zero as the bound concentration, c_b, reaches a saturation value, $c_{b,sat}$; the rate of reverse binding is proportional to the bound concentration, c_b.

Since $c_{b,sat}$ is the saturation concentration of the analyte (an upper limit on the bound concentration), c_b, the ratio $\theta = (c_b/c_{b,sat})$ is the fractional coverage in the antibody interface with the limits $0 \leq \theta \leq 1$; this range or interval for θ can be observed (and used as a check) on the numerical solutions discussed subsequently. This check on θ is an example of a basic diagnostic that can be used to evaluate a numerical solution. Other possibilities would be the physical or chemical constraints $c(z,t) \geq 0, c_b(t) \geq 0$. The idea that concentrations must be nonnegative is obvious, yet these constraints could be useful; for example, the concentrations could become negative through something as simple as a sign error in the model equations or in the programming of the equations. Thus, we are suggesting that the analyst always look at the numerical solution critically and thoroughly as a form of basic error analysis; this is especially important when an analytical solution is not available as a check of the numerical solution, which is the case in most realistic applications.

Equation (2.3) indicates that at a sufficiently large distance from the antibody interface, $z = h$, the analyte concentration has the constant value c_{bulk}. In fact, this value of c_{bulk} drives the model away from the ICs of eqs. (2.4) and (2.6) (discussed next).

Since eq. (2.1) is first order in t it requires one initial condition (IC), which is taken as

$$c(z,t=0) = c_0, \tag{2.4}$$

where c_0 is a prescribed initial concentration of analyte (which could be a function of z).

$c_b(t)$, the concentration of the analyte bound on the antibody, is given by the ODE

$$\frac{dc_b}{dt} = k_f c(z=0,t)(c_{b,sat} - c_b) - k_r c_b. \tag{2.5}$$

Table 2.1. Dependent and independent variables of eqs. (2.1) to (2.6)

Variable	Brief description
c	analyte concentration, mole/m^3
z	distance from antibody interface, m
t	time, s
c_b	concentration of the bound analyte, mole/m^2

Table 2.2. Parameters and numerical values for eqs. (2.1) to (2.6)

Parameter	Units, numerical value
D	1×10^{-10} m^2/s
k_f	1×10^5 $\text{M}^{-1}\text{s}^{-1}$ ($\text{M} = \text{molarity} = \text{mole/m}^3$)
k_r	1×10^{-2} s^{-1}
$c_{b,sat}$	2.66×10^{-8} mole/m^2
c_{bulk}	4.48×10^{-5} mole/m^3
h	5.0×10^{-5} m
c_0	0 mole/m^3
c_{b0}	0 mole/m^2

The IC for eq. (2.5) is

$$c_b(t = 0) = c_{b0}, \tag{2.6}$$

where c_{b0} is a prescribed initial concentration.

Another possibility for an apparent, but readily available, test of the numerical solution is to observe whether the solution starts out at the initial condition, e.g., eqs. (2.4) and (2.6). This check seems obvious, but might still be useful in finding an error, especially in the programming of the model equations.

Equations (2.1) to (2.6) constitute the complete ODE/PDE model. The model variables and parameters are summarized in Tables 2.1 and 2.2.

Note that we have used the SI (MKS) system of units. Also, the concentration of the bound component at the antibody interface is expressed through an area concentration (e.g., c_b is in mole/m^2) while the diffusing analyte is expressed through a volume (or bulk) concentration (e.g., c is in mole/m^3).

An important first step in developing or analyzing a new mathematical model is to check the units of each term in the model equations. We next illustrate this process through eqs. (2.1) to (2.6).

2.2 Units check

The units in a system of equations for a physical or chemical problem are checked for the following reasons:

- The units throughout each equation must be consistent. That is, different terms in an equation cannot have different units (in a sense, it cannot be an "equation" under conditions of inconsistent units, e.g., LHS cannot have the units of apples while the RHS has the units of oranges).
- The units give valuable insight into the physical and chemical significance of each term in the equation.
- Parameters taken from the literature used in an equation can have a variety of units depending on their source. Therefore it is necessary to check the units and convert them if necessary for consistency throughout the equation.
- This process of checking and possibly converting units often provides insight into the relative magnitude of the various terms in an equation, and thus, may indicate which terms are most significant when using the equation. In other words, we may gain some insight into why the equation solutions have particular features and characteristics.

To illustrate the process of unit checking, we start with eq. (2.1). The units are

$$\frac{\text{mole/m}^3}{\text{s}} = \frac{\text{m}^2}{\text{s}} \frac{\text{mole/m}^3}{\text{m}^2} \tag{2.7}$$

We observe from this result that the diffusivity, D, has the units of m^2/s; the numerical value 1×10^{-10} from Table 2.2 is typical for large molecules in an aqueous solution. Alternative length units that are typically used for a diffusivity are centimeters (cm) $= 1 \times 10^{-2}$ m, millimeters (mm) $= 1 \times 10^{-3}$ m and micrometers (microns, μm, or just μ) $= 1 \times 10^{-6}$ m. The relationship between the various units for D in Table 2.2 is:

$$1 \times 10^{-10}\,\text{m}^2/\text{s} = 1 \times 10^{-6}\,\text{cm}^2/\text{s} = 1 \times 10^{-4}\,\text{mm}^2/\text{s} = 1 \times 10^{2}\,\mu^2/\text{s}. \tag{2.8}$$

The units of eq. (2.7) are consistent throughout the equation ($\text{mole/m}^3/\text{s}$). The LHS represents the volumetric accumulation or depletion of the analyte in a differential volume while the RHS represents the net diffusion of the analyte into or out of the differential volume. If accumulation occurs (the LHS is positive), the net diffusion is into the differential volume (the RHS is positive). While this analysis is perhaps obvious, something as simple as a sign error, e.g., the RHS has a negative sign, would produce an unstable solution to eq. (2.1).

The units of eq. (2.2) are (refer to Table 2.2)

$$\frac{\text{m}^2}{\text{s}} \frac{\text{mol/m}^3}{\text{m}} = \frac{1}{\text{mole/m}^3\text{s}} \left(\frac{\text{mole}}{\text{m}^3}\right) \left(\frac{\text{mole}}{\text{m}^2}\right) - \frac{1}{\text{s}} \frac{\text{moles}}{\text{m}^2}. \tag{2.9}$$

The net units of eq. (2.9) (LHS and RHS) are ($\text{mole/m}^2\text{s}$), which is a flux, that is, moles transferred per unit area per unit time. To repeat some of the previous discussion, on the LHS, the flux is for diffusion according to Fourier's first law or Fick's first law (also discussed subsequently). The RHS is the flux of the analyte onto or off of the antibody interface. This flux is made up of two components: (1) the flux onto the antibody interface is

$$k_\text{f} c(z = 0, t)(c_\text{b,sat} - c_\text{b})$$

where k_f is the forward mass transfer coefficient, (2) the flux off of the antibody interface is

$$-k_r c_b$$

where k_r is the reverse mass transfer coefficient. In other words, a net flux onto the antibody interface corresponds to a positive value of $k_f c(z=0,t)(c_{b,sat}-c_b)-k_r c_b$ and a net flux off of the antibody interface corresponds to a negative value of $k_f c(z=0,t)(c_{b,sat}-c_b)-k_r c_b$; note that according to eq. (2.5), these conditions correspond to a positive or negative value of (dc_b/dt), as expected (the bound concentration c_b is increasing or decreasing with t).

To continue the units analysis, eqs. (2.3) and (2.4) obviously have consistent units, i.e. (mole/m^3) on the LHS and RHS. The units of eq. (2.5) are

$$\frac{\text{mole}}{\text{m}^2}\frac{1}{\text{s}}=\frac{\text{mole}}{\text{m}^2\text{s}}, \tag{2.10}$$

where we have made use of eq. (2.9) in the RHS of eq. (2.10). Note that the RHS of eq. (2.2) is the same as that of eq. (2.5). This indicates that the diffusion flux of the analyte at $z=0$ equals the flux at the antibody interface (refer to Fig. 2.1); this equality of the two fluxes is an example of a continuity condition. Equation (2.6) obviously has consistent units, i.e. (mole/m^2) on the LHS and RHS.

This completes the units check for eqs. (2.1) to (2.6) with the inclusion of the units in Tables 2.1 and 2.2. As some additional introductory discussion concerning terminology, eq. (2.3) is termed a Dirichlet BC since it defines the dependent variable of eq. (2.1), $c(z,t)$, at the boundary $z=h$. A BC that defines the spatial derivative of the dependent variable is termed a Neumann BC. In heat transfer (conduction), if the spatial derivative is zero, the Neumann BC is termed an insulated BC, since from Fourier's first law,

$$-k\frac{\partial T(z=0,t)}{\partial z}=q, \tag{2.11a}$$

where the flux q (with typical units (cal/sm^2)) is zero (k is the thermal conductivity). In mass transfer (diffusion), if the spatial derivative is zero, the Neumann BC is termed a no-flux, zero gradient or impermeable BC, since from Fick's first law,

$$-D\frac{\partial c(z=0,t)}{\partial z}=m, \tag{2.11b}$$

the flux m (with typical units $(\text{mole}/\text{sm}^2)$) is zero ($D$ is the diffusivity discussed previously).

Since eq. (2.2) includes the derivative $(\partial c(z=0,t)/\partial z)$, it would seem that it is Neumann. Note, however, that it also includes the dependent variable, $c(z=0,t)$ in the RHS $k_f c(z=0,t)(c_{b,sat}-c_b)-k_r c_b$. Thus, eq. (2.2) is termed a third type or Robin BC (it includes both the dependent variable $c(z=0,t)$ and its spatial derivative, $\partial c(z=0,t)/\partial z$).

Also, eq. (2.2) is a nonlinear BC since the RHS includes the term $c(z=0,t)c_b$, that is the product of the dependent variable of eq. (2.1), $c(z=0,t)$, and the dependent variable of eq. (2.5), $c_b(t)$. While this may seem like a minor detail, this nonlinearity probably precludes finding an analytical solution to eqs. (2.1) to (2.6). However, as we shall observe, including this nonlinearity in a numerical (MOL) solution is easily accomplished. This example illustrates one of the major advantages of the numerical (rather than the analytical) approach; nonlinearities (which naturally arise in many applications) can easily be accommodated.

To consider this nonlinear term a little further, the forward rate of transfer to the antibody interface, $k_f c(z=0,t)(c_{b,sat} - c_b)$ consists of two basic components: (1) the concentration $c(z=0,t)$ corresponds to an increasing rate of forward transfer (as expected, this rate increases with increasing $c(z=0,t)$ because of the multiplication by $c(z=0,t)$), and (2) the concentration c_b corresponds to a decreasing rate of forward transfer because of the multiplication by $c_{b,sat} - c_b$ (as expected, this rate decreases with increasing c_b, with the decreasing rate limited by the difference $c_{b,sat} - c_b$ with $c_b \leq c_{b,sat}$). Thus, the net forward rate of transfer to the antibody interface is a balance between these two effects. This type of nonlinear rate ($k_f c(z=0,t)(c_{b,sat} - c_b)$) is usually termed logistic and eqs. (2.2) and (2.5) can be termed logistic equations. Of course, other forms of the transfer rate to the antibody interface could be considered and included in the computer analysis that follows. In other words, experimentation with the model equations is easily accomplished with the numerical approach and this facilitates an iterative approach to model development to arrive at a set of model equations that meets a specific criterion, usually a good fit to experimental data or some explanation of an observed phenomenon.

Finally, the reverse rate of transfer from the antibody interface is always negative through the term $-k_r c_b$ (with $k_r \geq 0, c_b \geq 0$), and as expected, this negative rate increases (becomes more negative) with increasing c_b.

In summary, eq. (2.2) can be classified as a nonlinear, third type BC while eq. (2.3) can be classified as Dirichlet. Additionally, eq. (2.2) would be no-flux Neumann if $k_f = k_r = 0$ since the transfer to the antibody interface would be zero.

2.3 MOL routines

We now consider a series of MATLAB routines for the implementation of eqs. (2.1) to (2.6). These routines generally are based on the MOL analysis of ODE/PDE systems.

2.3.1 ODE/PDE routine

First, the routine in which the PDE, eq. (2.1), is converted into a set of ODEs that are then combined with the model ODE, eq. (2.5), is listed (Listing 2.1).

```
  function ut=pde_1(t,u)
%
% Problem parameters
```

```
  global zl zu z dz dz2 D kf cbsat kr n cbulk ndss ncall
%
% ODE and PDE
  for i=1:n
    c(i)=u(i);
  end
  cb=u(n+1);
%
% BCs
  cf=c(2)-(2*dz/D)*(kf*c(1)*(cbsat-cb)-kr*cb);
  c(n)=cbulk;
%
% PDE
  for i=1:n
    if(i==1)      ct(1)=D*(c(2)-2*c(1)+cf)/dz2;
    elseif(i==n) ct(n)=0;
    else          ct(i)=D*(c(i+1)-2*c(i)+c(i-1))/dz2;
    end
  end
%
% ODE
  cbt=kf*c(1)*(cbsat-cb)-kr*cb;
%
% Derivative vector
  for i=1:n
    ut(i)=ct(i);
  end
  ut(n+1)=cbt;
%
% Transpose for ODE integrator
  ut=ut';
%
% Increment calls to pde_1
  ncall=ncall+1;
```

Listing 2.1 ODE routine pde_1

We can note the following details about pde_1.

- The function is defined and parameters and variables are declared global so that they can be shared with other routines. Most of these global variables are defined numerically in the main program, pde_1_main.

```
  function ut=pde_1(t,u)
%
% Problem parameters
  global zl zu z dz dz2 D kf cbsat kr n cbulk ndss ncall
```

The input arguments to pde_1 are the ODE/PDE independent variable, t, and a dependent variable vector, u. These input arguments are available (set numerically) coming into pde_1 and can therefore be used in the programming of eqs. (2.1) and

(2.5); this point cannot be fully confirmed until the programming in the other routines is explained.

The output argument of pde_1 is the derivative vector, ut, of length $n+1$ (n is set in the main program and passed as a global variable). All of the elements of ut must be defined numerically in pde_1 before the execution of pde_1 is complete (as explained subsequently). In other words, the ODE/PDE mathematical model of eqs. (2.1) to (2.3) and (2.5) is basically programmed in pde_1 (eqs. (2.4) and (2.6) are ICs used in the main program pde_1_main discussed next).

- The input vector, u, is transferred to two variables; c, which is the dependent variable of eq. (2.1), and cb, which is the dependent variable of eq. (2.5). Thus, pde_1 defines the RHS of $n+1$ ODEs. This change of variables is used primarily so that the subsequent programming can be done in terms of problem-oriented variables, i.e., c and cb are more convenient to use than u.

```
%
% ODE and PDE
  for i=1:n
    c(i)=u(i);
  end
  cb=u(n+1);
```

Note that $c(z,t)$ of eq. (2.1) is defined on a spatial grid in z with values

$$z(1), z(2), ..., z(i), ..., z(n),$$

as depicted in Fig. 2.2.

Thus, the code for c(i),i=1,2,...,n corresponds to the n values

$$c(z=z(1),t), c(z=z(2),t), ..., c(z=z(i),t), ..., c(z=z(n),t),$$

with $z(1)=0, z(n)=h$ corresponding to the boundary values of z of eqs. (2.2) and (2.3). This spatial grid is set up in the main program pde_1_main and provides the important feature of eq. (2.1) that the dependent variable, $c(z,t)$, is a function of both space (z) and time (t).

The initial values

$$c(z=z(1),t=0), c(z=z(2),t=0), ..., c(z=z(i),t=0), ..., c(z=z(n),t=0)$$

of IC (2.4) are defined in the main program and are used to start the numerical solution.

The solution values

$$c(z=z(1),t), c(z=z(2),t), ..., c(z=z(i),t), ..., c(z=z(n),t)$$

are computed as the solution of a set of n ODEs programmed in pde_1. The programming of these ODEs is discussed later as part of the discussion of pde_1. Note that we have now achieved the requirement that the solution of eq. (2.1), $c(z,t)$, is a function of z (defined at the discrete points $z(1), z(2), ..., z(n)$) and t.

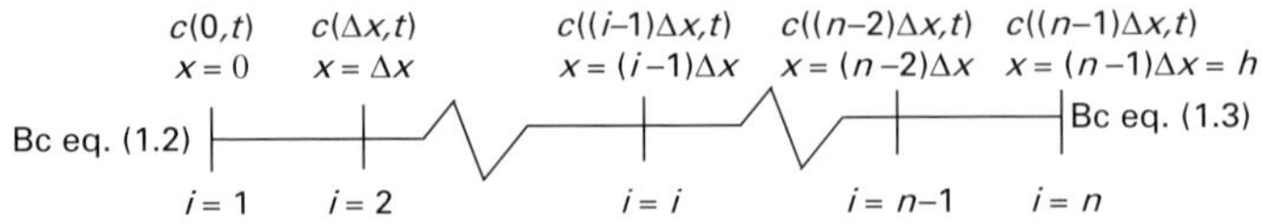

Figure 2.2 Finite difference grid for eq. (2.1)

- Boundary conditions (2.2) and (2.3) are programmed.

```
%
% BCs
  cf=c(2)-(2*dz/D)*(kf*c(1)*(cbsat-cb)-kr*cb);
  c(n)=cbulk;
```

For BC (2.2), the derivative $(\partial c(z=0,t)/\partial z)$ is approximated with a two point, second order finite difference (FD)

$$\frac{\partial c(z,t)}{\partial z} \approx \frac{c(z+\Delta z,t)-c(z-\Delta z,t)}{2\Delta z}+O(\Delta z^2), \tag{2.12a}$$

where Δz is the interval in z (for the FD grid in z); this interval is computed in the main program as `dz` and is passed to `pde_1` as a global variable, and thus is available to use in the programming. In other words, the spatial grid is uniformly spaced with

$$z(1)=0, z(2)=\Delta z, ..., z(i)=(i-1)\Delta z, ..., z(n)=(n-1)\Delta z=h.$$

Note that $z(i)=(i-1)\Delta z, i=1,2,...,n$ is used to accommodate the MATLAB limitation that subscripts such as i must be positive integers (0 cannot be used as a subscript).

Substitution of the FD approximation of eq. (2.12a) in eq. (2.2) with $z=0$ (at the boundary of eq. (2.2)) gives (disregard for a moment the term $O(\Delta z^2)$, which is discussed as the next item)

$$D\frac{c(z=\Delta z,t)-c(z=-\Delta z,t)}{2\Delta z}=k_{\mathrm{f}}c(z=0,t)(c_{\mathrm{b,sat}}-c_{\mathrm{b}})-k_{\mathrm{r}}c_{\mathrm{b}}. \tag{2.12b}$$

However, $c(-\Delta z,t)$ in the LHS of eq. (2.12b) is a value outside the domain in z (the leftmost value of z is `z(1)=0` so $z=-\Delta z$ is beyond this leftmost point). In other words, $c(-\Delta z,t)$ is a fictitious value, designated `cf` in the preceding code. Solving eq. (2.12b) for this fictitious value $c_{\mathrm{f}}=c(-\Delta z,t)$ gives

$$c_{\mathrm{f}}=c(z=\Delta z,t)-\frac{2\Delta z}{D}(k_{\mathrm{f}}c(z=0,t)(c_{\mathrm{b,sat}}-c_{\mathrm{b}})-k_{\mathrm{r}}c_{\mathrm{b}}), \tag{2.12c}$$

which is programmed as

```
cf=c(2)-(2*dz/D)*(kf*c(1)*(cbsat-cb)-kr*cb);
```

Note that the requirement of setting numerically everything that is used in a calculation applies to all quantities in the RHS calculation of `cf`; that is, `c(1)`, `c(2)`, and cb are defined numerically by the preceding code while dz, D, kf, cbsat, and kr are defined in the main program prior to the first call to pde_1. In other words, we must ensure an executable sequence in all of the coding that is used, which means all parameters and variables must be defined numerically before they are first used; while this may seem obvious, failure to do so is a common source of programming errors.

The programming of BC (2.3) is straightforward (cbulk is set numerically in the main program and passed as a global variable to pde_1).

```
c(n)=cbulk;
```

- The RHS of eq. (2.12a) has the term $O(\Delta z^2)$, which signifies that the truncation error of the FD approximation of eq. (2.12a) is second order. In other words, the error of this approximation to the derivative $(\partial c(z,t)/\partial z)$ varies as Δz^2 and the approximation of eq. (2.12a) can be termed a second order, centered finite difference; centered indicates that the functional values $c(z+\Delta z,t)$ and $c(z-\Delta z,t)$ are centered or symmetric with respect to the point of the approximation of the derivative, z.

  The term truncation error originates with the use of a Taylor series to derive eq. (2.12a) that is truncated after the Δz^2 term (also previously discussed as eq. (1.14) and programmed in dss002 of Listing 1.12). The truncation error should not be confused with roundoff error, which originates from the finite number of bits used to represent a number; typically this number is 32 or 64 bits in a word that represents a number or character digitally. Also, as a practical matter, the truncation error is a more serious source of error than the roundoff error in most scientific computations, such as the numerical solution of ODEs and PDEs; in fact, controlling the truncation error is an essential part of an error analysis of computed results as will be discussed subsequently.
- The derivative $(\partial c/\partial t)$ in eq. (2.1) is computed as ct over the grid of n points.

```
%
% PDE
  for i=1:n
    if(i==1)       ct(1)=D*(c(2)-2*c(1)+cf)/dz2;
    elseif(i==n) ct(n)=0;
    else           ct(i)=D*(c(i+1)-2*c(i)+c(i-1))/dz2;
    end
  end
```

We can note the following points about this code:

– At grid point i=1 corresponding to $z=0$, the fictitious value cf is used to calculate ct(1). The line of code

```
if(i==1)       ct(1)=D*(c(2)-2*c(1)+cf)/dz2;
```

is based on the second order, centered finite difference approximation for a second derivative (discussed as part of dss042 in Listing 1.18)

$$\frac{\partial^2 c(z,t)}{\partial z^2} \approx \frac{c(z+\Delta z,t)-2c(z,t)+c(z-\Delta z,t)}{\Delta z^2} + O(\Delta z^2). \tag{2.13a}$$

Again, this approximation is termed centered because the three functional values of the dependent variable, $c(z+\Delta z,t), c(z,t), c(z-\Delta z,t)$ are symmetric with respect to the point of the approximation, z. The order term $O(\Delta z^2)$ has the same interpretation as in eq. (2.12a).

For $z=0$, eq. (2.8a) becomes

$$\frac{\partial^2 c(z=0,t)}{\partial z^2} \approx \frac{c(z=\Delta z,t) - 2c(z=0,t) + c(z=-\Delta z,t)}{\Delta z^2} + O(\Delta z^2), \quad (2.13b)$$

where $c(z=-\Delta z,t)$ is a fictitious value that can be replaced by c_f of eq. (2.12c), as reflected in the preceding line of code for i=1. Thus, eq. (2.13b) includes BC (2.2) (through eq. (2.12c)).

- BC (2.3) at i=n is programmed as

```
elseif(i==n) ct(n)=0;
```

This code merely reflects that since $c(z=h,t) = c_{\text{bulk}}$, the derivative of this constant value with respect to t, ct(n), is zero.

- The remaining interior points (not i=1 or i=n) are programmed according to eqs. (2.1) and (2.13a)

```
else          ct(i)=D*(c(i+1)-2*c(i)+c(i-1))/dz2;
```

- This completes the MOL programming for eq. (2.1). The only other derivative in t is from eq. (2.5)

```
%
% ODE
  cbt=kf*c(1)*(cbsat-cb)-kr*cb;
```

- We now have the derivatives in t for $n+1$ ODEs. This set of derivatives is put into array ut that is the output argument of pde_1.

```
%
% Derivative vector
  for i=1:n
    ut(i)=ct(i);
  end
  ut(n+1)=cbt;
```

In other words, the calculation of the derivative vector ut must be complete before exiting pde_1.

- To complete pde_1, a transpose of ut is required by the ODE integrator, e.g., ode15s called in the main program.

```
%
% Transpose for ODE integrator
  ut=ut';
%
% Increment calls to pde_1
  ncall=ncall+1;
```

Also, the counter for the calls to pde_1 is incremented; its final value is displayed by the main program as an indication of the total computational effort required in the numerical integration of the $n+1$ ODEs (ncall is global and is therefore returned to the main program).

The main program pde_1_main that calls pde_1 of Listing 2.1 is considered next (to conserve space, a set of documentation comments for eqs. (2.1) to (2.6) is not included, as was done in the main programs of Chapter 1, but the following discussion relates the coding to these equations).

2.3.2 Main program

A basic main program follows (extensions will be considered subsequently).

```
%
% Clear previous files
  clear all
  clc
%
% Parameters shared with the ODE routine
  global zl zu z dz dz2 D kf cbsat kr n cbulk ndss ncall
%
% Parameter numerical values
  D=1.0e-10; kf=1.0e+05; cbulk=4.48e-05;
  h=5.0e-05; c0=0; cb0=0;
%
% Variation in interface binding saturation
  cbsat=1.66e-08;
  cbsat=1.66e-09;
%
% Variation in interface unbinding rate
  kr=1.0e-01;
  kr=1.0e+01;
%
% Spatial grid
  zl=0; zu=5.0e-05; n=21; dz=(zu-zl)/(n-1); dz2=dz^2;
%
% Initial condition
  for i=1:n
    u0(i)=c0;
  end
  u0(n+1)=cb0;
%
% Independent variable for ODE integration
  t0=0.0;
  tf=100;
  tout=(t0:2:tf);
  nout=51;
  ncall=0;
%
```

```
% ODE integration
%
% Variation in error tolerances
  reltol=1.0e-06; abstol=1.0e-06;
  reltol=1.0e-07; abstol=1.0e-07;
  options=odeset('RelTol',reltol,'AbsTol',abstol);
  mf=1;
  if(mf==1) % explicit FDs
    [t,u]=ode15s(@pde_1,tout,u0,options); end
  if(mf==2) ndss=4; % ndss = 2, 4, 6, 8 or 10 required
    [t,u]=ode15s(@pde_2,tout,u0,options); end
  if(mf==3) ndss=44; % ndss = 42, 44, 46, 48 or 50 required
    [t,u]=ode15s(@pde_3,tout,u0,options); end
%
% Store numerical solutions at z = 0
  for it=1:nout
    c_plot(it)=u(it,1);
    cb_plot(it)=u(it,n+1);
    theta_plot(it)=cb_plot(it)/cbsat;
    rate_plot(it)=kf*c_plot(it)*(cbsat-cb_plot(it))-kr*cb_plot(it);
  end
%
% Display selected output
  fprintf('\n mf = %2d   abstol = %8.1e   reltol = %8.1e\n',...
          mf,abstol,reltol);
  fprintf('\n      t       c(0,t)        cb(t)        theta         rate\n');
  for it=1:nout
    fprintf('%6.0f%12.3e%12.3e%12.3e%12.3e\n',...
            t(it),c_plot(it),cb_plot(it),theta_plot(it),rate_plot(it));
  end
  fprintf('\n ncall = %4d\n',ncall);
%
% Plot numerical solutions at z = 0
  figure(1);
  subplot(2,2,1)
  plot(t,c_plot); axis tight
  title('c(0,t) vs t'); xlabel('t'); ylabel('c(0,t)')
  subplot(2,2,2)
  plot(t,cb_plot); axis tight
  title('cb(t) vs t'); xlabel('t'); ylabel('cb(t)')
  subplot(2,2,3)
  plot(t,theta_plot); axis tight
  title('theta(t) vs t'); xlabel('t'); ylabel('theta(t)')
  subplot(2,2,4)
  plot(t,rate_plot); axis tight
  title('rate(t) vs t'); xlabel('t'); ylabel('rate(t)')
%
% Store numerical solution for 3D plot
  for it=1:nout
  for i=1:n
    c_3D(it,i)=u(it,i);
```

```
    end
    end
    z=[zl:dz:zu];
    figure(2)
    surf(z,t,c_3D)
    xlabel('z (m)'); ylabel('t (s)'); zlabel('c(z,t)
            (moles/m^3)');
    title('c(z,t) (moles/m^3), z=0,2.5\times10^{-6},...,
          5\times10^{-5} (m),t=0,2,...,100 (s)')
  % print -deps pde.eps; print -dps pde.ps
```

Listing 2.2 Main program pde_1_main

We can note the following details about pde_1_main.

- Previous files are cleared and selected parameters and variables are declared global so that they can be shared with other routines.

```
%
% Clear previous files
  clear all
  clc
%
% Parameters shared with the ODE routine
  global zl zu z dz dz2 D kf cbsat kr n cbulk ndss ncall
```

- Certain parameters that appear in the model equations, eqs. (2.1) to (2.6), are defined numerically. Most of these parameters are used in pde_1 of Listing 2.1 through the global declaration.

```
%
% Parameter numerical values
  D=1.0e-10; kf=1.0e+05; cbulk=4.48e-05;
  h=5.0e-05; c0=0; cb0=0;
```

- Multiple values of cbsat and kr are programmed. This reflects some of the experimentation that was done in developing the routines. In particular, the values of $c_{\mathrm{b,sat}}$ and k_{r} in eqs. (2.2) and (2.5) are sensitive parameters in determining the features of the numerical solution as discussed subsequently. As programmed, the last values are used in the calculations. Other values can be selected through the use of commenting (with %), with an if construction or with a case construction.

```
%
% Variation in interface binding saturation
  cbsat=1.66e-08;
  cbsat=1.66e-09;
%
% Variation in interface unbinding rate
  kr=1.0e-01;
  kr=1.0e+01;
```

- A spatial grid over the interval

$$z_{\mathrm{l}} \le z \le z_{\mathrm{u}} = 0 \le z \le 5 \times 10^{-5}\mathrm{m}$$

is defined on 21 points (see eq. (2.12a) for the use of Δz) with an interval

$$\Delta z = \frac{5 \times 10^{-5} - 0}{21 - 1} = 2.5 \times 10^{-6}\text{m}.$$

```
%
% Spatial grid
  zl=0; zu=5.0e-05; n=21; dz=(zu-zl)/(n-1); dz2=dz^2;
```

Δz^2 is also computed (see eq. (2.13a) for the use of Δz^2) and passed as a global variable to `pde_1`.

The number of grid points (e.g., $n = 21$) is usually determined by trial and error to achieve reasonable spatial resolution (in z) without excessive numbers of points; this resolution usually becomes clear when the numerical solution is plotted (as discussed subsequently).

The number of grid points to achieve acceptable resolution will increase when the solution changes rapidly in space. This often occurs when the solution displays a steep moving front or discontinuity. In the present case the variation of $c(z,t)$ with z is quite smooth and therefore only a modest number of grid points (21) is required (front resolution is discussed in some detail in Section (1.2.4)).

Also, the accuracy of the solution with respect to space can be inferred by changing the number of grid points and observing the effect on the numerical output. For example, if the solution does not change in the fourth figure (or beyond) as n is changed, we can infer that the solution is accurate to at least four figures. Of course, this type of result is not a proof of spatial convergence. But this approach does have the advantage that it can be used in essentially all applications (including when an analytical solution is not available to check on the spatial accuracy). Since in the numerical analysis literature the grid spacing is often given the symbol h (rather than Δz as used here), this experimentation with the number of grid points is often termed h refinement (see also Table 1.2 and the associated discussion concerning h refinement). The reader could easily use this technique with the present routines by changing the value of n and observing the effect on the numerical solution. Briefly, $n = 21$ was observed as adequate for reasonable spatial accuracy.

- Initial conditions (2.4) and (2.6) are programmed for the $n + 1$ ODEs and the initial values are placed in a single, one dimensional array, `u0` (`c0` and `cb0` were previously set to zero).

```
%
% Initial condition
  for i=1:n
    u0(i)=c0;
  end
  u0(n+1)=cb0;
```

The array `u0` is then an input to the ODE integrator to start the solution.

- The interval in t (of eqs. (2.1) and (2.5)) is defined as

$$0 \le t \le t_f \text{ or } 0 \le t \le 100 \text{ s}$$

with the solution to be displayed every 2 s.

```
%
% Independent variable for ODE integration
  t0=0.0;
  tf=100;
  tout=(t0:2:tf);
  nout=51;
  ncall=0;
```

Thus, there will be $(100 - 0/2) + 1 = 51$ output points (including the ICs at $t = 0$) or `nout=51`; these 51 values of t are placed in array `tout` (their values could be verified by removing the ; from `tout=(t0:2:tf);` which is a quick and convenient way to look at intermediate numerical results. Warning: this procedure may display more numerical output than you wish to view).

Also, the counter for the number of calls to `pde_1`, `ncall`, is initialized to zero (recall that this counter is incremented by 1 each time `pde_1` of Listing 2.1 is executed).

- The $n + 1 = 21$ ODEs are then integrated by a call to a MATLAB ODE integrator, `ode15s`.

```
%
% ODE integration
%
% Variation in error tolerances
  reltol=1.0e-06; abstol=1.0e-06;
  reltol=1.0e-07; abstol=1.0e-07;
  options=odeset('RelTol',reltol,'AbsTol',abstol);
  mf=1;
  if(mf==1) % explicit FDs
    [t,u]=ode15s(@pde_1,tout,u0,options); end
  if(mf==2) ndss=4; % ndss = 2, 4, 6, 8 or 10 required
    [t,u]=ode15s(@pde_2,tout,u0,options); end
  if(mf==3) ndss=44; % ndss = 42, 44, 46, 48 or 50 required
    [t,u]=ode15s(@pde_3,tout,u0,options); end
```

`ode15s` will attempt to integrate the ODEs numerically with an accuracy set by the two error tolerances, `reltol` (a relative error tolerance) and `abstol` (an absolute error tolerance). If `ode15s` cannot achieve the specified accuracy, it will display an error message (additional discussion of `ode15s` follows `pde_1_main` of Listing 1.6).

The two tolerances were first set to 1.0×10^{-6} and a solution was produced. They were then reset to 1.0×10^{-7} and a second solution was computed that could be compared (by visual inspection) with the first. In this case, the two solutions agreed to acceptable accuracy (e.g., three to four significant figures), which infers that convergence in time t was achieved. Thus, by varying the number of spatial grid points n and the error tolerances for the t integration, a basic error analysis gave some assurance that the numerical solutions would have acceptable accuracy in space and time. This is a basic diagnostic that usually can easily be performed.

Incidentally, if the error tolerances were increased much above 1.0×10^{-6}, such as 1.0×10^{-4}, the numerical solutions changed substantially (the reader could confirm this by changing the two error tolerances `reltol` and `abstol` to 1.0×10^{-4}). Fortunately, even with a stringent tolerance, such as 1.0×10^{-6} or 1.0×10^{-7}, the number of calls to `pde_1` remained quite modest (`ncall` typically has a final value of a few hundreds as will be observed in the subsequent discussion of the numerical output). A tradeoff between accuracy and the total computational effort (as reflected in the final value of `ncall`) is rather typical. In other words, as the accuracy is increased (through a tighter or smaller error tolerance), the computational effort frequently increases (as a larger final value of `ncall`).

`ode15s` is a sophisticated ODE integrator that not only changes the integration interval (it performs h refinement) but also changes the order of the integration formulas from first to fifth as it attempts to achieve the specified accuracy (which is the significance of 15 in the name of the integrator). Since in the numerical analysis literature the order of an approximation is often given the symbol p (e.g., in the order of the FD approximation of eq. (2.12a), $O(\Delta z^p)$ with $p = 2$), changing the order of the approximation is usually termed p refinement. In other words, `ode15s` performs h and p refinement simultaneously as it attempts to compute a solution with the accuracy specified with `reltol` and `abstol`; `ode15s` can therefore be termed a variable step, variable order integrator. The `s` in the name `ode15s`, refers to stiff; stiffness is discussed in Section 1.2.3.3 and subsequently (it is important in determining the performance of ODE integrators).

One of three approaches to the programming of the ODE routine is selected according to the value of the method flag, `mf`. For `mf=1`, `pde_1` of Listing 2.1 is called by `ode15s` (note that the first argument of `ode15s` is `@pde_1` where the `@` indicates the name of a routine is used as an input argument). For `mf=2,3`, the ODE routines called by `ode15s` are `pde_2` and `pde_3`, respectively. These routines will be discussed subsequently; they basically provide alternative programming of the $n + 1 = 22$ ODEs, as reflected in the explanatory comments.

In summary, for the coding

```
mf=1;
if(mf==1) % explicit FDs
  [t,u]=ode15s(@pde_1,tout,u0,options); end
```

the `ode15s` input arguments are

- `@pde_1`: the ODE routine called by `ode15s`; this routine must be available as a file with the name `pde_1`
- `tout`: the 1D array or vector of values of t at which the solution is to be displayed (both numerically and graphically as explained subsequently); in the present case, there will be `nout` values in `tout`
- `u0`: the 1D array or vector of initial values of $c(z,t=0), c_b(z,t=0)$ according to ICs (2.4) and (2.6). `ode15s` knows how many ODEs it should integrate by the length

of the IC vector u0; in other words, the number of ODEs ($n = 22$) is not an input argument to ode15s

- options: the options that define the operation of ode15s, in this case, the two tolerances, reltol and abstol; ode15s has an extensive set of options, some of which will be discussed subsequently.

The ode15s output arguments are

- t: a 1D array or vector of output (display) values of t; if the ODE integration proceeds as expected, the contents of t after ode15s computes a complete solution will be the same as in tout
- u: a 2D array of the ODE solution values of size u(nout,n+1) (total size is $n_{\text{out}} \times (n+1)$). Thus, the first dimension of u corresponds to t(it), it=1,2,...,nout or $t = 0, 2, ..., 100$. The second dimension of u corresponds to values of the $n+1$ ODE-dependent variables at each value of t(it). For example, u(4,1) corresponds to the solution $c(z=0, t=3(2))$, u(5,21) corresponds to $c(z=h, t=4(2))$ and u(6,22) corresponds to $c_{\text{b}}(t=5(2))$; note that the values of u are ordered with respect to the second dimension in the same way as in the initial condition vector u0 and the programming of the ODEs in pde_1 (using the subscript i in c(i)).

- The solution array u is sampled to store selected values of $c(z,t), c_{\text{b}}(t)$ for numerical and graphical output.

```
%
% Store numerical solutions at z = 0
  for it=1:nout
    c_plot(it)=u(it,1);
    cb_plot(it)=u(it,n+1);
    theta_plot(it)=cb_plot(it)/cbsat;
    rate_plot(it)=kf*c_plot(it)*(cbsat-cb_plot(it))-kr*cb_plot(it);
  end
```

c_plot(it) contains $c(z=0,t)$ at t(it) (note that the second subscript of u is 1 corresponding to $z=0$). cb_plot(it) contains $c_{\text{b}}(t)$ at t(it) (note the second subscript of u is n+1 corresponding to $c_{\text{b}}(t)$). theta_plot(it) contains $c_{\text{b}}(t)/c_{\text{b,sat}}$ (fractional antibody coverage) and rate_plot(it) contains the RHS of BC (2.2) and eq. (2.5), $k_{\text{f}}c(z=0,t)(c_{\text{b,sat}}-c_{\text{b}})-k_{\text{r}}c_{\text{b}}$; this net rate of binding or unbinding is plotted to gain some insight into the response of the model of eqs. (2.1) to (2.6), and illustrates how the dependent variables $(c(z,t), c_{\text{b}}(t))$ can be used to compute and display any of the terms of the model equations. Note also that since $k_{\text{f}}c(z=0,t)(c_{\text{b,sat}}-c_{\text{b}})-k_{\text{r}}c_{\text{b}}$ equals $(\text{d}c_{\text{b}}/\text{d}t)$ according to eq. (2.5), the derivatives in t can easily be displayed to further understand the response of the model, e.g., this diagnostic procedure also applies to $(\partial c/\partial t)$ of eq. (2.1).

- The numerical solution is then displayed numerically for the nout values of t through a for loop.

```
%
% Display selected output
```

```
fprintf('\n mf = %2d   abstol = %8.1e   reltol = %8.1e\n',...
        mf,abstol,reltol);
fprintf('\n     t       c(0,t)       cb(t)       theta        rate\n');
for it=1:nout
  fprintf('%6.0f%12.3e%12.3e%12.3e%12.3e\n',...
       t(it),c_plot(it),cb_plot(it),theta_plot(it),rate_plot(it));
end
fprintf('\n ncall = %4d\n',ncall);
```

At the end of this output, the final value of `ncall` is displayed as an indication of the total computational effort required to calculate the solution.

- These solution values are also plotted.

```
%
% Plot numerical solutions at z = 0
  figure(1);
  subplot(2,2,1)
  plot(t,c_plot); axis tight
  title('c(0,t) vs t'); xlabel('t'); ylabel('c(0,t)')
  subplot(2,2,2)
  plot(t,cb_plot); axis tight
  title('cb(t) vs t'); xlabel('t'); ylabel('cb(t)')
  subplot(2,2,3)
  plot(t,theta_plot); axis tight
  title('theta(t) vs t'); xlabel('t'); ylabel('theta(t)')
  subplot(2,2,4)
  plot(t,rate_plot); axis tight
  title('rate(t) vs t'); xlabel('t'); ylabel('rate(t)')
```

The MATLAB `subplot` utility is used to produce a 2×2 array of plots (a total of four plots, each drawn with the `plots` and basic labeling utilities), which are shown in Fig. 2.3a.

- One of the principal advantages of PDE analysis is the computation of a solution in both time and space. In the present case, this is the analyte concentration $c(z,t)$ defined by eq. (2.1). The preceding plotting gives only $c(z=0,t)$, the analyte concentration at the antibody interface at $z=0$. However, we can easily plot the analyte profiles in z as demonstrated by the following code for 3D plotting.

```
%
% Store numerical solution for 3D plot
  for it=1:nout
  for i=1:n
    c_3D(it,i)=u(it,i);
  end
  end
  z=[zl:dz:zu];
  figure(2)
  surf(z,t,c_3D)
  xlabel('z (m)'); ylabel('t (s)'); zlabel('c(z,t)
        (moles/m^3)');
  title('c(z,t) (moles/m^3), z=0,2.5\times10^{-6},...,
```

```
        5\times10^{-5} (m),t=0,2,...,100 (s)')
% print -deps pde.eps; print -dps pde.ps
```

We can note the following details.

- The solution array `u(it,i)` from `ode15s` is transferred to the array `c_3D(it,i)` for `nout = 51` points in t and `n = 21` point in z.
- The grid in z is defined with `z=[zl:dz:zu]`.
- The 3D plot is produced with a call to `surf`.
- Labels for the z and t axes are included with calls to `xlabel` and `ylabel`, respectively. A label for $c(z,t)$ is added with a call to `zlabel`.
- A title for the 3D plot is added with `title`. Note the use of coding for $\times^{-6}$ and $\times^{-5}$ to enhance the title.
- The commented `print` line demonstrates how output files in `eps` and `ps` formats can be produced. This can also be accomplished within MATLAB using the `save as...` menu and selecting the file format.

The 3D plot produced by this code is subsequently discussed as Fig. 2.3b.

This completes the discussion of the basic MATLAB routines, `pde_1` and `pde_1_main` of Listings 2.1 and 2.2, respectively. We now consider the output from these routines (with `mf=1` in the main program; the output for `mf=2,3` is considered subsequently).

2.4 Model output

A sample of the numerical output from `pde_1_main` and `pde_1` of Listings 2.1 and 2.2 follows.

We can note the following details about this output.

- The solutions starts at the ICs of eq. (2.4) and (2.6).

```
t       c(0,t)        cb(t)        theta         rate
0   0.000e+000   0.000e+000   0.000e+000   0.000e+000
```

  While this may seem like an obvious result, it is actually an important check, particularly as the number of ICs increases with the number of ODE/PDEs. In the present case, since there are 22 ODEs, a check on all 22 ICs would be worthwhile (if even one of the ICs is incorrect, the numerical solution will in general be incorrect).
- For $t > 0$, the concentrations $c(z,t)$ and $c_b(t)$ assume increasing, positive values as expected; for example, the values at $t = 2$ are

```
t       c(0,t)        cb(t)        theta         rate
2   3.735e-007   5.121e-012   3.085e-003   1.060e-011
```

  If any of these values were negative, this would be an immediate indication that the solution is in error (based on physical considerations, not mathematical analysis); such a result could be due to something as simple as a sign error in the RHS of one of the ODEs.

Table 2.3. Sample of output from `pde_1_main` and `pde_1`

```
  mf =   1    abstol = 1.0e-007    reltol = 1.0e-007

    t       c(0,t)        cb(t)         theta          rate
    0   0.000e+000   0.000e+000   0.000e+000   0.000e+000
    2   3.735e-007   5.121e-012   3.085e-003   1.060e-011
    4   3.050e-006   4.645e-011   2.798e-002   2.772e-011
    6   7.035e-006   1.063e-010   6.403e-002   3.014e-011
    8   1.121e-005   1.648e-010   9.927e-002   2.757e-011
   10   1.516e-005   2.165e-010   1.304e-001   2.301e-011
          .                                           .
          .                                           .
             output for t = 12 to 88 removed
          .                                           .
          .                                           .
   94   4.473e-005   5.130e-010   3.090e-001   8.640e-013
   96   4.474e-005   5.131e-010   3.091e-001   4.094e-013
   94   4.473e-005   5.130e-010   3.090e-001   8.640e-013
   96   4.474e-005   5.131e-010   3.091e-001   4.094e-013
   98   4.474e-005   5.131e-010   3.091e-001   2.026e-013
  100   4.475e-005   5.132e-010   3.092e-001   3.637e-014

ncall =   135
```

- For large t, e.g., $t > 88$, the solution approaches a steady-state or equilibrium condition.

```
    t       c(0,t)        cb(t)         theta          rate
   90   4.470e-005   5.127e-010   3.089e-001   1.430e-012
   92   4.472e-005   5.129e-010   3.089e-001   1.262e-012
   94   4.473e-005   5.130e-010   3.090e-001   8.640e-013
   96   4.474e-005   5.131e-010   3.091e-001   4.094e-013
   98   4.474e-005   5.131e-010   3.091e-001   2.026e-013
  100   4.475e-005   5.132e-010   3.092e-001   3.637e-014
```

This equilibrium condition results from the derivatives in t, $(\partial c/\partial t)$ and $(\mathrm{d}c_\mathrm{b}/\mathrm{d}t)$, approaching zero. This is clear from the values of `rate`; for example, `rate = 1.060e-011` at `t = 2` while `rate = 3.637e-014` at `t = 100`, a reduction by a factor of

$$\frac{3.637 \times 10^{-14}}{1.060 \times 10^{-11}} = 0.0034.$$

In other words, as `rate` $\rightarrow 0$, or

$$k_\mathrm{f}\, c(z=0,t)(c_{\mathrm{b,sat}} - c_\mathrm{b}) - k_\mathrm{r} c_\mathrm{b} \rightarrow 0,$$

eqs. (2.1) and (2.5) become

$$0 = \frac{\mathrm{d}^2 c}{\mathrm{d}z^2}, \tag{2.14a}$$

$$0 = k_\mathrm{f}\, c(z=0,t)(c_{\mathrm{b,sat}} - c_\mathrm{b}) - k_\mathrm{r} c_\mathrm{b}. \tag{2.14b}$$

Note that eq. (2.14a) is now an ODE (rather than a PDE) and eqs. (2.14a), (2.2), and (2.3) constitute a two point, boundary value ODE (BVODE) problem. In fact, this is an effective approach to the solution of a BVODE, that is, state it as a time-dependent PDE, then integrate the PDE to equilibrium; this approach can be applied to systems of BVODEs (not just a single BVODE). Also, this approach can be applied to nonlinear BVODEs (and not just linear BVODEs as eq. (2.14a)).

As a check on the numerical solution (of Table 2.3), since eq. (2.14a) is linear, it can easily be integrated analytically subject to BCs (2.2) and (2.3); this independent steady-state analytical solution, $c(z, t = \infty)$, could then be used as a check on the numerical solution, $c(z,t)$ for large t.

Also, eq. (2.14b) is algebraic and this result suggests an effective approach to the solution of nonlinear algebraic equations (NAE), that is, convert the NAEs to ODEs, then integrate the ODEs to equilibrium; this approach can be applied to systems of NAEs (not just a single NAE).

The fractional coverage, `theta` approaches $\theta = 0.309$ (30.9% coverage), a value in the interval $0 \leq \theta \leq 1$. This is another rather obvious, but important, check.

- `rate` has its largest values for small t; for example the largest value, `3.014e-011`, is at $t = 6$:

```
t      c(0,t)        cb(t)        theta        rate
6   7.035e-006   1.063e-010   6.403e-002   3.014e-011
```

This is rather typical of unsteady-state, transient or dynamic systems; the rate of change (or the derivatives in t) is largest at the beginning of the solution. As an explanation in the present case, the model equations are moved away from their initial values (as set by eqs. (2.4) and (2.6)) by c_{bulk} in eq. (2.3). In other words, c_{bulk} is the driving term for the model equations and it will have it largest effect for small t; as the system approaches the equilibrium condition of Table 2.3 for large t, the effect of c_{bulk} diminishes and approaches zero for large t.

Another way to look at this is to consider using the equilibrium solution as the initial condition; now the derivatives in t, $(\partial c/\partial t)$ and $(\mathrm{d}c_{\text{b}}/\mathrm{d}t)$, will be zero and the solution will not change with t.

- The approach to equilibrium and the maximum values of `rate` for small t are clearly indicated in the graphical output of Fig. 2.3a.

Note how $c(z = 0, t)$, $c_{\text{b}}(t)$ and $\theta = c(z = 0, t)/c_{\text{b,sat}}$ approach their equilibrium values and how `rate` peaks at small values of t. Also, the jagged appearance of `rate` is not unexpected or unusual since it is computed as the nonlinear sum of a series of terms, `rate` = $k_{\text{f}} c(z = 0, t)(c_{\text{b,sat}} - c_{\text{b}}) - k_{\text{r}} c_{\text{b}}$, with differences that can rapidly change value. Fortunately, the ODE integration process tends to smooth such behavior, as reflected in the smooth responses of $c(z = 0, t)$ and $c_{\text{b}}(t)$ (which have `rate` as their derivatives in t). In other words, the ODE integrator `ode15s` is not particularly upset by the jagged appearance of `rate` and computes an ODE solution with reasonable effort (modest final values of `ncall`) without any reported computational problems (error messages); however, this might explain why error tolerances of 1.0×10^{-7} rather than 1.0×10^{-4} were required to produce consistent (reproducible) solutions when the error tolerances were changed, e.g., 1.0×10^{-6} gives essentially the same solution as 1.0×10^{-7}. The success of `ode15s` in computing a solution is also an indication of its effectiveness in adjusting the integration step, h, using smaller values when the solution changes rapidly and larger values where the solution is smoother; in other words, h refinement is producing good results.

- The 3D plot from `surf` is in Fig. 2.3b.

  We can note the following details about Fig. 2.3b.

  - The axes in t and z are for the intervals $0 \le t \le 100$ s and $0 \le z \le 5 \times 10^{-5}$ m, respectively.
  - The interval in the analyte concentration, $c(z,t)$, is $0 \le c(z,t) \le c_{\mathrm{bulk}} = 4.48 \times 10^{-5}$ mole/m^3.
  - Initially $c(z,t)$ has the value $c(z,t=0) = c_0 = 0$ according to IC (2.4).
  - At $z = h = 5 \times 10^{-5}$ m, $c(z = h,t)$ moves almost immediately to $c(z = h,t) \approx c_{\mathrm{bulk}} = 4.48 \times 10^{-5}$ (not exactly 4.48×10^{-5} because of the mass transfer resistance reflected in BC (2.2)). $c(z = 0,t = 0)$ remains near IC (2.4), $c(z = 0,t = 0) \approx 0$, until the effect of $c_{\mathrm{bulk}} = 4.48 \times 10^{-5}$ begins to take effect through the diffusion from $z = h$ to $z = 0$.
  - For large t the entire solution approaches the value $c(z,t) = c_{\mathrm{bulk}} = 4.48 \times 10^{-5}$.

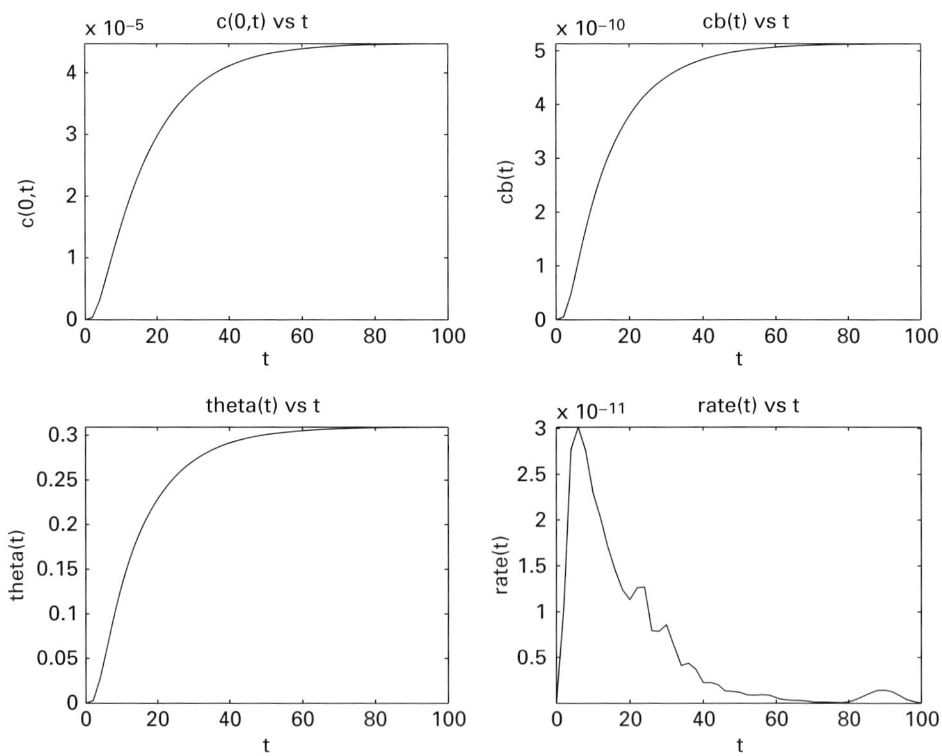

Figure 2.3a Plots of $c(z=0,t)$, $c_b(t)$, $\theta = c(z=0,t)/c_{b,\mathrm{sat}}$, `rate`

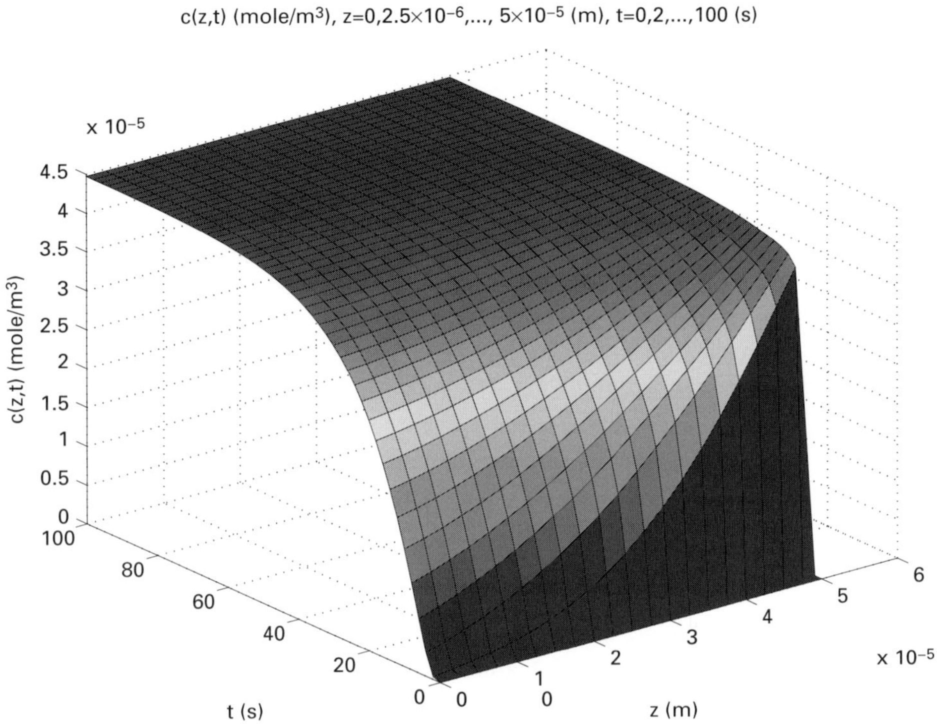

Figure 2.3b 3D Plot of $c(z,t)$ vs z and t

Thus, Fig. 2.3b reflects the expected properties of the solution of eq. (2.1) and provides a clear perspective of the entire solution for $c(z,t)$.

2.5 ODE stiffness

The preceding discussion indicates that the error tolerances specified for the ODE integrator (e.g., `reltol, abstol` = 1.0×10^{-7}) can be an important factor in determining the overall accuracy of the MOL solution of an ODE/PDE model (the other important source of errors is the spatial approximation that can be studied through h and p refinement). Varying the ODE error tolerances (`relerr, abserr`) is a form of h refinement since the ODE integrator, in this case `oed15s`, will adjust the integration interval to achieve the specified accuracy; as noted previously, `ode15s` also performs p refinement since it changes the order of the integration algorithm from one to five (and thus the 15 in the name of the integrator).

Another possibility for an ODE error analysis is to change the integrator. Here we consider replacing `ode15s` with another MATLAB library integrator, `ode45`. This is easily accomplished by simply changing the integrator name in the calling statement, that is, by using the following statements in the main program.

```
mf=1;
if(mf==1) % explicit FDs
  [t,u]=ode45(@pde_1,tout,u0,options); end
```

Our expectation, then, would be to produce a numerical solution that could be compared with the previous numerical solutions produced by `ode15s`. In fact, when this modification with the call to `ode45` is executed, the calculation fails (no solution is produced with a reasonable computer run time). `ode45` is a well-established ODE integrator and this unexpected result requires some explanation.

The principal difference between `ode15s` and `ode45` is that `ode15s` is intended for stiff ODEs (hence the "s" in the name of this integrator) while `ode45` is intended for nonstiff ODEs. Therefore, the failure of `ode45` is most likely due to the stiffness of the 22 ODEs of the MOL approximation of eqs. (2.1) to (2.6). This naturally then leads to the question of what is meant by "stiffness". This is an important area within numerical analysis that has an extensive literature. Here we discuss just a few details pertaining to the stiffness of the ODEs approximating eq. (2.1) to (2.6). Additional discussion of stiffness is given in Appendix 2 in terms of a 2×2 ODE system. Additional information on ODE integration and stiffness is available in the articles by Shampine and Thompson ([5, 6] and Appendix C of the book by Lee and Schiesser ([3])).

To investigate the stiffness of the ODEs approximating eq. (2.1) to (2.6), a fixed-step explicit (nonstiff) integrator, `rk4` of Listing 1.5, was used in place of `ode15s` (see Section 1.2.3.2 concerning the use of `rk4`). By trial and error, a stable solution could be computed with `nsteps = 100, h = 0.02, nout = 51` (used in `pde_1_main` of Listing 1.1). The number of calls to ODE routine `pde_1` of Listing 2.1 was therefore `ncall = (51 - 1)(100)(4) = 20000`; the factor 4 comes from four derivative evaluations (calls to `pde_1` in `rk4` of Listing 1.5) for each step of length `h = 0.02`. This figure (`ncall = 20000`) contrasts with `ncall = 135` of Table 2.3 and clearly demonstrates the computational efficiency of `ode15s`. With the `rk4` parameters changed to `nsteps = 50, h = 0.04, nout = 51` (the integration step is doubled), the numerical solution was unstable, which demonstrates the stability constraint of the explicit `rk4`.

In summary, if an explicit ODE integrator requires a large computational effort, e.g., large `ncall`, stiffness is probably a problem, and a stiff (implicit) integrator should be used. The latter will require more computations for each step, but much larger integration steps can be used, and the overall result is better computational efficiency, e.g., `135` vs `20000` steps.

2.6 Parameter sensitivity analysis

The preceding discussion of the characteristics of `rate` suggests that some additional numerical investigation is possible to enhance our understanding of the model solutions. Specifically, if we look at the individual RHS terms in `rate =` $k_f c(z=0,t)(c_{b,sat} - c_b) - k_r c_b$, we can better understand the relative rates of binding, $k_f c(z=0,t)(c_{b,sat} - c_b)$, and unbinding, $-k_r c_b$. To this end, `pde_1_main` of Listing 2.2 was modified slightly to `pde_1a_main`. The coding that was changed follows in Listing 2.2a.

```
                    .
                    .
                    .
%
% Store numerical solutions at z = 0
  for it=1:nout
    c_plot(it)=u(it,1);
    cb_plot(it)=u(it,n+1);
    theta_plot(it)=cb_plot(it)/cbsat;
    for_plot(it)= kf*c_plot(it)*(cbsat-cb_plot(it));
    rev_plot(it)=-kr*cb_plot(it);
    rate_plot(it)=kf*c_plot(it)*(cbsat-cb_plot(it))-kr*cb_plot(it);
  end
                    .
                    .
                    .
%
% RHS terms at z = 0
  figure(1);
  subplot(2,2,1)
  plot(t,theta_plot); axis tight
  title('\theta vs t'); xlabel('t'); ylabel('\theta(t)')
  subplot(2,2,2)
  plot(t,for_plot); axis tight
% axis([0 100 0 5e-09]);
  title('forward rate vs t'); xlabel('t'); ylabel('forward rate')
  subplot(2,2,3)
  plot(t,rev_plot); axis tight
% axis([0 100 -5e-09 0]);
  title('reverse rate vs t'); xlabel('t'); ylabel('reverse rate')
  subplot(2,2,4)
  plot(t,rate_plot); axis tight
  title('net rate vs t'); xlabel('t'); ylabel('net rate')
```

Listing 2.2a `pde_1a_main` with modifications to `pde_1_main` of Listing 2.2 to investigate the binding and unbinding rates

We can note the following details about this revised code.

- The forward binding rate is stored as `for_plot(it)`.

```
    for_plot(it)= kf*c_plot(it)*(cbsat-cb_plot(it));
    rev_plot(it)=-kr*cb_plot(it);
    rate_plot(it)=kf*c_plot(it)*(cbsat-cb_plot(it))-kr*cb_plot(it);
```

  The reverse unbinding rate is stored as `rev_plot(it)` and the net binding rate is stored as `rate_plot(it)` (the difference between the forward and reverse binding rates).
- These three rates are then available for plotting with the following code.

```
%
% RHS terms at z = 0
  figure(1);
```

```
  subplot(2,2,1)
  plot(t,theta_plot); axis tight
  title('\theta vs t'); xlabel('t'); ylabel('\theta(t)')
  subplot(2,2,2)
  plot(t,for_plot); axis tight
% axis([0 100 0 5e-09]);
  title('forward rate vs t'); xlabel('t'); ylabel('forward rate')
  subplot(2,2,3)
  plot(t,rev_plot); axis tight
% axis([0 100 -5e-09 0]);
  title('reverse rate vs t'); xlabel('t'); ylabel('reverse rate')
  subplot(2,2,4)
  plot(t,rate_plot); axis tight
  title('net rate vs t'); xlabel('t'); ylabel('net rate')
```

We can note the following details about this code for plotting.

- The fractional coverage, θ, is first plotted (as `subplot(2,2,1)`) to provide a point of reference for the other three plots. As noted previously, θ is constrained to $0 \leq \theta \leq 1$ corresponding to no bounded analyte ($\theta = 0$) to saturation of the antibody interface ($\theta = 1$); these constraints provide an important test of the numerical solution (if they are not observed, an error can be investigated in the model, in the computer code, or possibly both).
- The forward binding rate is then plotted (as `subplot(2,2,2)`). The `% axis([0 100 0 5e-09]);` was an attempt to improve the scaling of this plot, but was not particularly successful so it was converted to a comment – the reader might activate (decomment) this statement to observe the effect on the second plot.
- The reverse binding rate is next plotted (as `subplot(2,2,3)`). Again, the `% axis([0 100 -5e-09 0]);` was an attempt to improve the scaling of this plot, but was not particularly successful so it was converted to a comment – again, the reader might activate (decomment) this statement to observe the effect on the second plot.
- The net binding rate is finally plotted (as `subplot(2,2,4)`) to observe the effect of subtracting the reverse binding rate from the forward binding rate.

The numerical output from this modified main program is the same as in Table 2.3 and is therefore not presented here. The four plots are in Fig. 2.4.

We can note the following details about the plots of Fig. 2.4.

- The plot of $\theta = c_{\text{b}}(t)/c_{\text{b,sat}}$ gives an indication of the transition from no bound analyte at $t = 0$ ($\theta = 0$) to an unsaturated condition of $\theta = 0.309$ at approximately $t > 50$ s. This increasing binding is reflected in the other three plots.
- The plot of the binding rate $k_{\text{f}}c(z=0,t)(c_{\text{b,sat}} - c_{\text{b}})$ closely follows the preceding plot of $\theta = c_{\text{b}}(t)/c_{\text{b,sat}}$. This is expected since the binding rate is proportional to θ,

$$k_{\text{f}}c(z=0,t)(c_{\text{b,sat}} - c_{\text{b}}) = k_{\text{f}}c_{\text{b,sat}}c(z=0,t)(1 - c_{\text{b}}/c_{\text{b,sat}}) = k_{\text{f}}c_{\text{b,sat}}c(z=0,t)(1-\theta)$$

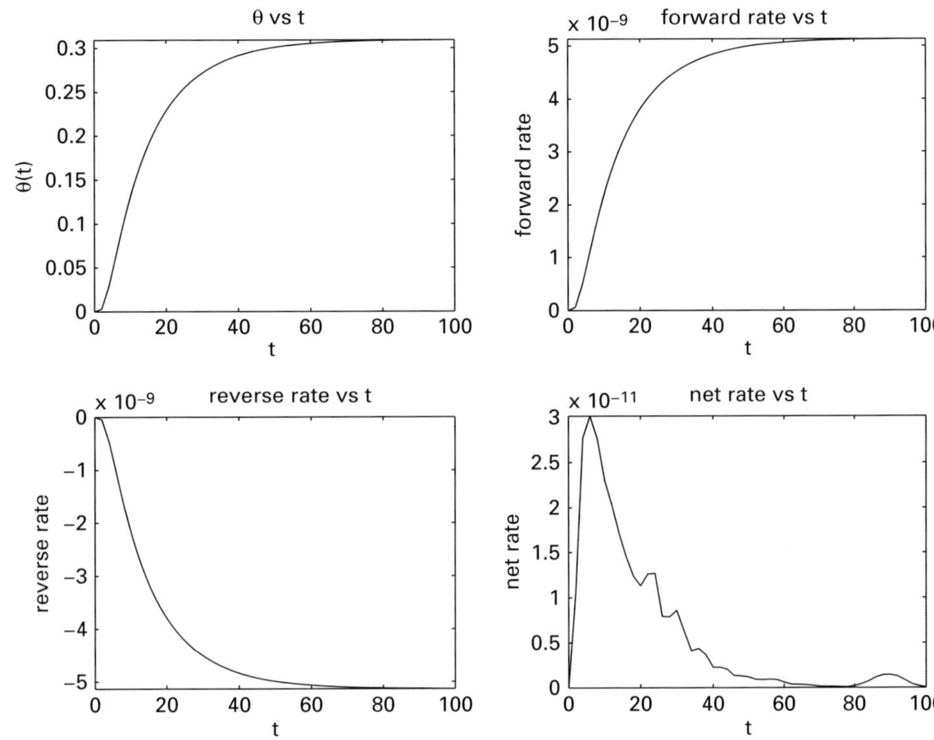

Figure 2.4 Plots of (1) $\theta = c_{\rm b}(t)/c_{\rm b,sat}$, (2) $k_{\rm f} c(z=0,t)(c_{\rm b,sat} - c_{\rm b})$,(3) $-k_{\rm r} c_{\rm b}$, (4) `rate` = $k_{\rm f} c(z=0,t)$ $(c_{\rm b,sat} - c_{\rm b}) - k_{\rm r} c_{\rm b}$

In other words, $c(z = 0,t)$ and θ approach equilibrium values and therefore $c(z = 0,t)(1-\theta)$ also approaches an equilibrium value. For example, from Table. 2.3, $c(z = 0, t \rightarrow \infty) = 4.475 \times 10^{-5}$, $\theta(t \rightarrow \infty) = 0.3092$, and $c(z = 0,t)(1-\theta(t)) = 4.475 \times 10^{-5}(1-0.3092) = 3.019 \times 10^{-5}$

- The plot of the unbinding rate $-k_{\rm r} c_{\rm b}$ also closely follows the preceding plot of $\theta = c_{\rm b}(t)/c_{\rm b,sat}$. This is expected since the unbinding rate is proportional to $c_{\rm b}(t) = \theta c_{\rm b,sat}$.
- The plot of `rate` = $k_{\rm f} c(z=0,t)(c_{\rm b,sat} - c_{\rm b}) - k_{\rm r} c_{\rm b}$ indicates that this net rate is of the order 3×10^{-11}, which is two orders of magnitude (10^{-2}) below the forward binding rate in the second plot or the reverse unbinding rate of the third plot (both of these rates are of the order of 3×10^{-9}). In other words, the net rate equals the difference of two nearly equal rates. This subtraction of two nearly equal quantities can be prone to error (even with the high precision of computer arithmetic), as illustrated by the irregular (jagged) fourth plot. In fact, if we again note that this rate is the RHS of eq. (2.5), $c_{\rm b}(t)$ is computed through the integration of this rate and we might then conclude that $c_{\rm b}(t)$ is unexpectedly well-behaved (smooth). This comes about through the smoothing of the numerical integration (by `ode15s`), that is, sharp increases and decreases in the

rate tend to cancel to some extent and thus produce a smooth integrated result (as exhibited in the second plot of Fig 2.3a, $c_b(t)$ vs t).

The preceding discussion of the forward and reverse binding rates, and in particular, their small differences, suggests that the forward and reverse rate constants, k_f and k_r, may be sensitive parameters, especially since small changes in their values may have large effects on the net binding rate, `rate`. This sensitivity could be investigated mathematically by considering the parameter sensitivity functions, for example $(\partial c_b(t)/\partial k_f)$ and $(\partial c_b(t)/\partial k_r)$. These partial derivatives are available from the model equations and could be computed as part of the numerical solution (how these functions change with t). However, for our purpose of a brief introduction to parameter sensitivity, we will merely change the parameter values and observe the effect on the numerical solutions. This is a basic procedure that can always be applied at the beginning of a computer-based PDE analysis. More sophisticated approaches ([1, 4]) could be well worth the effort to gain enhanced insight, for example, into how the rate constants affect the solution.

As an example of investigating parameter sensitivity, we consider the case where the reverse unbinding rate constant, k_r, is reduced by a factor of 10^{-2}. This is programmed in the main program of Listing 2.2 as

Table 2.4. Sample of output from `pde_1_main` and `pde_1` for `kr=1.0e-01`

```
mf =  1   abstol = 1.0e-007   reltol = 1.0e-007

      t      c(0,t)        cb(t)        theta          rate
      0  0.000e+000   0.000e+000   0.000e+000   0.000e+000
      2  9.435e-008   6.855e-012   4.130e-003   1.491e-011
      4  3.666e-007   7.471e-011   4.501e-002   5.064e-011
      6  6.119e-007   1.978e-010   1.191e-001   6.970e-011
      8  8.583e-007   3.470e-010   2.091e-001   7.799e-011
     10  1.146e-006   5.073e-010   3.056e-001   8.143e-011
           .                                      .
           .                                      .
              output for t = 12 to 88 removed
           .                                      .
           .                                      .
     90  4.473e-005   1.624e-009   9.781e-001  -5.749e-014
     92  4.474e-005   1.624e-009   9.782e-001  -1.036e-013
     94  4.475e-005   1.624e-009   9.782e-001  -1.705e-013
     96  4.476e-005   1.624e-009   9.782e-001  -2.599e-013
     98  4.476e-005   1.624e-009   9.782e-001  -2.697e-013
    100  4.478e-005   1.624e-009   9.782e-001  -4.040e-014

 ncall =  234
```

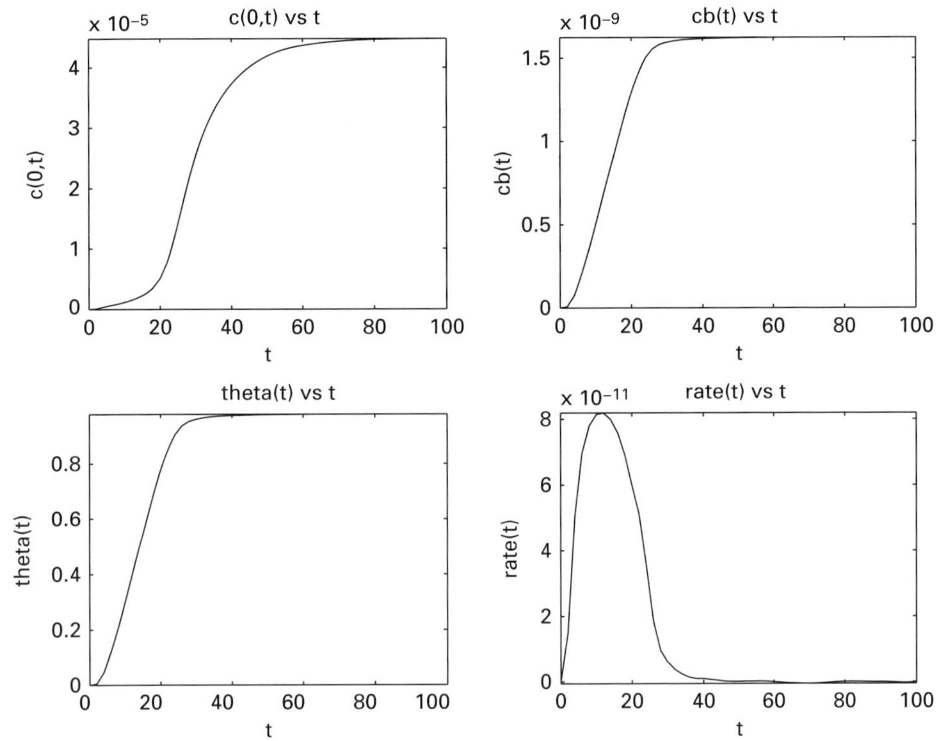

Figure 2.5 Plots of (1) $\theta = c_{\rm b}(t)/c_{\rm b,sat}$, (2) $k_{\rm f}c(z=0,t)(c_{\rm b,sat} - c_{\rm b})$, (3) $-k_{\rm r}c_{\rm b}$, (4) `rate` $= k_{\rm f}c(z=0,t)$ $(c_{\rm b,sat} - c_{\rm b}) - k_{\rm r}c_{\rm b}$

```
%
% Variation in interface unbinding rate
  kr=1.0e-01;
% kr=1.0e+01;
```

Note the use of a comment (%) to deactivate the second value of `kr` and thereby activate the first (smaller) value.

A portion of the numerical output follows in Table 2.4.

We can note the following details about this output.

- The equilibrium value $\theta = 0.9782$ indicates close to a saturation value for $c_{\rm b}$. This increase from the previous value $\theta = 0.3092$ (see Table 2.3) is to be expected since the rate at which the analyte leaves the antibody surface has been reduced (`kr=1.0e+01` reduced to `kr=1.0e-01`).
- The net rate of binding goes through a maximum, then decreases to essentially zero. This is reflected in Fig. 2.5 (bottom right plot), and is a marked departure from Fig. 2.4. The approach of `rate` to zero is due to the near saturation of the antibody binding, that is, `rate` $\rightarrow 0$ as $\theta \rightarrow 1$ with a small value of $k_{\rm r}$ (from `rate` $= k_{\rm f}c(z=0,t)c_{\rm b,sat}(1 - \theta) - k_{\rm r}c_{\rm b}$).

- `ncall` has increased from `135` (Table 2.3) to `234`; this is still a modest computational requirement (but as a word of caution, the computational effort could be substantially increased, depending on the sensitivity to parameter values, or changes in the model structure).

The intention of this example is to demonstrate the feasibility of changing parameters in the model. Typically, this would be done to estimate model parameters by comparing the computed solutions with experimental data, or perhaps to test a hypothesis. For example, if the coverage θ could be measured experimentally, the distinction between Figs. 2.4 and 2.5 could possibly give an indication of the value of k_r.

2.7 Spatial derivatives by stagewise differentiation

We now conclude this chapter with a discussion of two variations on function `pde_1` of Listing 2.1 for the calculation of the spatial derivative $(\partial^2 c/\partial z^2)$ in eq. (2.1) and the derivative $(\partial c(z=0,t)/\partial z)$ in eq. (2.2). Recall that in `pde_1` these derivatives were calculated by finite differences (FDs) that were programmed explicitly. We now consider how these derivatives can be calculated by library routines.

As the first variation of `pde_1`, we consider the following routine, `pde_2` (Listing 2.3).

```
  function ut=pde_2(t,u)
%
% Problem parameters
  global zl zu z dz dz2 D kf cbsat kr n cbulk ndss ncall
%
% ODE and PDE
  for i=1:n
    c(i)=u(i);
  end
  cb=u(n+1);
%
% BC
  c(n)=cbulk;
%
% cz
  cz=dss004(zl,zu,n,c);
%
% BC
  cz(1)=(1/D)*(kf*c(1)*(cbsat-cb)-kr*cb);
%
% czz
  czz=dss004(zl,zu,n,cz);
%
% PDE
  ct=D*czz;
  ct(n)=0;
%
% ODE
```

```
  cbt=kf*c(1)*(cbsat-cb)-kr*cb;
%
% Derivative vector
  for i=1:n
    ut(i)=ct(i);
  end
  ut(n+1)=cbt;
%
% Transpose for ODE integrator
  ut=ut';
%
% Increment calls to pde_2
  ncall=ncall+1;
```

Listing 2.3 ODE routine pde_2

We can note the following details about pde_2 (with emphasis on the differences from pde_1).

- The function is first defined followed by a global area as in pde_1.
- The composite solution vector u (the second input argument to pde_2) is placed in two arrays, c,cb, to facilitate programming in terms of problem-oriented variables as in pde_1.
- BC (2.3) is imposed.

```
%
% BC
  c(n)=cbulk;
```

- The derivative $(\partial c(z,t)/\partial z)$ is calculated by library routine dss004.

```
%
% cz
  cz=dss004(zl,zu,n,c);
```

  Note that c, the variable to be differentiated, is an input to dss004. The use of dss004 has the following advantages over the explicit programing of the first derivative in pde_1 of Listing 2.1.

  - The calculated derivative cz is fourth order correct (because of the five point FDs in dss004) rather than second order correct (because of the three point FDs used in pde_1.). A higher order derivative is generally a major improvement in the accuracy of the numerical derivative (cz).
  - The use of fictitious points as in pde_1 is avoided since the FDs of dss004 are noncentered at the boundaries and therefore do not require a separate analysis for the boundaries (see Listing 1.17 and eqs. (2.13) for additional discussion of this point).
  - The use of a library routine (dss004) simplifies the programming (compared with pde_1).

- Boundary condition (2.2) is used to reset the first derivative at $z = 0$ (grid point 1) from dss004, $(\partial c(z = 0, t)/\partial z)$

```
%
% BC
  cz(1)=(1/D)*(kf*c(1)*(cbsat-cb)-kr*cb);
```

Note the use of $c(z = 0, t)$ and $c_b(t)$ according to eq. (2.2); these concentrations vary with t as the integration proceeds via ode15s and the previous programming based on u.

- The second derivative in eq. (2.1), $(\partial^2 c/\partial z^2)$, is calculated with dss004 (by differentiating cz).

```
%
% czz
  czz=dss004(zl,zu,n,cz);
```

This two-step differentiation is an example of stagewise differentiation.

- Equation (2.1) is programmed.

```
%
% PDE
  ct=D*czz;
  ct(n)=0;
```

Note the use of the MATLAB vector facility (subscripting is not required). Also, BC (2.3) is enforced by setting $(\partial c(z = h, t)/\partial z) = 0$.

- Equation (2.5) is programmed.

```
%
% ODE
  cbt=kf*c(1)*(cbsat-cb)-kr*cb;
```

Integration of this ODE provides $c_b(t)$, which is then used in the other parts of the programming.

- The $n(= 22)$ ODEs are now programmed and a single derivative vector can be formed (and returned from pde_2 as a RHS output argument).

```
%
% Derivative vector
  for i=1:n
    ut(i)=ct(i);
  end
  ut(n+1)=cbt;
```

- Finally, a transpose of ut is required by ode15s and the counter for the number of calls to pde_2 is incremented.

```
%
% Transpose for ODE integrator
  ut=ut';
%
```

```
% Increment calls to pde_2
  ncall=ncall+1;
```

To use pde_2, the method flag mf in the main program of Listing 2.2 is changed from mf=1 to mf=2. Note how ode15s calls pde_2 with mf=2.

This completes the alternative programming of the MOL/ODEs based on the use of dss004. The numerical and graphical outputs are essentially identical to the output from pde_1 and are therefore not discussed here to conserve space.

2.8 Spatial derivatives by direct calculation

We now consider a third alternative to the programming of the MOL/ODEs based on the direct calculation of the second derivative ($\partial^2 c/\partial z^2$) of eq. (2.1) (rather than the stagewise differentiation of pde_2). The routine, pde_3, is given in Listing 2.4.

```
  function ut=pde_3(t,u)
%
% Problem parameters
  global zl zu z dz dz2 D kf cbsat kr n cbulk ndss ncall
%
% ODE and PDE
  for i=1:n
    c(i)=u(i);
  end
  cb=u(n+1);
%
% BCs
  c(n)=cbulk;
  cz(1)=(1/D)*(kf*c(1)*(cbsat-cb)-kr*cb);
  nu=1; nl=2;
%
% czz
  czz=dss044(zl,zu,n,c,cz,nl,nu);
%
% PDE
  ct=D*czz;
  ct(n)=0;
%
% ODE
  cbt=kf*c(1)*(cbsat-cb)-kr*cb;
%
% Derivative vector
  for i=1:n
    ut(i)=ct(i);
  end
  ut(n+1)=cbt;
%
% Transpose for ODE integrator
```

```
  ut=ut';
%
% Increment calls to pde_3
  ncall=ncall+1;
```

Listing 2.4 ODE routine pde_3

We can note the following details about pde_3, with emphasis on the differences from pde_2.

- The function and a global area are defined, and the composite-dependent variable vector u is placed in two arrays, c,cb, as in pde_2.
- Boundary conditions (2.2) and (2.3) are programmed. Note that BC (2.2) is declared Neumann with nl=2 (from the derivative $(\partial c(z=0,t)/\partial z)$) and BC (2.3) is declared Dirichlet with nu=1 (from the dependent variable $c(z=h,t)$).

```
%
% BCs
  c(n)=cbulk;
  cz(1)=(1/D)*(kf*c(1)*(cbsat-cb)-kr*cb);
  nu=1; nl=2;
```

- The second derivative $(\partial^2 c/\partial z^2)$ of eq. (2.1) is calculated directly (as czz) from c(z,t) (as c).

```
%
% czz
  czz=dss044(zl,zu,n,c,cz,nl,nu);
```

  The first derivative $(\partial c(z=0,t)/\partial z)$ = cz(1) is an input to dss044 and is used in the calculation of czz because nl=2.
- Equations (2.1) and (2.5) are programmed in the same way as in pde_2 to give ct,cbt.
- These two vectors are then placed in the single composite array ut, followed by a transpose and incrementing of the derivative counter as in pde_2.

To use pde_3, the method flag mf in the main program of Listing 2.2 is changed from mf=1 to mf=3. The numerical and graphical output is essentially identical to the output from pde_1 and is therefore not discussed here to conserve space (dss044 is also based on fourth order FDs). The intent in providing three ODE routines, pde_1,pde_2,pde_3, is to give alternative programming that might be useful in other applications.

In summary, this chapter has demonstrated through the example of analyte binding the construction of an ODE/PDE model, the MOL solution of the model, an investigation of the numerical solution with regard to the sensitivity to parameter values, and alternative programming of the MOL/ODEs. This example and associated procedures are intended to illustrate the development of a model and code, and the interpretation of the output (e.g., for comparison with experimental data) as important steps in research to better understand the relevant phenomena in a physical or chemical system.

References

[1] Brenan, K. E., Campbell, S. L., and Petzold, L. R. (1996), *Numerical Solution of Initial-Value Problems in Differential-Algebraic Equations*, SIAM, Philadelphia, 136

[2] Klapper, J. and Dockery, J. (2010), Mathematical description of microbial biofilms, *SIAM Rev.*, **52** (2), 221–265

[3] Lee, H. J. and Schiesser, W. E. (2004), *Ordinary and Partial Differential Equation Routines in C, C++, Fortran, Java, Maple and MATLAB*, Boca Raton, FL: Chapman & Hall/CRC

[4] Li, S. and Petzold, L. R. (2004), Adjoint sensitivity analysis for time-dependent partial differential equations with adaptive mesh refinement, *J. Comp. Phys.*, **198** (1), 310–325

[5] Shampine, L. F. and Thompson, S. (2007), Initial value problems, *Scholarpedia*, **2** (3), 2861; www.scholarpedia.org/article/Initial_value_problems

[6] Shampine, L. F. and Thompson, S. (2007), Stiff systems, *Scholarpedia*, **2** (3), 2855; www.scholarpedia.org/article/Stiff_systems

[7] Vijayendran, R. A., Ligler, F. S., and Leckband, D. E. (1999), A computational reaction-diffusion model for the analysis of transport-limited kinetics, *Anal. Chem.*, **71**, 5405–5412

3 Acid-mediated tumor growth

Recent research into the environment for tumor growth has identified acidity as an important factor. We now consider a PDE model for acid-mediated tumor growth (ATG) discussed in several recent studies, starting with the following dimensional equations formulated in spherical coordinates to reflect the approximately spherical geometry of tumors. Specifically, as tumor cell density increases with time, metabolism (anaerobic glycolysis) produces H^+ (as lactic acid) that leads to destruction of normal cells surrounding the tumor and thus a reduction in normal cell density. These interacting phenomena are included in a model first proposed by Gatenby and Gawlinski [3]; a series of studies gives experimental support to the model, e.g., [4]. The model is presented in the following set of PDEs.

3.1 Tumor growth PDE model

$$\frac{\partial N_n}{\partial t} = r_{n1} N_n \left(1 - \frac{N_n}{K_n}\right) - r_{n2} C_h N_n, \tag{3.1a}$$

$$\frac{\partial N_t}{\partial t} = r_{t1} N_t \left(1 - \frac{N_t}{K_t}\right) + \frac{1}{r^2}\frac{\partial}{\partial r}\left[r^2 D(N_n)\frac{\partial N_t}{\partial r}\right]; \; D(N_n) = D_t \left(1 - \frac{N_n}{K_n}\right), \tag{3.1b}$$

$$\frac{\partial C_h}{\partial t} = r_{h1} N_t - r_{h2} C_h + D_h \frac{1}{r^2}\frac{\partial}{\partial r}\left(r^2 \frac{\partial C_h}{\partial r}\right). \tag{3.1c}$$

The variables of these equations are summarized in Table 3.1 (subscripts "n,t" refer to normal and tumor cells, respectively).

M refers to molar concentration in g-mol/liter = g-mol/1000 cm^3. The physical and chemical significance of the terms in eqs. (3.1) is discussed subsequently. But first, we complete the definition of the model.

The parameters of eqs. (3.1) are summarized in Table 3.2. Numerical values of the parameters given in [2, 3] are tabulated in Table 3.3.

Equations (3.1) are first order in time, t, and therefore each equation requires an initial condition (IC).

$$N_n(r, t = 0) = f_n(r), \tag{3.2a}$$

$$N_t(r, t = 0) = f_t(r), \tag{3.2b}$$

$$C_h(r, t = 0) = f_h(r), \tag{3.2c}$$

Table 3.1. Variables of the model eqs. (3.1)

N_{n}	population of normal cells (cells/cm^3)
N_{t}	population of tumor cells (cells/cm^3)
C_{h}	concentration of excess H^+ ($\mathrm{M} = \mathrm{g\,mol}/1000\ \mathrm{cm}^3$)
r	radial coordinate (cm)
t	time coordinate (s)

Table 3.2. Parameters of the model eqs. (3.1)

r_{n1}	rate constant for normal cells (1/s)
r_{n2}	rate constant for normal cells ($1/\mathrm{M\,s} = 1000\ \mathrm{cm}^3/\mathrm{g\,mol\,s}$)
r_{t1}	rate constant for tumor cells (1/s)
r_{h1}	rate constant for excess H^+ ($\mathrm{M\,cm}^3/\mathrm{s} = \mathrm{g\,mol\,cm}^3/1000\ \mathrm{cm}^3\ \mathrm{s}$)
r_{h2}	rate constant for excess H^+ (1/s)
K_{n}	normal cell carrying capacity (cells/cm^3)
K_{t}	tumor cell carrying capacity (cells/cm^3)
D_{t}	tumor cell diffusivity (cm^2/s)
D_{h}	H^+ diffusivity (cm^2/s)

Table 3.3. Numerical values of the parameters in Table 3.2

Parameter	Units
r_{n1}	1×10^{-6}/s
r_{n2}	0–10/M s
r_{t1}	1×10^{-6}/s
r_{h1}	2.2×10^{-17} M cm^3/s
r_{h2}	1.1×10^{-4}/s
K_{n}	5×10^{7} cells/cm^3
K_{t}	5×10^{7} cells/cm^3
D_{t}	2×10^{-10} cm^2/s
D_{h}	5×10^{-6} cm^2/s

where $f_{\mathrm{n}}(r)$,$f_{\mathrm{t}}(r)$,$f_{\mathrm{h}}(r)$ are functions to be specified. In particular, $f_{\mathrm{t}}(r)$ defines an initial distribution of tumor cells and the model then projects the growth of the tumor and decline of the surrounding normal tissue.

Equations (3.1b) and (3.2c) are second order in radial position, r, and therefore each equation requires two boundary conditions (BCs). The first BC at $r = 0$ reflects symmetry.

$$\frac{\partial N_{\mathrm{t}}(r=0,t)}{\partial r} = \frac{\partial C_{\mathrm{h}}(r=0,t)}{\partial r} = 0. \tag{3.3a,b}$$

The second BCs for eqs. (3.1b) and (3.1c) specify that at a sufficiently large distance, the solution does not change with r.

$$\frac{\partial N_{\mathrm{t}}(r \to \infty, t)}{\partial r} = \frac{\partial C_{\mathrm{h}}(r \to \infty, t)}{\partial r} = 0 \tag{3.3c,d}$$

The nonlinear diffusion term in eq. (3.1b) requires additional analysis, particularly at $r = 0$.

$$\frac{1}{r^2}\frac{\partial}{\partial r}\left[r^2 D(N_{\mathrm{n}})\frac{\partial N_{\mathrm{t}}}{\partial r}\right],$$

where $D(N_{\mathrm{n}})$ is given by the second eq. (3.1b), $D(N_{\mathrm{n}}) = D_{\mathrm{t}}(1 - N_{\mathrm{n}}/K_{\mathrm{n}})$. Expanding the derivative of the product, we have

$$\begin{aligned}
&\frac{1}{r^2}\frac{\partial}{\partial r}\left[r^2 D(N_{\mathrm{n}})\frac{\partial N_{\mathrm{t}}}{\partial r}\right] \\
&= \frac{1}{r^2}\left[r^2\frac{\partial}{\partial r}\left(D(N_{\mathrm{n}})\frac{\partial N_{\mathrm{t}}}{\partial r}\right)\right] + \frac{1}{r^2}\left[2rD(N_{\mathrm{n}})\frac{\partial N_{\mathrm{t}}}{\partial r}\right] \\
&= \frac{\partial}{\partial r}\left(D(N_{\mathrm{n}})\frac{\partial N_{\mathrm{t}}}{\partial r}\right) + \frac{2}{r}D(N_{\mathrm{n}})\frac{\partial N_{\mathrm{t}}}{\partial r} \\
&= D(N_{\mathrm{n}})\frac{\partial^2 N_{\mathrm{t}}}{\partial r^2} + \frac{\mathrm{d}D(N_{\mathrm{n}})}{\mathrm{d}N_{\mathrm{n}}}\frac{\partial N_{\mathrm{n}}}{\partial r}\frac{\partial N_{\mathrm{t}}}{\partial r} + \frac{2}{r}D(N_{\mathrm{n}})\frac{\partial N_{\mathrm{t}}}{\partial r} \\
&= D(N_{\mathrm{n}})\frac{\partial^2 N_{\mathrm{t}}}{\partial r^2} + \left(\frac{-D_{\mathrm{t}}}{K_{\mathrm{n}}}\right)\frac{\partial N_{\mathrm{n}}}{\partial r}\frac{\partial N_{\mathrm{t}}}{\partial r} + \frac{2}{r}D(N_{\mathrm{n}})\frac{\partial N_{\mathrm{t}}}{\partial r}
\end{aligned} \tag{3.4a}$$

The third term is indeterminate at $r = 0$, and application of l'Hospital's rule gives

$$\begin{aligned}
&\lim_{r \to 0}\left[\frac{2}{r}D(N_{\mathrm{n}})\frac{\partial N_{\mathrm{t}}}{\partial r}\right] \\
&= 2D(N_{\mathrm{n}})\frac{\partial^2 N_{\mathrm{t}}}{\partial r^2} + 2\frac{\mathrm{d}D(N_{\mathrm{n}})}{\mathrm{d}N_{\mathrm{n}}}\frac{\partial N_{\mathrm{n}}}{\partial r}\frac{\partial N_{\mathrm{t}}}{\partial r} \\
&= 2D(N_{\mathrm{n}})\frac{\partial^2 N_{\mathrm{t}}}{\partial r^2} + 2\left(\frac{-D_{\mathrm{t}}}{K_{\mathrm{n}}}\right)\frac{\partial N_{\mathrm{n}}}{\partial r}\frac{\partial N_{\mathrm{t}}}{\partial r}.
\end{aligned} \tag{3.4b}$$

Combining eqs. (3.4a) and (3.4b), and using BCs (3.3a) and (3.3b) gives

$$\frac{1}{r^2}\frac{\partial}{\partial r}\left[r^2 D(N_{\mathrm{n}})\frac{\partial N_{\mathrm{t}}}{\partial r}\right]_{r=0} = 3D(N_{\mathrm{n}})\frac{\partial^2 N_{\mathrm{t}}}{\partial r^2}. \tag{3.5}$$

We now consider the origin of the individual terms in eqs. (3.1).

3.1.1 Normal cell balance

Equation (3.1a) is a conservation balance for normal cells in spherical coordinates starting with the terms:

LHS-1: $(4\pi r^2 dr)\partial N_n/\partial t$ – Accumulation of normal cells in a differential volume $4\pi r^2 dr$. Note that the units of this term are (cm^3)(normal cells/cm^3)(1/s) = normal cell-s/s, that is, the accumulation of normal cells per second (or the depletion of normal cells if the derivative in t is negative).

RHS-1: $(4\pi r^2 dr)r_{n1}N_n(1 - N_n/K_n)$ – A logistic rate for the increase in the number of normal cells, N_n, in a differential volume $4\pi r^2 dr$. Note that as $N_n/K_n \to 1$, this rate approaches zero (see Tables 3.2 and 3.3 for information about K_n); again, the net units are normal cells/s, as in LHS-1.

RHS-2: $(4\pi r^2 dr)r_{n2}C_h N_n$ – Rate of reduction in the number of normal cells, N_n, in a differential volume $4\pi r^2 dr$. Note that this rate is proportional to the product of two dependent variables, C_h and N_n, and is therefore nonlinear. The net units are normal cells/s, as in LHS-1 and RHS-1.

If these three terms are placed in a balance for N_n,

$$(4\pi r^2 dr)\frac{\partial N_n}{\partial t} = (4\pi r^2 dr)r_{n1}N_n\left(1 - \frac{N_n}{K_n}\right) - (4\pi r^2 dr)r_{n2}C_h N_n,$$

eq. (3.1a) results.

3.1.2 Tumor cell balance

Equation (3.1b) is a conservation balance for tumor cells in spherical coordinates starting with the terms:

LHS-1: $(4\pi r^2 dr)\partial N_t/\partial t$ – Accumulation of tumor cells in a differential volume $4\pi r^2 dr$. Note that the units of this term are (cm^3)(tumor cells/cm^3)(1/s) = normal cells/s, that is, the accumulation of tumor cells per second (or the depletion of tumor cells if the derivative in t is negative)

RHS-1: $(4\pi r^2 dr)r_{t1}N_t(1 - N_t/K_t)$ – A logistic rate for the increase in the number of tumor cells, N_t, in a differential volume $4\pi r^2 dr$. Note that as $N_t/K_t \to 1$, this rate approaches zero (see Tables 3.2 and 3.3 for information about K_t); again, the net units are tumor cells/s, as in LHS-1.

RHS-2: $-(4\pi r^2)D_t(1 - N_n/K_n)\partial N_t/\partial r|_r$ – Rate of diffusion of tumor cells into the differential volume $4\pi r^2 dr$ at r. This is an application of Fick's first law for diffusion. The net units are tumor cells/s, as in LHS-1 and RHS-1. Note that the diffusivity for N_t is a function of N_n, to reflect the decrease in the rate of diffusion of tumor cells as the number of normal cells increases; this is a nonlinear effect that can be accommodated within the numerical approach to the solution of eq. (3.1b), to be discussed subsequently.

RHS-3: $-(4\pi(r+\mathrm{d}r)^2)D_\mathrm{t}(1-N_\mathrm{n}/K_\mathrm{n})\,\partial N_\mathrm{t}/\partial r|_{r+\mathrm{d}r}$ – Rate of diffusion of tumor cells out of a differential volume $4\pi r^2\mathrm{d}r$ at $r+\mathrm{d}r$. The net units are tumor cells/s, as in LHS-1, RHS-1, and RHS-2.

If these terms are combined into a conservation equation for N_t (with $D(N_\mathrm{n}) = D_\mathrm{t}(1-N_\mathrm{n}/K_\mathrm{n})$),

$$(4\pi r^2\mathrm{d}r)\frac{\partial N_\mathrm{t}}{\partial t} = (4\pi r^2\mathrm{d}r) r_{\mathrm{t1}} N_\mathrm{t}\left(1-\frac{N_\mathrm{t}}{K_\mathrm{t}}\right) - (4\pi r^2)D(N_\mathrm{n})\left.\frac{\partial N_\mathrm{t}}{\partial r}\right|_r + (4\pi(r+\mathrm{d}r)^2)D(N_\mathrm{n})\left.\frac{\partial N_\mathrm{t}}{\partial r}\right|_{r+\mathrm{d}r}.$$

Division of this equation by $4\pi r^2\mathrm{d}r$ and minor rearrangement gives

$$\frac{\partial N_\mathrm{t}}{\partial t} = r_{\mathrm{t1}} N_\mathrm{t}\left(1-\frac{N_\mathrm{t}}{K_\mathrm{t}}\right) + \frac{((r+\mathrm{d}r)^2)D(N_\mathrm{n})\left.\frac{\partial N_\mathrm{t}}{\partial r}\right|_{r+\mathrm{d}r} - (r^2)D(N_\mathrm{n})\left.\frac{\partial N_\mathrm{t}}{\partial r}\right|_r}{r^2\mathrm{d}r}.$$

In the limit $r \to 0$, the second RHS term becomes

$$\frac{1}{r^2}\frac{\partial}{\partial r}\left[r^2 D(N_\mathrm{n})\frac{\partial N_\mathrm{t}}{\partial r}\right]$$

and thus, eq. (3.1b) results,

$$\frac{\partial N_\mathrm{t}}{\partial t} = r_{\mathrm{t1}} N_\mathrm{t}\left(1-\frac{N_\mathrm{t}}{K_\mathrm{t}}\right) + \frac{1}{r^2}\frac{\partial}{\partial r}\left[r^2 D(N_\mathrm{n})\frac{\partial N_\mathrm{t}}{\partial r}\right].$$

3.1.3 H^+ balance

Equation (3.1c) is a conservation balance for H^+ in spherical coordinates starting with the terms:

LHS-1: $(4\pi r^2\mathrm{d}r)\partial C_\mathrm{h}/\partial t$ - Accumulation of H^+ in a differential volume $4\pi r^2\mathrm{d}r$. Note that the units of this term are $(\mathrm{cm}^3)(H^+/\mathrm{cm}^3)(1/\mathrm{s}) = H^+/\mathrm{s}$, that is, the accumulation of H^+ per second (or the depletion of H^+ if the derivative in t is negative).

RHS-1: $(4\pi r^2\mathrm{d}r) r_{\mathrm{t1}} C_\mathrm{h}(1-C_\mathrm{h}/K_h)$ – A logistic rate for the increase in the number of H^+, in a differential volume $4\pi r^2\mathrm{d}r$. Note that as $C_\mathrm{h}/K_\mathrm{h} \to 1$, this rate approaches zero (see Tables 3.2 and 3.3 for information about K_h). The net units are H^+/s as in LHS-1.
RHS-2: $-(4\pi r^2)D_\mathrm{h}\partial C_\mathrm{h}/\partial r|_r$ – Rate of diffusion of H^+ into the differential volume $4\pi r^2\mathrm{d}r$ at r. The net units are H^+/s, as in LHS-1 and RHS-1.

RHS-3: $-(4\pi(r+\mathrm{d}r)^2)D_\mathrm{h}\partial C_\mathrm{h}/\partial r|_{r+\mathrm{d}r}$ – Rate of diffusion of H^+ out of a differential volume $4\pi r^2\mathrm{d}r$ at $r+\mathrm{d}r$. The net units are H^+/s, as in LHS-1, RHS-1, and RHS-2.

If these terms are combined into a conservation equation for C_h,

$$(4\pi r^2 \mathrm{d}r)\frac{\partial C_\mathrm{h}}{\partial t} = (4\pi r^2 \mathrm{d}r) r_{\mathrm{t1}} C_\mathrm{h}\left(1-\frac{C_\mathrm{h}}{K_\mathrm{t}}\right) - (4\pi r^2) D_\mathrm{h}\frac{\partial C_\mathrm{h}}{\partial r}|_r$$
$$+ (4\pi(r+\mathrm{d}r)^2) D_\mathrm{h}\frac{\partial C_\mathrm{h}}{\partial r}|_{r+\mathrm{d}r}.$$

Division of this equation by $4\pi r^2 \mathrm{d}r$ and some minor rearrangement gives

$$\frac{\partial C_\mathrm{h}}{\partial t} = r_{\mathrm{t1}} C_\mathrm{h}\left(1-\frac{C_\mathrm{h}}{K_\mathrm{t}}\right) + \frac{((r+\mathrm{d}r)^2) D_\mathrm{h}\frac{\partial C_\mathrm{h}}{\partial r}|_{r+\mathrm{d}r} - (r^2) D_\mathrm{h}\frac{\partial C_\mathrm{h}}{\partial r}|_r}{r^2 \mathrm{d}r}.$$

In the limit $r \rightarrow 0$, the second RHS term becomes

$$\frac{1}{r^2}\frac{\partial}{\partial r}\left[r^2 D_\mathrm{h}\frac{\partial C_\mathrm{h}}{\partial r}\right]$$

and thus, eq. (3.1c) results (for constant D_h),

$$\frac{\partial C_\mathrm{h}}{\partial t} = r_{\mathrm{t1}} C_\mathrm{h}\left(1-\frac{C_\mathrm{h}}{K_\mathrm{t}}\right) + D_\mathrm{h}\frac{1}{r^2}\frac{\partial}{\partial r}\left[r^2\frac{\partial C_\mathrm{h}}{\partial r}\right].$$

3.2 MOL routines

We now consider the MATLAB routines for eqs. (3.1) to (3.5), starting with the ODE routine, pde_1 (Listing 3.1).

3.2.1 ODE routine

```
  function ut=pde_1(t,u)
%
% Function pde_1 defines the ODEs in the MOL solution of three
% PDEs for the ATG model
%
  global      Nn        Nt        Ch...
               rl        ru         r         n...
              rn1       rn2        Kn...
              rt1        Dt        Kt...
              rh1       rh2        Dh...
            ncall     ncase
%
% One vector to three vectors
  for i=1:n
    Nn(i)=u(i);
    Nt(i)=u(i+n);
    Ch(i)=u(i+2*n);
```

```
  end
%
% First order spatial derivatives
  Nnr=dss004(rl,ru,n,Nn);
  Ntr=dss004(rl,ru,n,Nt);
  Chr=dss004(rl,ru,n,Ch);
%
% BCs
  Ntr(1)=0; Ntr(n)=0;
  Chr(1)=0; Chr(n)=0;
%
% Second order spatial derivatives
  nl=2; nu=2;
  Ntrr=dss044(rl,ru,n,Nt,Ntr,nl,nu);
  Chrr=dss044(rl,ru,n,Ch,Chr,nl,nu);
%
% PDEs
  for i=1:n
    D=Dt*(1-Nn(i)/Kn);
    if(D<0)D=0;end
    if(i==1)
      Nnt(i)=rn1*Nn(i)*(1-Nn(i)/Kn)-rn2*Ch(i)*Nn(i);
      Ntt(i)=rt1*Nt(i)*(1-Nt(i)/Kt)+3*D*Ntrr(i);
      Cht(i)=rh1*Nt(i)-rh2*Ch(i)+3*Dh*Chrr(i);
    else
      Nnt(i)=rn1*Nn(i)*(1-Nn(i)/Kn)-rn2*Ch(i)*Nn(i);
      Ntt(i)=rt1*Nt(i)*(1-Nt(i)/Kt)...
            +D*(Ntrr(i)+2/r(i)*Ntr(i))+(-Dt/Kn)*Nnr(i)*Ntr(i);
      Cht(i)=rh1*Nt(i)-rh2*Ch(i)+Dh*(Chrr(i)+2/r(i)*Chr(i));
    end
  end
%
% Three vectors to one vector
  for i=1:n
    ut(i)    =Nnt(i);
    ut(i+n)  =Ntt(i);
    ut(i+2*n)=Cht(i);
  end
  ut=ut';
%
% Increment calls to pde_1
  ncall=ncall+1;
```

Listing 3.1 ODE routine pde_1

We can note the following points about this routine.

- The function and some global variables are defined.

```
  function ut=pde_1(t,u)
%
% Function pde_1 defines the ODEs in the MOL solution of three
```

```
% PDEs for the ATG model
%
  global     Nn       Nt       Ch...
             rl       ru       r        n...
            rn1      rn2       Kn...
            rt1       Dt       Kt...
            rh1      rh2       Dh...
          ncall    ncase
```

- The single ODE-dependent variable vector, u, is placed in three vectors, Nn,Nt,Ch, which facilitates programming in terms of problem-oriented variables, the dependent variables of eqs. (3.1).

```
%
% One vector to three vectors
  for i=1:n
    Nn(i)=u(i);
    Nt(i)=u(i+n);
    Ch(i)=u(i+2*n);
  end
```

- The first order derivatives in r are computed by dss004. Then BCs (3.3a,b,c,d) are applied.

```
%
% First order spatial derivatives
  Nnr=dss004(rl,ru,n,Nn);
  Ntr=dss004(rl,ru,n,Nt);
  Chr=dss004(rl,ru,n,Ch);
%
% BCs
  Ntr(1)=0; Ntr(n)=0;
  Chr(1)=0; Chr(n)=0;
```

- The second order derivatives in r are computed by dss044. Note that Neumann BCs are specified with nl=2,nu=2 according to eqs. (3.3).

```
%
% Second order spatial derivatives
  nl=2; nu=2;
  Ntrr=dss044(rl,ru,n,Nt,Ntr,nl,nu);
  Chrr=dss044(rl,ru,n,Ch,Chr,nl,nu);
```

- This completes the calculation of the derivatives in r in eqs. (3.1). These PDEs can then be programmed.

```
%
% PDEs
  for i=1:n
    D=Dt*(1-Nn(i)/Kn);
    if(D<0)D=0;end
    if(i==1)
      Nnt(i)=rn1*Nn(i)*(1-Nn(i)/Kn)-rn2*Ch(i)*Nn(i);
```

```
      Ntt(i)=rt1*Nt(i)*(1-Nt(i)/Kt)+3*D*Ntrr(i);
      Cht(i)=rh1*Nt(i)-rh2*Ch(i)+3*Dh*Chrr(i);
    else
      Nnt(i)=rn1*Nn(i)*(1-Nn(i)/Kn)-rn2*Ch(i)*Nn(i);
      Ntt(i)=rt1*Nt(i)*(1-Nt(i)/Kt)...
            +D*(Ntrr(i)+2/r(i)*Ntr(i))+(-Dt/Kn)*Nnr(i)*Ntr(i);
      Cht(i)=rh1*Nt(i)-rh2*Ch(i)+Dh*(Chrr(i)+2/r(i)*Chr(i));
    end
  end
```

We can note the following details about this coding for eqs. (3.1), which is accomplished by stepping along the grid in r using a `for` loop. Two sections of code apply at $r = 0$ and $r \neq 0$; in both cases, the variable diffusivity, $D(N_n)$ = `D` is first computed.

- For $r = 0$, `i=1`, and eqs. (3.1) are programmed. The three vectors of derivatives in t that result are the LHS of eqs. (3.1), that is $\partial N_n/\partial t$ = `Nnt`, $\partial N_t/\partial t$ = `Ntt`, $\partial C_h/\partial t$ = `Cht`.

```
%
% PDEs
  for i=1:n
    D=Dt*(1-Nn(i)/Kn);
    if(D<0)D=0;end
    if(i==1)
      Nnt(i)=rn1*Nn(i)*(1-Nn(i)/Kn)-rn2*Ch(i)*Nn(i);
      Ntt(i)=rt1*Nt(i)*(1-Nt(i)/Kt)+3*D*Ntrr(i);
      Cht(i)=rh1*Nt(i)-rh2*Ch(i)+3*Dh*Chrr(i);
```

The factor `3*D` follows from the application of eq. (3.5) to the diffusion term of eq. (3.1b). Similar reasoning leads to the factor `3*Dh` in eq. (3.1c).

Note the important detail that $D(N_n)$ of (algebraic) eq. (3.1b) is constrained to be nonnegative. This is required in order that the diffusion of `Nt` based on the diffusivity $D(N_n)$ is in the correct direction (in the direction of negative concentration gradient). Mathematically, if $D(N_n)$ assumes a negative value ($N_n/K_n > 1$ in eq. (3.1b)), N_t from PDE eq. (3.1b) is unstable; in other words, the integration of $\partial N_t/\partial t$ = `Ntt` in t to give N_t is unstable and is manifest by a failure of the ODE integration in `ode15s`.

The diffusivity $D(N_n) =$ `D` of eq. (3.1b) is used in the second PDE (for `Ntt`) and the diffusivity $D_h =$ `Dh` (a constant) is used in the third PDE (for `Cht`) according to eqs. (3.1b) and (3.1c).

- For $r \neq 0$, `i=2...n`, and eqs. (3.1) are programmed. The three vectors of derivatives in t follow from the LHS of eqs. (3.1), that is `Nnt,Ntt,Cht` (for $r \neq 0$).

```
    else
      Nnt(i)=rn1*Nn(i)*(1-Nn(i)/Kn)-rn2*Ch(i)*Nn(i);
      Ntt(i)=rt1*Nt(i)*(1-Nt(i)/Kt)...
            +D*(Ntrr(i)+2/r(i)*Ntr(i))+(-Dt/Kn)*Nnr(i)*Ntr(i);
      Cht(i)=rh1*Nt(i)-rh2*Ch(i)+Dh*(Chrr(i)+2/r(i)*Chr(i));
    end
```

The MOL approximation of eqs. (3.1) is used, including eq. (3.4a) (the expansion of the products in r) for eq. (3.1b). Again, the diffusivity $D(N_n) =$ `D` of eq. (3.1b) is used in the second PDE (for Ntt) and the diffusivity D_h = Dh (a constant) is used in the third PDE (for Cht) according to eqs. (3.1b) and (3.1c).

- The MOL for loop (i=1...n) is terminated with an end. This completes the programming of the MOL/ODEs over the full grid in r. The three derivative vectors in t are then placed in a single vector, ut, to be returned from PDE_1 to ode15s after the required transpose. Finally, the counter for the calls to pde_1 is incremented.

```
  end
%
% Three vectors to one vector
  for i=1:n
    ut(i)    =Nnt(i);
    ut(i+n)  =Ntt(i);
    ut(i+2*n)=Cht(i);
  end
  ut=ut';
%
% Increment calls to pde_1
  ncall=ncall+1;
```

This programming of the PDEs in pde_1 is straightforward considering the complexity of eqs. (3.1) and the special requirements at $r = 0$.

The initial condition routine of Listing 3.2, inital_1, implements ICs (3.2).

```
  function u=inital_1(t0)
%
% Function inital_1 is called by the main program to define the
% initial conditions of the 3-PDE ATG model
%
  global rl ru r n ncall ncase
%
% Model parameters
  global     Nn       Nt        Ch...
             rl       ru        r        n...
            rn1      rn2       Kn...
            rt1       Dt       Kt...
            rh1      rh2       Dh...
          ncall    ncase
%
% Initial conditions
  for i=1:n
    u(i)    =Nn_1(i);
    u(i+n)  =Nt_1(i);
    u(i+2*n)=Ch_1(i);
  end
%
% Initialize calls to inital_1
  ncall=0;
```

Listing 3.2 IC routine inital_1 for eqs. (3.2)

We can note the following details about `inital_1`.

- The function and some global variables are defined.

```
  function u=inital_1(t0)
%
% Function inital_1 is called by the main program to define the
% initial conditions of the 3-PDE ATG model
%
  global rl ru r n ncall ncase
%
% Model parameters
  global      Nn       Nt       Ch...
              rl       ru        r        n...
             rn1      rn2       Kn...
             rt1       Dt       Kt...
             rh1      rh2       Dh...
           ncall    ncase
```

- The ICs (3.2) are defined individually for eqs. (3.1) over the grid in r by a `for` loop in which functions `Nn_1,Nt_1,Ch_1` are called (discussed next).

```
%
% Initial conditions
  for i=1:n
    u(i)      =Nn_1(i);
    u(i+n)   =Nt_1(i);
    u(i+2*n)=Ch_1(i);
  end
%
% Initialize calls to inital_1
  ncall=0;
```

These initial condition values are then stored in a single vector, `u`, and returned to the main program (discussed subsequently) for use by the ODE integrator, `ode45` or `ode15s`. Finally, the counter for the calls to `pde_1` is initialized.

The IC functions in eqs. (3.2), f_n, f_t, f_h, (Listing 3.3) have a similar structure based on the hyperbolic tangent function $\tanh(r)$ as explained next.

```
  function u0=Nn_1(i)
%
% Function u0 computes the IC for the Nn PDE ATG model
%
  global      Nn       Nt       Ch...
              rl       ru        r        n...
             rn1      rn2       Kn...
             rt1       Dt       Kt...
             rh1      rh2       Dh...
           ncall    ncase
%
% IC function
  rs=50;
```

```
  num=exp(rs*(r(i)-r(21)))-exp(-rs*(r(i)-r(21)));
  den=exp(rs*(r(i)-r(21)))+exp(-rs*(r(i)-r(21)));
  tanhr=num/den;
  u0=5.0e+07*(1-tanhr)/2+1.0e+08*(1+tanhr)/2;

  function u0=Nt_1(i)
%
% Function u0 computes the IC for the Nt PDE ATG model
%
  global   Nn      Nt      Ch...
           rl      ru       r       n...
          rn1     rn2      Kn...
          rt1      Dt      Kt...
          rh1     rh2      Dh...
        ncall   ncase
%
% IC function
  rs=50;
  num=exp(rs*(r(i)-r(21)))-exp(-rs*(r(i)-r(21)));
  den=exp(rs*(r(i)-r(21)))+exp(-rs*(r(i)-r(21)));
  tanhr=num/den;
  u0=1.0e+05*(1-tanhr)/2+1.0e+03*(1+tanhr)/2;

  function u0=Ch_1(i)
%
% Function u0 computes the IC for the Ch PDE ATG model
%
  global   Nn      Nt      Ch...
           rl      ru       r       n...
          rn1     rn2      Kn...
          rt1      Dt      Kt...
          rh1     rh2      Dh...
        ncall   ncase
%
% IC function
  rs=50;
  num=exp(rs*(r(i)-r(11)))-exp(-rs*(r(i)-r(11)));
  den=exp(rs*(r(i)-r(11)))+exp(-rs*(r(i)-r(11)));
  tanhr=num/den;
  u0=1.0e-09*(1-tanhr)/2+0*(1+tanhr)/2;
```

Listing 3.3 Functions f_n, f_t, f_h = `Nn_1, Nt_1, Ch_1` for ICs (3.2)

We can note the following details about `Nn_1, Nt_1, Ch_1`.

- Each starts with a function definition and specification of some global variables; for example, for `Nn_1`.

```
  function u0=Nn_1(i)
%
% Function u0 computes the IC for the Nn PDE ATG model
%
```

```
global     Nn       Nt       Ch...
           rl       ru        r        n...
          rn1      rn2       Kn...
          rt1       Dt       Kt...
          rh1      rh2       Dh...
        ncall    ncase
```

- $\tanh(r)$ is used to define the IC function of eqs. (3.2). For example, in Nn_1

```
%
% IC function
  rs=50;
  num=exp(rs*(r(i)-r(21)))-exp(-rs*(r(i)-r(21)));

 den=exp(rs*(r(i)-r(21)))+exp(-rs*(r(i)-r(21)));
  tanhr=num/den;
  u0=5.0e+07*(1-tanhr)/2+1.0e+08*(1+tanhr)/2;
```

To further explain the details of this code:

- Two functions of exponentials are first computed,

$$\text{num} = e^{r_s(r-r_0)} - e^{r_s(r-r_0)},$$

$$\text{den} = e^{r_s(r-r_0)} + e^{r_s(r-r_0)},$$

where r is the radial independent variable in eqs. (3.1), r_0 (= r(21)) is the radial position for the transition from one limiting value of the $\tanh(r)$ to a second limiting value, and r_s is a scaling factor (positive constant) that determines the rate of variation of the $\tanh(r)$ with r.
- For $r \ll r_0$, the limiting value is tanhr=-1; For $r \gg r_0$, the limiting value is tanhr=1.
- The function is then computed as a linear combination of two terms depending on $\tanh(r)$. For example, for Nn_1,

```
tanhr=num/den;
u0=5.0e+07*(1-tanhr)/2+1.0e+08*(1+tanhr)/2;
```

Thus, for $r \ll r_0$, the limiting value is uanal=5.0e+07; For $r \gg r_0$, the limiting value is uanal=1.0e+08. In between (in the neighborhood of r_0 = r(21)), u0 varies smoothly between the two limiting values. These limiting values are selected in accordance with the physical situation for $r \ll r_0$, $r \gg r_0$.
- The value r(21) (= r_0) was selected for $n = 101$ and $0 \le r \le 0.5$ cm (defined in the main program). Thus, r(21) corresponds to $r = 0.1$ cm = 1 mm, which is considered the initial radius of the tumor (for the transition from tumor cells to the left of 1 mm to normal cells to the right of 1 mm).

- In summary, $\tanh(r)$ is used to define the initial configuration (distribution) normal cells, tumor cells, and H^+ in the interval $0 \le r \le 0.5$ cm (note that the model parameters in Table (3.2) are defined in terms of a length scale in cm).
- The limiting values are different in Nn_1, Nt_1, Ch_1 of Listing 3.3, depending on the physical situation for the three dependent variables of eqs. (3.1), N_n, N_t, C_h. The

effect of these limiting values will be clearer when the plotted output is considered subsequently (in Figs. 3.1 to 3.4).

Function `jpattern_num_1` called by `ode15s` for the sparse matrix integration of the $3n$ ODEs will not be considered in detail here. It is set up for the three PDEs of eqs. (3.1) by the following code:

```
%
% Set independent, dependent variables for the calculation
% of the sparsity pattern
  tbase=0;
  for i=1:3*n
    ybase(i)=0.5;
  end
  ybase=ybase';
%
% Compute the corresponding derivative vector
  ytbase=pde_1(tbase,ybase);
  fac=[];
  thresh=1e-16;
  vectorized='on';
  [Jac,fac]=numjac(@pde_1,tbase,ybase,ytbase,thresh,fac,vectorized);
%
```

Note in particular the use in two places of `pde_1` of Listing 3.1 to define the sparsity pattern of the ODE Jacobian matrix.

3.2.2 Main program

The main program, `pde_1_main` is similar to the main program of Chapter 2, but it is listed here to provide a complete discussion.

```
%
% Three-PDE ATG model
%
% Clear previous files
  clear all
  clc
%
% Model parameters shared with other routines
  global    Nn      Nt      Ch...
            rl      ru       r       n...
           rn1     rn2      Kn...
           rt1      Dt      Kt...
           rh1     rh2      Dh...
          ncall   ncase
%
% Case
%
%   ncase = 1 - four 2D plots of dependent variables
%               Nn, Nt, Ch, pH vs t
```

```
%
%   ncase = 2 - four 3D plots of dependent variables
%               Nn, Nt, Ch, pH vs t
%
%   ncase = 3 - case = 1 with 17 supplemental plots for
%               the derivatives in t and the individual
%               PDE RHS terms
  ncase=1;
%
% Radial grid
  rl=0; ru=0.5; n=101;
  for i=1:n
    r(i)=rl+(ru-rl)*(i-1)/(n-1);
  end
%
% Nn PDE
  rn1=1.0e-06; rn2=1; Kn=5.0e+07;
%
% Nt PDE
  rt1=1.0e-06; Dt=2.0e-10; Kt=5.0e+07;
%
% Ch PDE
  rh1=2.2e-17; rh2=1.1e-04; Dh=5.0e-06;
%
% Independent variable t for ncase = 1, 3
  if(ncase==1 | ncase==3)
    t0=0.0;
    tf=5.0e+06;
    tout=[t0:1.0e+06:tf]';
    nout=6;
  end
%
% Independent variable t for ncase = 2 (to give additional
% resolution in t)
  if(ncase==2)
    t0=0.0;
    tf=5.0e+06;
    tout=[t0:0.25e+06:tf]';
    nout=21;
  end
%
% Initial condition
  u0=inital_1(t0);
%
% ODE integration
  mf=2;
  reltol=1.0e-06; abstol=1.0e-05;
  options=odeset('RelTol',reltol,'AbsTol',abstol);
%
% Explicit (nonstiff) integration
  if(mf==1)[t,u]=ode45(@pde_1,tout,u0,options); end
```

```
%
% Implicit (sparse stiff) integration
  if(mf==2)
    S=jpattern_num_1;
%   pause
    options=odeset(options,'JPattern',S)
    [t,u]=ode15s(@pde_1,tout,u0,options);
  end
%
% One vector to three vectors
  for it=1:nout
  for i=1:n
    Nn(it,i)=u(it,i);
    Nt(it,i)=u(it,i+n);
    Ch(it,i)=u(it,i+2*n);
  end
  end
%
%   Display selected output
    for it=1:nout
      fprintf('\n      t         r        Nn(it,i)        Nt(it,i)
                 Ch(it,i)\n');
      for i=1:10:n
        fprintf('%6.1f%8.3f%15.4e%15.4e%15.4e\n',...
          t(it)/(60*60*24),r(i),Nn(it,i),Nt(it,i),Ch(it,i));
      end
    end
    fprintf('\n    ncall = %4d\n',ncall);
%
% 2D plots
%
% ncase = 1, 3: 2D Nn, Nt, Ch, pH plots in t (figures 1 - 4)
  if(ncase==1 | ncase==3)
    pH=-log10(4.0e-08+Ch);
    figure(1)
    plot(r,Nn,'-');
    xlabel('r (cm)'); ylabel('Nn (cells/cm^3)');
    title('Nn (normal); 3-PDE ATG model');
    figure(2)
    plot(r,Nt,'-');
    xlabel('r (cm)'); ylabel('Nt (cells/cm^3)');
    title('Nt (tumor); 3-PDE ATG model')
    figure(3)
    plot(r,Ch,'-');
    xlabel('r (cm)'); ylabel('Ch (M = gm mols H^+/liter)');
    title('Ch (excess H^+); 3-PDE ATG model');
    figure(4)
    plot(r,pH,'-');
    xlabel('r (cm)'); ylabel('pH');
    title('pH; 3-PDE ATG model');
  end
```

```
%
% ncase = 2: 3D Nn, Nt, Ch, pH plots in t (figures 1 - 4)
  if(ncase==2)
    tp=t/(60*60*24);
    pH=-log10(4.0e-08+Ch);
    figure(1)
    surf(r,tp,Nn)
    view(-40,50);
    xlabel('r (cm)'); ylabel('t (days)');
    zlabel('Nt (normal cells/cm^3)');
    figure(2)
    surf(r,tp,Nt)
    view(-25,50)
    xlabel('r (cm)'); ylabel('t (days)');
    zlabel('Nt (tumor cells/cm^3)');
    figure(3)
    surf(r,tp,Ch)
    xlabel('r (cm)'); ylabel('t (days)');
    zlabel('Ch (excess gm mols H^+/liter)');
    figure(4)
    surf(r,tp,pH)
    view(-37.5,60);
    xlabel('r (cm)'); ylabel('t (days)');
    zlabel('pH');
  end
%
% case = 3 supplemental 2D plots for derivatives in t
  (figures 5 - 7)
  if(ncase==3)
    for it=1:nout
      u1d=u(it,:);
      ut=pde_1(t(it),u1d);
      Nnt(it,:)=ut(1:n);
      Ntt(it,:)=ut(n+1:2*n);
      Cht(it,:)=ut(2*n+1:3*n);
    end
    figure(5)
    plot(r,Nnt,'-');
    xlabel('r (cm)'); ylabel('Nnt (cells/cm^3-s)');
    title('Nnt (normal); 3-PDE ATG model');
    figure(6)
    plot(r,Ntt,'-');
    xlabel('r (cm)'); ylabel('Ntt (cells/cm^3-s)');
    title('Ntt (normal); 3-PDE ATG model');
    figure(7)
    plot(r,Cht,'-');
    xlabel('r (cm)'); ylabel('Cht (M/s = gm mols H^+/liter-s)');
    title('Cht (excess H^+); 3-PDE ATG model');
%
% Supplemental 2D plots for RHS terms in derivatives in t
% (figures 8 - 21)
```

```
    for it=1:nout
      u1d=u(it,:);
      [ut,term]=pde_1(t(it),u1d);
      RHS1(it,:)=term(1,1:n);
      RHS2(it,:)=term(2,1:n);
      RHS3(it,:)=term(3,1:n);
      RHS4(it,:)=term(4,1:n);
      RHS5(it,:)=term(5,1:n);
      RHS6(it,:)=term(6,1:n);
      RHS7(it,:)=term(7,1:n);
      RHS8(it,:)=term(8,1:n);
    end
%
%   Nn PDE
    figure(8)
    plot(r,RHS1,'-');
    xlabel('r (cm)'); ylabel('Nn PDE RHS term 1');
    title('Nn PDE RHS term 1; Nn PDE');
    figure(9)
    plot(r,RHS2,'-');
    xlabel('r (cm)'); ylabel('Nn PDE RHS term 2');
    title('Nn PDE RHS term 2; Nn PDE');
    figure(10)
    plot(r,RHS1(1,:),'+',r,RHS2(1,:),'o',r,Nnt(1,:),'-');
    xlabel('r (cm)'); ylabel('Nn PDE RHS terms 1,2,sum; t=t0');
    title('term 1 - +, term 2 - o, sum = solid; t = t0; Nn PDE');
    figure(11)
    plot(r,RHS1(nout,:),'+',r,RHS2(nout,:),'o',r,Nnt(nout,:),
         '-');
    xlabel('r (cm)'); ylabel('Nn PDE RHS terms 1,2,sum; t=tf');
    title('term 1 - +, term 2 - o, sum = solid; t = tf; Nn PDE');
%
%   Nt PDE
    figure(12)
    plot(r,RHS3,'-');
    xlabel('r (cm)'); ylabel('Nt PDE RHS term 1');
    title('Nt PDE RHS term 1; Nt PDE');
    figure(13)
    plot(r,RHS4,'-');
    xlabel('r (cm)'); ylabel('Nt PDE RHS term 2');
    title('Nt PDE RHS term 2; Nt PDE');
    figure(14)
    plot(r,RHS5,'-');
    xlabel('r (cm)'); ylabel('Nt PDE RHS term 3');
    title('Nt PDE RHS term 3; Nt PDE');
    figure(15)
    plot(r,RHS3(1,:),'+',r,RHS4(1,:),'o',r,RHS5(1,:),'x',r,
         Ntt(1,:),'-');
    xlabel('r (cm)'); ylabel('Nt PDE RHS terms 1,2,3,sum;
           t = t0');
    title('term 1 - +, term 2 - o, term 3 = x; sum = solid;
```

```
             t = t0; Nt PDE');
      figure(16)
      plot(r,RHS3(nout,:),'+',r,RHS4(nout,:),'o',r,RHS5(nout,:),
           'x',r,Ntt(nout,:),'-');
      xlabel('r (cm)'); ylabel('Nt PDE RHS terms 1,2,sum; t = tf');
      title('term 1 - +, term 2 - o, term 3 - x, sum = solid;
            t = tf; Nt PDE');
%
%     Ch PDE
      figure(17)
      plot(r,RHS6,'-');
      xlabel('r (cm)'); ylabel('Ch PDE RHS term 1');
      title('Ch PDE RHS term 1; Ch PDE');
      figure(18)
      plot(r,RHS7,'-');
      xlabel('r (cm)'); ylabel('Ch PDE RHS term 2');
      title('Ch PDE RHS term 2; Ch PDE');
      figure(19)
      plot(r,RHS8,'-');
      xlabel('r (cm)'); ylabel('Ch PDE RHS term 3');
      title('Ch PDE RHS term 3; Ch PDE');
      figure(20)
      plot(r,RHS6(1,:),'+',r,RHS7(1,:),'o',r,RHS8(1,:),'x',r,
           Cht(1,:),'-');
      xlabel('r (cm)'); ylabel('Ch PDE RHS terms 1,2,3,sum; t = t0');
      title('term 1 - +, term 2 - o, term 3 = x; sum = solid; t = t0;
             Ch PDE');
      figure(21)
      plot(r,RHS6(nout,:),'+',r,RHS7(nout,:),'o',r,RHS8(nout,:),'x',r,
           Cht(nout,:),'-');
      xlabel('r (cm)'); ylabel('Ch PDE RHS terms 1,2,sum; t = tf');
      title('term 1 - +, term 2 - o, term 3 - x, sum = solid; t = tf;
             Ch PDE');
    end
```

Listing 3.4 Main program pde_1_main for eqs. (3.1) to (3.5)

We can note the following details about pde_1_main.

- After previous files are cleared, selected global variables are defined.

```
%
% Three-PDE ATG model
%
% Clear previous files
  clear all
  clc
%
% Model parameters shared with other routines
  global   Nn     Nt     Ch...
           rl     ru      r      n...
          rn1    rn2     Kn...
          rt1     Dt     Kt...
```

```
          rh1     rh2      Dh...
        ncall   ncase
```

- One of three cases is selected; these differ primarily in the graphical display of the computed solution.

```
%
% Case
%
%   ncase = 1 - four 2D plots of dependent variables
%               Nn, Nt, Ch, pH vs t
%
%   ncase = 2 - four 3D plots of dependent variables
%               Nn, Nt, Ch, pH vs t
%
%   ncase = 3 - case = 1 with 17 supplemental plots for
%               the derivatives in t and the individual
%               PDE RHS terms
  ncase=1;
```

- A radial grid for r in eqs. (3.1) of `101` points is defined over the interval $0 \leq r \leq 0.5$ cm (for $r_l \leq r \leq r_u$).

```
%
% Radial grid
  rl=0; ru=0.5; n=101;
  for i=1:n
    r(i)=rl+(ru-rl)*(i-1)/(n-1);
  end
```

- The parameter values for eqs. (3.1) from Table 3.2c are specified. These are taken from [2].

```
%
% Nn PDE
  rn1=1.0e-06; rn2=1; Kn=5.0e+07;
%
% Nt PDE
  rt1=1.0e-06; Dt=2.0e-10; Kt=5.0e+07;
%
% Ch PDE
  rh1=2.2e-17; rh2=1.1e-04; Dh=5.0e-06;
```

- An interval in t is defined as $0 \leq t \leq 5.0 \times 10^6$ with output displayed at intervals of 1.0×10^6 for a total of six outputs for `ncase = 1,3`, and intervals of 0.25×10^6 for a total of 21 outputs for `ncase = 2`. In the subsequent output, these values of t in seconds are converted to days by division by $60 \times 60 \times 24$.

```
%
% Independent variable t for ncase = 1, 3
  if(ncase==1 | ncase==3)
    t0=0.0;
```

```
    tf=5.0e+06;
    tout=[t0:1.0e+06:tf]';
    nout=6;
  end
%
% Independent variable t for ncase = 2 (to give additional
% resolution in t)
  if(ncase==2)
    t0=0.0;
    tf=5.0e+06;
    tout=[t0:0.25e+06:tf]';
    nout=21;
  end
```

```
% Initial condition
  u0=inital_1(t0);
```

The ICs of eqs. (3.2) are then defined by a call to `inital_1`.

- The ODE integration is performed by `ode45` (nonstiff) or `ode15s` (stiff), depending on the value of the method flag `mf`. For `mf=1`, a solution is not computed with a reasonable run time (by `ode45`) indicating that the 101 ODEs are apparently stiff.

```
%
% ODE integration
  mf=2;
  reltol=1.0e-06; abstol=1.0e-05;
  options=odeset('RelTol',reltol,'AbsTol',abstol);
%
% Explicit (nonstiff) integration
  if(mf==1)[t,u]=ode45(@pde_1,tout,u0,options); end
%
% Implicit (sparse stiff) integration
  if(mf==2)
    S=jpattern_num_1;
%   pause
    options=odeset(options,'JPattern',S)
    [t,u]=ode15s(@pde_1,tout,u0,options);
  end
```

- The single dependent variable vector `u` from the ODE integration is put into three vectors to facilitate interpretation of the solution in terms of the dependent variables of eqs. (3.1) and subsequent plotting.

```
%
% One vector to three vectors
  for it=1:nout
  for i=1:n
    Nn(it,i)=u(it,i);
    Nt(it,i)=u(it,i+n);
    Ch(it,i)=u(it,i+2*n);
  end
  end
```

3.3 Model output

- Tabulated numerical values for the solutions $N_n(r,t)$, $N_t(r,t)$, $C_h(r,t)$ of eqs. (3.1) is produced for the nout values of t (every 10th value of r is used to keep the output to a manageable size).

```
%
%   Display selected output
    for it=1:nout
      fprintf('\n      t       r      Nn(it,i)      Nt(it,i)      Ch(it,i)\n');
      for i=1:10:n
        fprintf('%6.1f%8.3f%15.4e%15.4e%15.4e\n',...
                t(it)/(60*60*24),r(i),Nn(it,i),Nt(it,i),Ch(it,i));
      end
    end
    fprintf('\n     ncall = %4d\n',ncall);
```

The value of ncall gives an indication of the total computational effort for the numerical solution of eqs. (3.1).

- For ncase=1 or 3, four plots of 2D profiles in r are produced for $N_n(r,t)$, $N_t(r,t)$, $C_h(r,t)$, pH(r,t) at six values of t (each array of dependent variables is 6×101 from the ODE integrator, for example Nn(6,101)).

```
%
% 2D plots
%
% ncase = 1, 3: 2D Nn, Nt, Ch, pH plots in t (figures 1 - 4)
  if(ncase==1 | ncase==3)
    pH=-log10(4.0e-08+Ch);
    figure(1)
    plot(r,Nn,'-');
    xlabel('r (cm)'); ylabel('Nn (cells/cm^3)');
    title('Nn (normal); 3-PDE ATG model');
    figure(2)
    plot(r,Nt,'-');
    xlabel('r (cm)'); ylabel('Nt (cells/cm^3)');
    title('Nt (tumor); 3-PDE ATG model')
    figure(3)
    plot(r,Ch,'-');
    xlabel('r (cm)'); ylabel('Ch (M = gm mols H^+/liter)');
    title('Ch (excess H^+); 3-PDE ATG model');
    figure(4)
    plot(r,pH,'-');
    xlabel('r (cm)'); ylabel('pH');
    title('pH; 3-PDE ATG model');
  end
```

Note that pH is first calculated from the array Ch based on a threshold value 4.0e-08. That is, C_h of eq. (3.1c) is defined as excess H^+ above 4.0×10^{-8}, which is the way C_h is reported elsewhere (e.g., [2]).

- For ncase=2, analogous 3D plots in r and t are produced by surf for 21 values of t (to give better resolution in t). The four dependent variable arrays are therefore 21×101.

```
%
% ncase = 2: 3D Nn, Nt, Ch, pH plots in t (figures 1 - 4)
  if(ncase==2)
    tp=t/(60*60*24);
    pH=-log10(4.0e-08+Ch);
    figure(1)
    surf(r,tp,Nn)
    view(-40,50);
    xlabel('r (cm)'); ylabel('t (days)');
    zlabel('Nt (normal cells/cm^3)');
    figure(2)
    surf(r,tp,Nt)
    view(-25,50)
    xlabel('r (cm)'); ylabel('t (days)');
    zlabel('Nt (tumor cells/cm^3)');
    figure(3)
    surf(r,tp,Ch)
    xlabel('r (cm)'); ylabel('t (days)');
    zlabel('Ch (excess gm mols H^+/liter)');
    figure(4)
    surf(r,tp,pH)
    view(-37.5,60);
    xlabel('r (cm)'); ylabel('t (days)');
    zlabel('pH');
  end
```

- Since the numerical solutions $N_n(r,t)$, $N_t(r,t)$, $C_h(z,t)$ are determined by their corresponding derivatives in t (that are integrated by the ODE integrator), these derivatives are also of interest. They are plotted for ncase=3.

```
%
% case = 3 supplemental 2D plots for derivatives in t
  (figures 5 - 7)
  if(ncase==3)
    for it=1:nout
      u1d=u(it,:);
      ut=pde_1(t(it),u1d);
      Nnt(it,:)=ut(1:n);
      Ntt(it,:)=ut(n+1:2*n);
      Cht(it,:)=ut(2*n+1:3*n);
    end
    figure(5)
    plot(r,Nnt,'-');
    xlabel('r (cm)'); ylabel('Nnt (cells/cm^3-s)');
    title('Nnt (normal); 3-PDE ATG model');
    figure(6)
    plot(r,Ntt,'-');
    xlabel('r (cm)'); ylabel('Ntt (cells/cm^3-s)');
    title('Ntt (normal); 3-PDE ATG model');
```

```
figure(7)
plot(r,Cht,'-');
xlabel('r (cm)'); ylabel('Cht (M/s = gm mols H^+/liter-s)');
title('Cht (excess H^+); 3-PDE ATG model');
```

- An important advantage of the numerical solution of PDEs is that individual terms in the PDE are readily available and can be displayed numerically and graphically. This is accomplished in the present example for `ncase=3` by calling `pde_1` with a second output argument, `term`, which contains individual terms of the PDEs. This revised form of `pde_1` is discussed subsequently. First, the RHS terms of eqs. (3.1) are placed in arrays `RHS1` to `RHS8`.

```
%
% Supplemental 2D plots for RHS terms in derivatives in t
    for it=1:nout
      u1d=u(it,:);
      [ut,term]=pde_1(t(it),u1d);
      RHS1(it,:)=term(1,1:n);
      RHS2(it,:)=term(2,1:n);
      RHS3(it,:)=term(3,1:n);
      RHS4(it,:)=term(4,1:n);
      RHS5(it,:)=term(5,1:n);
      RHS6(it,:)=term(6,1:n);
      RHS7(it,:)=term(7,1:n);
      RHS8(it,:)=term(8,1:n);
    end
```

- The RHS terms of eq. (3.1a), `RHS1,RHS2`, are plotted vs r as Figs. 8 and 9. Then `RHS1,RHS2,Nnt` are plotted at $t = 0$, $t = 5 \times 10^6$ vs r as Figs. 10,11.

```
%
%   Nn PDE
    figure(8)
    plot(r,RHS1,'-'); xlabel('r (cm)'); ylabel('Nn PDE RHS term 1')
    title('Nn PDE RHS term 1; Nn PDE')
    figure(9)
    plot(r,RHS2,'-'); xlabel('r (cm)'); ylabel('Nn PDE RHS term 2')
    title('Nn PDE RHS term 2; Nn PDE')
    figure(10)
    plot(r,RHS1(1,:),'+',r,RHS2(1,:),'o',r,Nnt(1,:),'-');
    xlabel('r (cm)'); ylabel('Nn PDE RHS terms 1,2,sum; t=t0')
    title('term 1 - +, term 2 - o, sum = solid; t = t0; Nn PDE')
    figure(11)
    plot(r,RHS1(nout,:),'+',r,RHS2(nout,:),'o',r,Nnt(nout,:),'-');
    xlabel('r (cm)'); ylabel('Nn PDE RHS terms 1,2,sum; t=tf')
    title('term 1 - +, term 2 - o, sum = solid; t = tf; Nn PDE')
```

- The RHS terms of eq. (3.1b) are plotted as Figs. 12 – 16.

```
%
%   Nt PDE
    figure(12)
    plot(r,RHS3,'-');
```

```
    xlabel('r (cm)'); ylabel('Nt PDE RHS term 1');
    title('Nt PDE RHS term 1; Nt PDE');
    figure(13)
    plot(r,RHS4,'-');
    xlabel('r (cm)'); ylabel('Nt PDE RHS term 2');
    title('Nt PDE RHS term 2; Nt PDE');
    figure(14)
    plot(r,RHS5,'-');
    xlabel('r (cm)'); ylabel('Nt PDE RHS term 3');
    title('Nt PDE RHS term 3; Nt PDE');
    figure(15)
    plot(r,RHS3(1,:),'+',r,RHS4(1,:),'o',r,RHS5(1,:),'x',r,
         Ntt(1,:),'-');
    xlabel('r (cm)'); ylabel('Nt PDE RHS terms 1,2,3,sum;
           t = t0');
    title('term 1 - +, term 2 - o, term 3 = x; sum = solid;
           t = t0; Nt PDE');
    figure(16)
    plot(r,RHS3(nout,:),'+',r,RHS4(nout,:),'o',r,RHS5(nout,:),
         'x',r,Ntt(nout,:),'-');
    xlabel('r (cm)'); ylabel('Nt PDE RHS terms 1,2,sum; t = tf');
    title('term 1 - +, term 2 - o, term 3 - x, sum = solid;
          t = tf; Nt PDE');
```

- The RHS terms of eq. (3.1c) are plotted as Figs. 17 – 21.

```
%
%   Ch PDE
    figure(17)
    plot(r,RHS6,'-');
    xlabel('r (cm)'); ylabel('Ch PDE RHS term 1');
    title('Ch PDE RHS term 1; Ch PDE');
    figure(18)
    plot(r,RHS7,'-');
    xlabel('r (cm)'); ylabel('Ch PDE RHS term 2');
    title('Ch PDE RHS term 2; Ch PDE');
    figure(19)
    plot(r,RHS8,'-');
    xlabel('r (cm)'); ylabel('Ch PDE RHS term 3');
    title('Ch PDE RHS term 3; Ch PDE');
    figure(20)
    plot(r,RHS6(1,:),'+',r,RHS7(1,:),'o',r,RHS8(1,:),'x',r,
         Cht(1,:),'-');
    xlabel('r (cm)'); ylabel('Ch PDE RHS terms 1,2,3,sum; t = t0');
    title('term 1 - +, term 2 - o, term 3 = x; sum = solid; t = t0;
           Ch PDE');
    figure(21)
    plot(r,RHS6(nout,:),'+',r,RHS7(nout,:),'o',r,RHS8(nout,:),'x',r,
         Cht(nout,:),'-');
    xlabel('r (cm)'); ylabel('Ch PDE RHS terms 1,2,sum; t = tf');
    title('term 1 - +, term 2 - o, term 3 - x, sum = solid; t = tf;
           Ch PDE');
  end
```

The end terminates the if for ncase=3.

The four plots produced with ncase=1 are reviewed next. The first plot displays the spatial profiles of the normal cells, $N_n(r,t)$.
We can note the following details about Fig. 3.1.

- The normal cells are more concentrated for $r > 1$ mm and as time evolves through the values $t = 0, 11.6, 23.1, 34.7, 46.3, 57.9$ days, the population of normal cells declines, as expected (since tumor cells become more dominant). In other words, the derivative $\partial N_n/\partial t$ in eq. (3.1a) is negative due to the RHS terms of eq. (3.1a).
- For $t = 0$, the IC of eq. (3.2a) implemented in Nn_1 of Listing 3.3 (as function $\tanh(r)$) provides the steepest profile. Then, as t evolves, this profile is smoothed by diffusion of the tumor cells through the domain $0 \le r \le 0.5$ cm, according to eq. (3.1b).
- Also, for $t = 0$, the left hand value in the neighborhood of $r = 0$ is 5×10^7, as expected from the statement

  ```
  u0=5.0e+07*(1-tanhr)/2+1.0e+08*(1+tanhr)/2;
  ```

  in Listing 3.3 for Nn_1. The right hand value in the neighborhood of $r = 0.5$ cm is 1.0×10^8, as expected from this statement.
- The solution displayed in Fig. 3.1 is not a traveling wave solution in the sense that any given solution curve at t cannot be obtained from the IC curve by a simple translation of the form $r - vt$, where v is a characteristic velocity for eqs. (3.1).

The second plot displays the spatial profiles of the tumor cells, $N_t(r,t)$.
We can note the following details about Fig. 3.2.

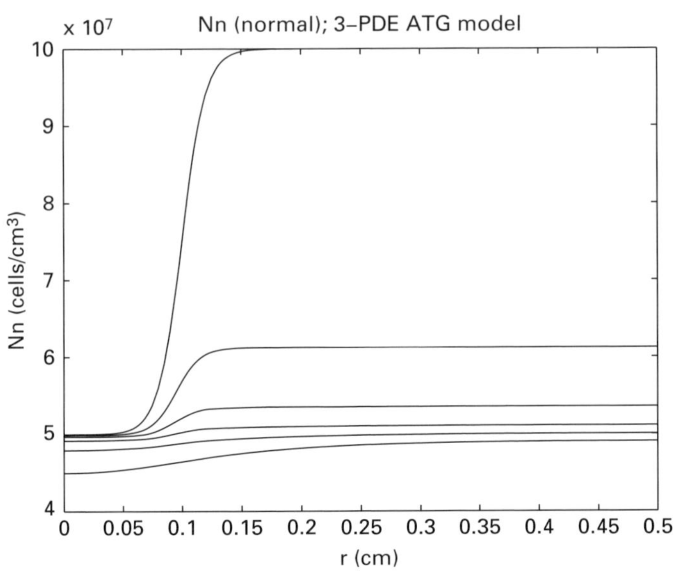

Figure 3.1 Numerical solution for $N_n(r,t)$ of eq. (3.1a) for $0 \le r \le 0.5$ cm $t = 0, 11.6, 23.1, 34.7, 46.3, 57.9$ days (top to bottom)

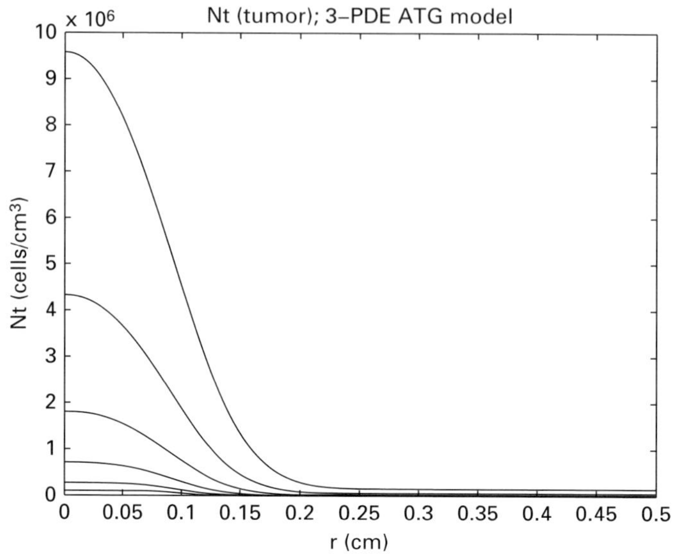

Figure 3.2 Numerical solution for $N_t(r,t)$ of eq. (3.1b) for $0 \le r \le 0.5$ cm $t = 0, 11.6, 23.1, 34.7, 46.3, 57.9$ days (bottom to top)

- The cancer cells are more concentrated for $r < 1$ mm and as time evolves through the values $t = 0, 11.6, 23.1, 34.7, 46.3, 57.9$ days, the population of tumor cells increases, as expected. In other words, the derivative $\partial N_t/\partial t$ in eq. (3.1b) is positive due to the RHS terms of eq. (3.1b).
- For $t = 0$, the IC of eq. (3.3b) implemented in `Nt_1` of Listing 3.3 (as function $\tanh(r)$) produces the smallest values of N_t. Then, as t evolves, the tumor cells increase substantially through the domain $0 \le r \le 0.5$ cm according to eq. (3.1b), particularly for $r < 1$ mm, but also, there is penetration of the tumor cells into the region $r > 1$ mm.
- For $t = 0$, the left hand value in the neighborhood of $r = 0$ is 1.0×10^5, as expected from the statement

```
u0=1.0e+05*(1-tanhr)/2+1.0e+03*(1+tanhr)/2;
```

  in Listing 3.3 for `Nt_1`. The right hand value in the neighborhood of $r = 0.5$ cm is 1.0×10^3, as expected from this statement. These limiting values are small compared with the initial values of N_n, so the growth in tumor cells in Fig. 3.2 is quite significant.
- The zero slope (homogeneous Neumann) BCs of eqs. (3.3a) and (3.3c) are maintained at $r = 0$ and $r = 5$ (the latter is essentially at infinity according to eq. (3.3c) for $t > 0$). The interpretation of these BCs is: (a) the slope (derivative in r) is zero at $r = 0$ mm due to symmetry, and (b) the slope is zero at $r = 5$ because this is far enough out in r that there is no departure of the solution from the IC ($t = 0$) condition. In other words, the zero slope BCs correspond to no flux BCs in the sense that there is no diffusion through the boundaries at $r = 0, 0.5$ cm.

- Again, the solution displayed in Fig. 3.2 is not a traveling wave solution in the sense that any given solution curve at t cannot be obtained from the IC curve by a simple translation of the form $r - vt$, where v is a characteristic velocity for eqs. (3.1).

The third plot displays the spatial profiles of the excess H^+, $C_h(r,t)$. We can note the following details about Fig. 3.3.

- The excess H^+ is more concentrated for $r < 1$ mm and as time evolves through the values $t = 0, 11.6, 23.1, 34.7, 46.3, 57.9$ days, this concentration of excess H^+ increases as expected (since H^+ is produced by the tumor cells).
- For $t = 0$, the IC of eq. (3.2c) implemented in `Ch_1` of Listing 3.3 (as function $\tanh(r)$) produces the smallest values of C_h. Then, as t evolves, the excess H^+ concentration increases substantially throughout the domain $0 \le r \le 0.5$ cm, according to eq. (3.1c). This spread of excess H^+ in turn leads to the reduction in normal cells.
- For $t = 0$, the left hand value in the neighborhood of $r = 0$ is 1.0×10^{-9}, as expected from the statement

```
u0=1.0e-09*(1-tanhr)/2+0*(1+tanhr)/2;
```

  in Listing 3.3 for `Ch_1`. The right hand value in the neighborhood of $r = 0.5$ cm is 0 (no excess H^+), as expected from this statement. These limiting values correspond to essentially no excess H^+ initially. Subsequent increases in excess H^+ for $t > 0$ are due to production by the tumor cells as reflected in eq. (3.1c).
- The zero slope (homogeneous Neumann) BCs of eqs. (3.3b) and (3.3d) are maintained at $r = 0$ and $r = 5$. The interpretation of these zero slope BCs is the same as for Fig. 3.2.

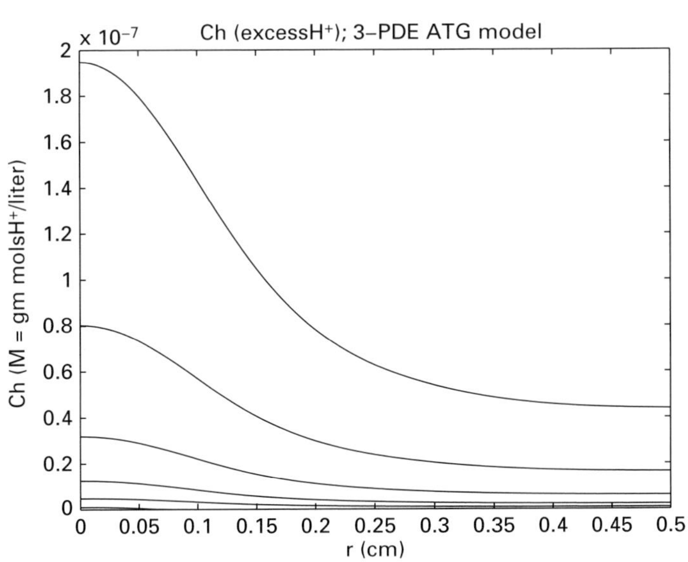

Figure 3.3 Numerical solution for $C_h(r,t)$ of eq. (3.1c) for $0 \le r \le 0.5$ cm $t = 0, 11.6, 23.1, 34.7, 46.3, 57.9$ days (bottom to top)

- Again, the solution displayed in Fig. 3.3 is not a traveling wave solution in the sense that any given solution curve at t cannot be obtained from the IC curve by a simple translation of the form $r - vt$, where v is a characteristic velocity for eqs. (3.1).

Finally, the fourth plot displays the spatial profiles of the excess pH, which follows directly from the C_h values of Fig. 3.3 through the relation $\text{pH} = -\log_{10}(C_h)$.
We can note the following details about Fig. 3.4.

- The pH decreases (greater acidity) as the excess H^+ increases, which follows from the way in which pH is calculated ($\text{pH} = -\log_{10}(C_h)$). This reduced pH in turn leads to a reduction of normal cells through a combination of eqs. (3.1a) and (3.1c).
- The pH starts (at $t = 0$) initially slightly basic (≈ 3.4) and becomes significantly more acidic for $t > 0$. This is the basis for the name *acid-mediated tumor invasion*.
- Again, the solution displayed in Fig. 3.4 is not a traveling wave solution in the sense that any given pH curve at t cannot be obtained from the inital ($t = 0$) curve by a simple translation of the form $r - vt$, where v is a characteristic velocity for eqs. (3.1).

Selected numerical output from the main program `atg_1_main` is listed in Table 3.4. We can note the following points about this output.

- The range of the dependent variables N_n, N_t, C_h is typically approximately 15 orders of magnitude, e.g.,

```
57.9    0.250      4.8609e+007      1.4798e+005      6.1053e-008
```

However, there was no difficulty in calculating a numerical solution. In other words, normalization or nondimensionalization was not required to compute the numerical solution.

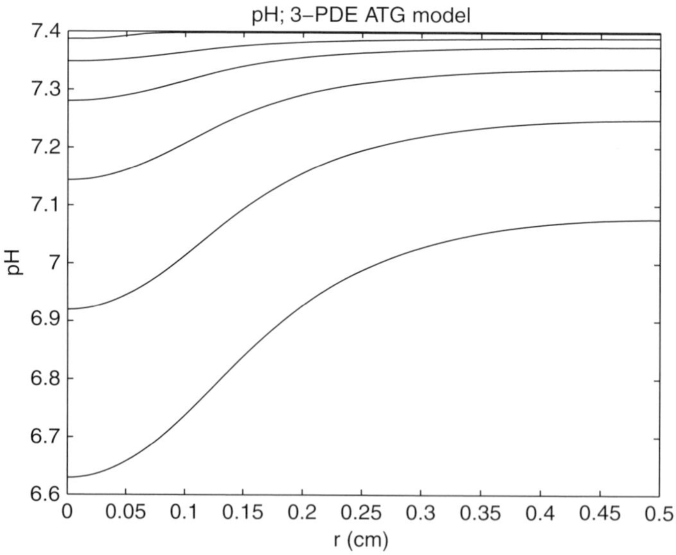

Figure 3.4 pH for $0 \le r \le 0.5$ cm, $t = 0, 11.6, 23.1, 34.7, 46.3, 57.9$ days (top to bottom)

Table 3.4. Abbreviated output from `atg_1_main`

```
   t         r          Nn(it,i)         Nt(it,i)         Ch(it,i)
  0.0     0.000      5.0002e+007      9.9996e+004      9.9331e-010
  0.0     0.050      5.0335e+007      9.9337e+004      5.0000e-010
  0.0     0.100      7.5000e+007      5.0500e+004      6.6929e-012
  0.0     0.150      9.9665e+007      1.6626e+003      4.5398e-014
  0.0     0.200      9.9998e+007      1.0045e+003      3.0590e-016
  0.0     0.250      1.0000e+008      1.0000e+003      2.0612e-018
  0.0     0.300      1.0000e+008      1.0000e+003      1.3888e-020
  0.0     0.350      1.0000e+008      1.0000e+003      9.3592e-023
  0.0     0.400      1.0000e+008      1.0000e+003      5.5511e-025
  0.0     0.450      1.0000e+008      1.0000e+003      0.0000e+000
  0.0     0.500      1.0000e+008      1.0000e+003      0.0000e+000

   t         r          Nn(it,i)         Nt(it,i)         Ch(it,i)
 11.6     0.000      4.9890e+007      2.7088e+005      5.1553e-009
 11.6     0.050      5.0021e+007      2.6912e+005      4.7056e-009
 11.6     0.100      5.6910e+007      1.5309e+005      3.4076e-009
 11.6     0.150      6.1173e+007      4.5285e+003      2.1677e-009
 11.6     0.200      6.1233e+007      2.7304e+003      1.5532e-009
 11.6     0.250      6.1241e+007      2.7183e+003      1.2293e-009
 11.6     0.300      6.1245e+007      2.7182e+003      1.0454e-009
 11.6     0.350      6.1248e+007      2.7182e+003      9.3829e-010
 11.6     0.400      6.1249e+007      2.7182e+003      8.7744e-010
 11.6     0.450      6.1250e+007      2.7182e+003      8.4691e-010
 11.6     0.500      6.1250e+007      2.7182e+003      8.3795e-010
               .                                           .
               .                                           .
               .                                           .
                 Output for t=23.1,34.7,46.3 deleted
               .                                           .
               .                                           .
               .                                           .
   t         r          Nn(it,i)         Nt(it,i)         Ch(it,i)
 57.9     0.000      4.4032e+007      1.1461e+007      2.3353e-007
 57.9     0.050      4.4509e+007      1.1385e+007      2.1465e-007
 57.9     0.100      4.6016e+007      7.2868e+006      1.5975e-007
 57.9     0.150      4.7496e+007      2.5264e+005      1.0410e-007
 57.9     0.200      4.8223e+007      1.4867e+005      7.5920e-008
 57.9     0.250      4.8609e+007      1.4798e+005      6.1053e-008
 57.9     0.300      4.8829e+007      1.4798e+005      5.2613e-008
 57.9     0.350      4.8957e+007      1.4798e+005      4.7696e-008
 57.9     0.400      4.9030e+007      1.4798e+005      4.4903e-008
 57.9     0.450      4.9067e+007      1.4798e+005      4.3501e-008
 57.9     0.500      4.9078e+007      1.4798e+005      4.3090e-008

   ncall =   496
```

- The computational effort was quite modest, as reflected in the value `ncall = 496`. Of course, this conclusion could change as the model and code are modified, but so far, the code has remained robust and efficient.

To conclude, the numerical integration of eqs. (3.1) subject to the ICs and BCs of eqs. (3.2) and (3.3) is straightforward. Also, because of the numerical procedure programmed in the ODE routine, `pde_1`, changing the PDEs to investigate additional effects is easily accomplished.

Two extensions of `pde_1` are discussed next.

1. The response of the model, as reflected in Figs. 3.1 to 3.4, is determined by the PDEs, eqs. (3.1), and the ICs and BCs, eqs. (3.2) and (3.3). Specifically, the RHS derivatives, $\partial N_n/\partial t, \partial N_t/\partial t, \partial C_h/\partial t$ of eqs. (3.1) determine how the dependent variables N_n, N_t, C_h vary with t, and since these derivatives in t also vary with r, the LHS derivatives of eqs. (3.1) also determine the solution variation with r.

   However, the LHS derivatives are, of course, equal to the RHS expressions of eqs. (3.1), and these RHS expressions are rather complicated. In particular, they are composed of a sum of terms that reflect various physical phenomena, such as generation (or depletion) and diffusion (additionally these terms are in some cases nonlinear, which generally precludes analytical or exact solutions to eqs. (3.1)).

   To facilitate an understanding of the variation of the LHS derivatives in t and r, the RHS terms can be examined individually, as discussed previously. In other words, if their values are computed and displayed, the contributions of the individual terms can be determined and their contribution to the total variation of the dependent variables in t and r can be assessed. This additional computation is easily accomplished through modification of the programming in the ODE routine `pde_1`.
2. In addition to the RHS terms of eqs. (3.1), further RHS terms can easily be added in `pde_1` to include other physical and chemical phenomena. For example, eq. (3.1a) does not have a diffusion term, yet diffusion of the normal cells would certainly be possible. Therefore, a term can be added to the RHS of eq. (3.1a) to investigate the effect of normal cell diffusion; this is illustrated subsequently by considering the extended statements in `pde_1`.

3.4 Supplemental output

Figures 3.1 to 3.4 provide the numerical solution to eqs. (3.1) as $N_n(r,t), N_t(r,t), C_h(r,t)$; $\mathrm{pH}(r,t)$ obtained from $C_h(r,t)$ is also plotted (Fig. 3.4). In a sense, these plots provide an overall picture of the solution of eqs. (3.1), which encompasses the effect of the individual RHS terms of eqs. (3.1). The contributions of these terms are quite significant in that they (1) represent various physical and chemical phenomena and (2) have relatively different magnitudes so that certain terms may determine the solution to the PDEs more than others. To elucidate the contribution of individual RHS terms of eqs. (3.1), some additional coding can be added to `pde_1` and `pde_1_main`, as discussed previously.

First, the individual RHS of eqs. (3.1) can be easily stored in arrays since they are computed as part of the coding for eqs. (3.1) in pde_1.

```
  function [ut,term]=pde_1c(t,u)
%
% Function pde_1c defines the RHS terms and ODEs in the MOL
% solution of three
% PDEs for the ATG model
%
  global    Nn      Nt      Ch...
             rl      ru      r       n...
            rn1     rn2     Kn...
            rt1      Dt     Kt...
            rh1     rh2     Dh...
          ncall   ncase
%
% One vector to three vectors
  for i=1:n
    Nn(i)=u(i);
    Nt(i)=u(i+n);
    Ch(i)=u(i+2*n);
  end
%
% First order spatial derivatives
  Nnr=dss004(rl,ru,n,Nn);
  Ntr=dss004(rl,ru,n,Nt);
  Chr=dss004(rl,ru,n,Ch);
%
% BCs
  Ntr(1)=0; Ntr(n)=0;
  Chr(1)=0; Chr(n)=0;
%
% Second order spatial derivatives
  nl=2; nu=2;
  Ntrr=dss044(rl,ru,n,Nt,Ntr,nl,nu);
  Chrr=dss044(rl,ru,n,Ch,Chr,nl,nu);
%
% PDEs
  for i=1:n
    D=Dt*(1-Nn(i)/Kn);
    if(D<0)D=0;end
    if(i==1)
      term(1,i)=rn1*Nn(i)*(1-Nn(i)/Kn);
      term(2,i)=-rn2*Ch(i)*Nn(i);
      Nnt(i)=term(1,i)+term(2,i);
      term(3,i)=rt1*Nt(i)*(1-Nt(i)/Kt);
      term(4,i)=+3*D*Ntrr(i);
      Ntt(i)=term(3,i)+term(4,i);
      term(6,i)=rh1*Nt(i);
      term(7,i)=-rh2*Ch(i);
      term(8,i)=+3*Dh*Chrr(i);
```

```
        Cht(i)=term(6,i)+term(7,i)+term(8,i);
      else
        term(1,i)=rn1*Nn(i)*(1-Nn(i)/Kn);
        term(2,i)=-rn2*Ch(i)*Nn(i);
        Nnt(i)=term(1,i)+term(2,i);
        term(3,i)=rt1*Nt(i)*(1-Nt(i)/Kt);
        term(4,i)=+D*(Ntrr(i)+2/r(i)*Ntr(i));
        term(5,i)=+(-Dt/Kn)*Nnr(i)*Ntr(i);
        Ntt(i)=term(3,i)+term(4,i)+term(5,i);
        term(6,i)=rh1*Nt(i);
        term(7,i)=-rh2*Ch(i);
        term(8,i)=+Dh*(Chrr(i)+2/r(i)*Chr(i));
        Cht(i)=term(6,i)+term(7,i)+term(8,i);
      end
    end
%
% Three vectors to one vector
  for i=1:n
    ut(i)     =Nnt(i);
    ut(i+n)   =Ntt(i);
    ut(i+2*n)=Cht(i);
  end
  ut=ut';
%
% Increment calls to pde_1c
  ncall=ncall+1;
```

Listing 3.5 pde_1 of Listing 3.1 modified to store the RHS terms of eqs. (3.1)

We can note the following points about routine pde_1c of Listing 3.5.

- pde_1c has a second return argument, term (see the first line of pde_1c) that contains the various RHS terms of eqs. (3.1), as computed in pde_1c.
- pde_1 of Listing 3.1 and pde_1c of Listing 3.5 are the same except for the for loop, which steps through the n grid points to calculate the RHSs of eqs. (3.1).

```
%
% PDEs
  for i=1:n
    D=Dt*(1-Nn(i)/Kn);
    if(D<0)D=0;end
    if(i==1)
      term(1,i)=rn1*Nn(i)*(1-Nn(i)/Kn);
      term(2,i)=-rn2*Ch(i)*Nn(i);
      Nnt(i)=term(1,i)+term(2,i);
      term(3,i)=rt1*Nt(i)*(1-Nt(i)/Kt);
      term(4,i)=+3*D*Ntrr(i);
      Ntt(i)=term(3,i)+term(4,i);
      term(6,i)=rh1*Nt(i);
      term(7,i)=-rh2*Ch(i);
      term(8,i)=+3*Dh*Chrr(i);
      Cht(i)=term(6,i)+term(7,i)+term(8,i);
```

```
    else
      term(1,i)=rn1*Nn(i)*(1-Nn(i)/Kn);
      term(2,i)=-rn2*Ch(i)*Nn(i);
      Nnt(i)=term(1,i)+term(2,i);
      term(3,i)=rt1*Nt(i)*(1-Nt(i)/Kt);
      term(4,i)=+D*(Ntrr(i)+2/r(i)*Ntr(i));
      term(5,i)=+(-Dt/Kn)*Nnr(i)*Ntr(i);
      Ntt(i)=term(3,i)+term(4,i)+term(5,i);
      term(6,i)=rh1*Nt(i);
      term(7,i)=-rh2*Ch(i);
      term(8,i)=+Dh*(Chrr(i)+2/r(i)*Chr(i));
      Cht(i)=term(6,i)+term(7,i)+term(8,i);
    end
  end
```

- This additional code might appear rather formidable, but it is actually just a minor extension of the code in Listing 3.1. For example, for $r = 0$ corresponding to `i=1`, eq. (3.1a) for $N_n(r,t)$ is programmed with a few additional lines.

```
  for i=1:n
    D=Dt*(1-Nn(i)/Kn);
    if(D<0)D=0;end
    if(i==1)
      term(1,i)=rn1*Nn(i)*(1-Nn(i)/Kn);
      term(2,i)=-rn2*Ch(i)*Nn(i);
      Nnt(i)=term(1,i)+term(2,i);
```

  The first RHS term of eq. (3.1a), $r_{n1}N_n(1 - N_n/K_n)$ is computed as `term(1,i)`. Similarly, the second RHS term of eq. (3.1a), $-r_{n2}C_hN_n$, is programmed as `term(2,i)`.
- These two terms are then added to make up the RHS of eq. (3.1a).

```
      Nnt(i)=term(1,i)+term(2,i);
```

- In the same way, the RHS terms of eqs. (3.1b) and (3.1c) are computed as `term(3,i)` to `term(8,i)`, then added to complete the coding for eqs. (3.1b) and (3.1c). Thus, all of the RHS terms are in array `term`, which is passed to the main program as the second return argument of `pde_1c` where it can be used in output statements.

The main program of Listing 3.4 is changed only at the end to include some additional plotting (for `ncase=3`). Clearly, a large number of plots (21) is produced with this additional code, but also, we gain a detailed picture of how the RHS terms of eqs. (3.1) determine the solutions $N_n(r,t), N_t(r,t), C_h(r,t)$. For example, the relative magnitudes of the various RHS terms are clear and therefore those terms that contribute most significantly to the solution of eqs. (3.1) are identified. To illustrate these points, we include just two additional plots, Figs. 3.5 (figure(5) in `pde_1_main` of Listing 3.4) and 3.6 (figure(8) in `pde_1_main` of Listing 3.4).

Figure 3.5 indicates that the derivative $\partial N_n/\partial t$ approaches small values with increasing t so that the solution to eq. (3.1a) is approaching a steady state (with little variation in t).

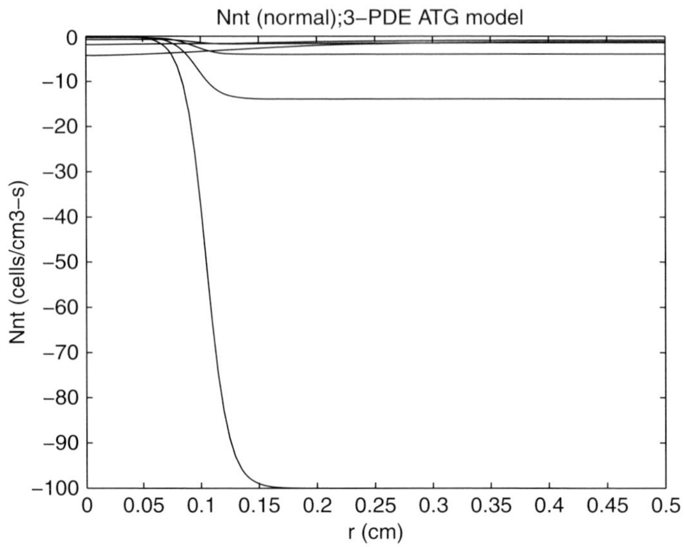

Figure 3.5 The derivative $\partial N_n/\partial t$ of eq. (3.1a) for $0 \le r \le 0.5$ cm $t = 0, 11.6, 23.1, 34.7, 46.3, 57.9$ (bottom to top)

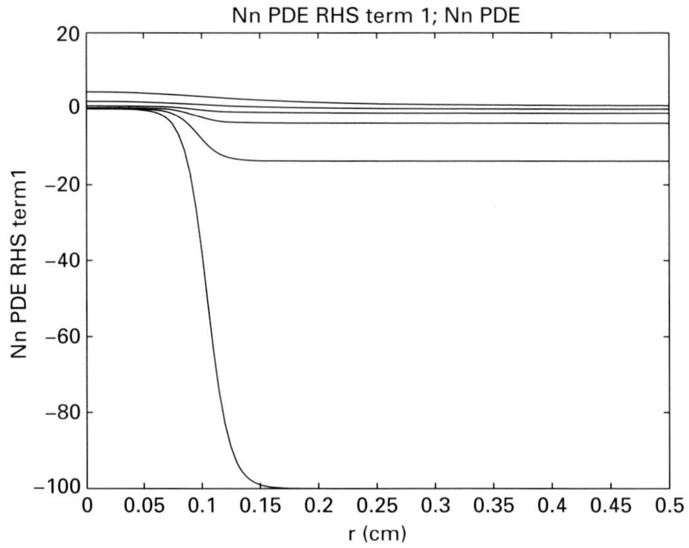

Figure 3.6 The first RHS term of eq. (3.1), $r_{n1}N_n\,(1 - N_n/K_n)$ for $0 \le r \le 0.5$ cm, $t = 0,11.6,23.1,34.7,$ 46.3,57.9 days (bottom to top)

Figure 3.6 indicates that the first RHS term of eq. (3.1a) decreases rapidly with increasing t, owing to the decreasing values of N_n with t in this term, $r_{n1}N_n\,(1 - N_n/K_n)$ (also signifying an approach to steady state).

In summary, we can gain a detailed explanation of the PDE solutions by observing the individual terms in the PDEs. These terms are readily available for display from the MOL ODE routine, e.g., pde_1c.

3.5 Extension of the model

Now that a code for eqs. (3.1) is available, we can easily modify it to reflect changes in the PDE model that might be of interest. For example, eq. (3.1a) does not have diffusion of N_n which is not entirely logical if eqs. (3.1b) and (3.1c) have diffusion terms for N_t and C_h, respectively. To add a diffusion term to eq. (3.1a), the code in pde_1 is easily modified. The only change is indicated next.

```
%
% PDEs
  for i=1:n
    D=Dt*(1-Nn(i)/Kn);
    if(D<0)D=0;end
    Dn=Dt;
    if(i==1)
      Nnt(i)=rn1*Nn(i)*(1-Nn(i)/Kn)-rn2*Ch(i)*Nn(i)+3*D*Nnrr(i);
      Ntt(i)=rt1*Nt(i)*(1-Nt(i)/Kt)+3*D*Ntrr(i);
      Cht(i)=rh1*Nt(i)-rh2*Ch(i)+3*Dh*Chrr(i);
    else
      Nnt(i)=rn1*Nn(i)*(1-Nn(i)/Kn)-rn2*Ch(i)*Nn(i)...
          +D*(Nnrr(i)+2/r(i)*Nnr(i))+(-Dn/Kn)*Nnr(i)*Nnr(i);
      Ntt(i)=rt1*Nt(i)*(1-Nt(i)/Kt)...
          +D*(Ntrr(i)+2/r(i)*Ntr(i))+(-Dt/Kn)*Nnr(i)*Ntr(i);
      Cht(i)=rh1*Nt(i)-rh2*Ch(i)+Dh*(Chrr(i)+2/r(i)*Chr(i));
    end
  end
```

Note that the diffusion terms for eq. (3.1b),

```
+3*D*Ntrr(i) (i=1)

+D*(Ntrr(i)+2/r(i)*Ntr(i))+(-Dt/Kn)*Nnr(i)*Ntr(i) (i not equal 1)
```

have been modified and added to the code for eq. (3.1a) as the terms

```
+3*D*Nnrr(i)

+D*(Nnrr(i)+2/r(i)*Nnr(i))+(-Dn/Kn)*Nnr(i)*Nnr(i)
```

The same diffusivities have been used for N_n and N_t (through Dn=Dt) but these could easily be made distinct.

We will not discuss here the effects of adding diffusion to eq. (3.1a). Rather, the intention is to illustrate how changes in the PDEs can be accomplished. Additionally, PDEs can be added to the model by additional programming in the ODE routine, pde_1. Thus, the numerical MOL procedure offers essentially unlimited opportunity for experimentation with the acid-mediated tumor growth PDE model.

In conclusion, the discussion in Sections 3.3 and 3.4 illustrates how the detailed structure of the model of eqs. (3.1) can be studied, and how this structure can be extended to include additional physical and chemical phenomena. Of course, extensions of the model might also include adding PDEs; this is the basis for ongoing research.

3.6 Additional references

The development of ATG models is an active area of research. Here are only a few selected references with extensive bibliographies for further study. Buffering control of tumor and normal cell environment pH is explored in [5] through the use of an ODE model. Other papers concerning ATG include [1, 6, 7, 8].

Acknowledgements

The contributions of Ms. Catherine M. Griffin and Ms. Yaas Bigdeli in researching the ATG literature are gratefully acknowledged.

References

[1] Bianchini, L. and Fasano, A. (2009), A model combining acid-mediated tumour invasion and nutrient dynamics, *Nonlinear Anal. Real*, **10**, 1955–1975

[2] Fasano, A., Herrero, M. A., and Rodrigo, M. R. (2009), Slow and fast invasion waves in a model of acid-mediated tumour growth, *Math. Biosci.*, **220**, 45–56

[3] Gatenby, R. A. and Gawlinski, E. T. (1996), A reaction-diffusion model of cancer invasion, *Cancer Res.*, **56**, 5745–5753

[4] Martin, G. R. and Jain, R. K. (1994), Noninvasive measurement of interstitial pH profiles in normal and neoplastic tissue using fluorescence ratio imaging spectroscopy, *Cancer Res.*, **54**, 5670–5674

[5] Martin, N. K. Gaffney, E. A., Gatenby R. A., *et al.* (2011), A mathematical model of tumour and blood pHe regulation: the HCO_3^-/CO_2 buffering system, *Math. Biosci.*, **230**, 1–11

[6] Patel, A. A. Gawlinski, E. T., Lemieux, S. K., and Gatenby, R. A. (2001), A cellular automation model of early tumor growth and invasion: the effects of native tissue vascularity and increased anaerobic tumor metabolism, *J. Theor. Biol.*, **213**, 315–331

[7] Singh, R. K. and Siegal, G. P. (1995), Amino acid transport systems modulate human tumor cell growth and invasion: a working hypothesis, *Med. Hypotheses*, **44**, 195–201

[8] Smallbone, K., Gatenby, R. A., and Maini, P. K. (2008), Mathematical modelling of tumour acidity, *J. Theor. Biol.*, **255**, 106–112

4 Retinal O_2 transport

The continuous transport of O_2 in the retina is essential for the functioning of the photoreceptor cells (rods and cones) that provide vision. The O_2 originates in the blood supply to the retina and is transported by diffusion through several layers of cells to the photoreceptors. In the model discussed next, the O_2 transport is considered through four layers with metabolism in each layer that consumes O_2. The model can be used to study how much O_2 arrives for use by the photoreceptors under varying conditions.

4.1 Four-section PDE model

The retinal O_2 transport model is explained in Fig. 4.1 primarily with words.

We can note the following details about the model represented in Fig. 4.1:

- The model has four sections, as discussed in [1, 2]:
  - Inner retina (IR),
  - Outer retina (OR),
  - Fluid layer (FL),
  - Choriocapillaris (CC).
- At the left boundary, $z = z_L$ (see Fig. 4.1), the O_2 pressure is specified. Since the dependent variable, O_2 pressure, $P_{IR}(z = z_L, t) = P_{IR\text{-}S}$, is specified, this is a Dirichlet BC as discussed in Section 1.3.1.
- At the right boundary, $z = z_{CC}$, the O_2 pressure is specified, typically normal breathing pressure. Since the dependent variable, O_2 pressure, $P_{CC}(z = z_{CC}, t) = P_{CC\text{-}S}$, is specified, this is a Dirichlet BC as discussed in Section 1.3.1.
- Within each of the four sections (IR, OR, FL, CC), O_2 transport is by time-dependent diffusion with depletion of O_2 by normal metabolism (specified by *Diffusion–depletion* in Fig. 4.1). Additionally, if the O_2 reaches a low level (hypoxia), vascular endothelial growth factor (VEGF) is produced that can result in neovascularization (and, in turn, age-related macular degeneration (AMD)).
- The diffusion is modeled by the classical 1D diffusion equation in Cartesian coordinates, eq. (1.18), with a constant diffusion coefficient (diffusivity).
- At the interface between adjacent sections, such as between the IR and OR at $z = z_{IR}$, two BCs are imposed.

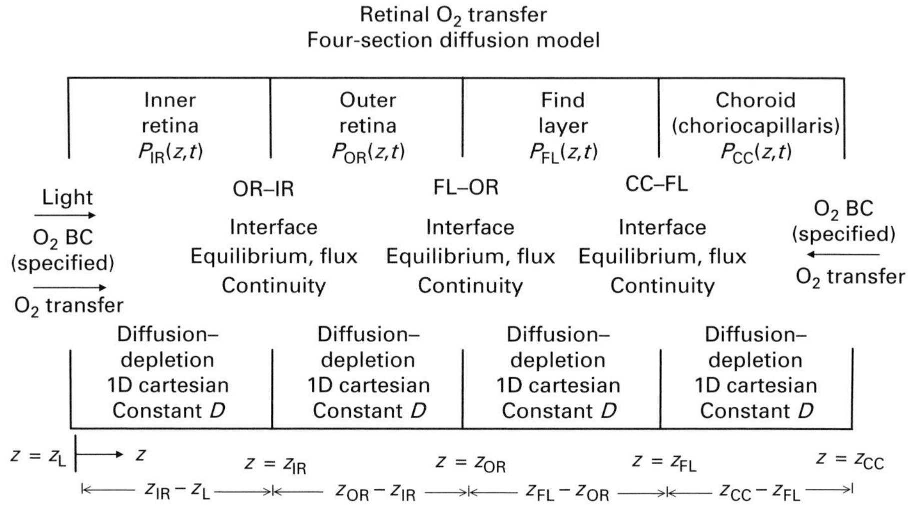

Figure 4.1 Diagram of the four-section O_2 transport model

– An equilibrium condition relating the two O_2 concentrations, such as O_2 pressures P_{IR} and P_{OR}. This condition provides a Dirichlet BC as will be discussed next.
– Continuity of O_2 flux, that is, the flux in the IR equals the flux in the OR. This condition provides a Neumann BC.

- Solution of the four-section PDE model equations provides $P_{IR}(z,t)$, $P_{OR}(z,t)$, $P_{FL}(z,t)$, and $P_{CC}(z,t)$. As a notational detail, since u is generally used in the numerical PDE literature to denote a PDE-dependent variable, the four pressures will be denoted as u_{IR}, u_{OR}, u_{FL} and u_{CC}, respectively, in the statement of the model equations that follows, and as `uir`, `uor`, `ufl`, and `ucc` in the MOL routines that follow.

The representation of the model in Fig. 4.1 is restated in Fig. 4.2 in terms of equations.

From Fig. 4.2, the model equations are now stated (at first, without photoreceptor cell density or VEGF concentration).

The IR diffusion equation with depletion is

$$\frac{\partial u_{IR}}{\partial t} = D_{IR}\frac{\partial^2 u_{IR}}{\partial z^2} - k_{IR}u_{IR},\ z_L \le z \le z_{IR}, \tag{4.1a}$$

with variables as listed in Table 4.1.

The initial condition (IC) and boundary conditions (BCs) for eq. (4.1a) are

$$u_{IR}(z,t=0) = f_{IR}(z), \tag{4.1b}$$

$$u_{IR}(z=z_L,t) = P_{IR\text{-}S}(t), \tag{4.1c}$$

$$u_{IR}(z=z_{IR},t) = k_{IR-OR}u_{OR}(z=z_{IR},t), \tag{4.1d}$$

where $P_{IR\text{-}S}(t)$ is a prescribed function.

Table 4.1. Variables and parameters of eq. (4.1a)

Variable	Interpretation and units
u_{IR}	O_2 concentration (mm Hg)
z	position in IC (μm)
t	time (s)
D_{IR}	diffusivity (μm^2/s)
k_{IR}	rate constant (1/s)

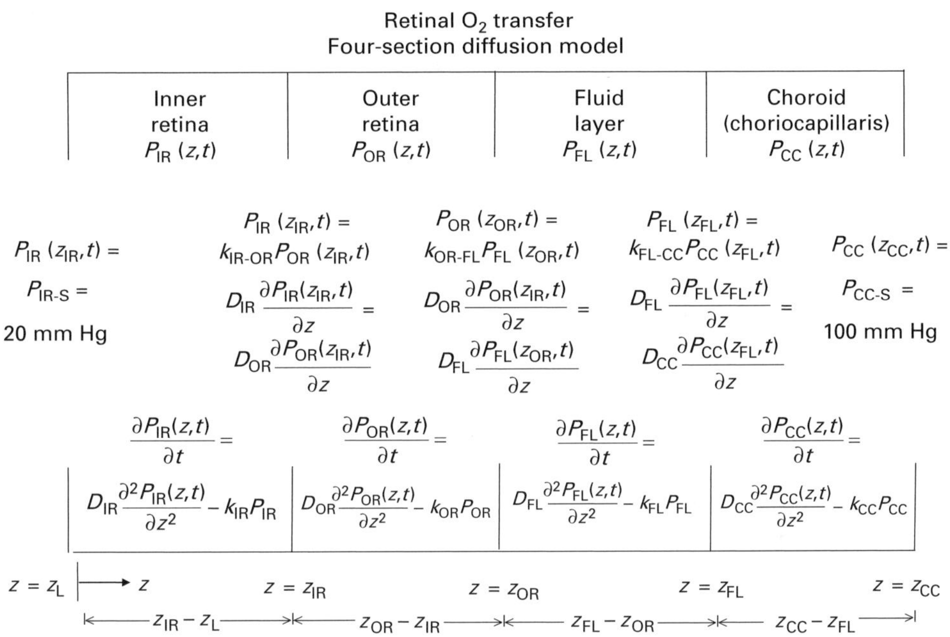

Figure 4.2 Equation summary for O_2 transport model

The variables in eqs. (4.1) correspond to Table 4.1 or are explained in Fig. 4.2. The IC function $f_{IR}(z)$ is specified, typically as a constant. Equation (4.1c) includes $P_{IR\text{-}S}(t)$, which specifies O_2 at the left end $z = z_L$. In eq. (4.1d), k_{IR-OR} is an equilibrium constant relating the two interfacial concentrations, $u_{IR}(z = z_{IR}, t)$ and $u_{OR}(z = z_{IR}, t)$.

The equations for the OR, FL and CC are analogous to eqs. (4.1). They are stated next without a detailed explanation. For OR,

$$\frac{\partial u_{OR}}{\partial t} = D_{OR}\frac{\partial^2 u_{OR}}{\partial z^2} - k_{OR}u_{OR}, \quad z_{IR} \le z \le z_{OR}, \tag{4.2a}$$

$$u_{OR}(z, t = 0) = f_{OR}(z), \tag{4.2b}$$

$$\frac{\partial u_{\mathrm{OR}}(z=z_{\mathrm{IR}},t)}{\partial z} = (D_{\mathrm{IR}}/D_{\mathrm{OR}})\frac{\partial u_{\mathrm{IR}}(z=z_{\mathrm{IR}},t)}{\partial z}, \tag{4.2c}$$

$$u_{\mathrm{OR}}(z=z_{\mathrm{OR}},t) = k_{\mathrm{OR-FL}}u_{\mathrm{FL}}(z=z_{\mathrm{OR}},t). \tag{4.2d}$$

For FL,

$$\frac{\partial u_{\mathrm{FL}}}{\partial t} = D_{\mathrm{FL}}\frac{\partial^2 u_{\mathrm{FL}}}{\partial z^2} - k_{\mathrm{FL}}u_{\mathrm{FL}},\ z_{\mathrm{OR}} \le z \le z_{\mathrm{FL}}, \tag{4.3a}$$

$$u_{\mathrm{FL}}(z,t=0) = f_{\mathrm{FL}}(z), \tag{4.3b}$$

$$\frac{\partial u_{\mathrm{FL}}(z=z_{\mathrm{OR}},t)}{\partial z} = (D_{\mathrm{OR}}/D_{\mathrm{FL}})\frac{\partial u_{\mathrm{OR}}(z=z_{\mathrm{OR}},t)}{\partial z}, \tag{4.3c}$$

$$u_{\mathrm{FL}}(z=z_{\mathrm{FL}},t) = k_{\mathrm{FL-CC}}u_{\mathrm{CC}}(z=z_{\mathrm{FL}},t). \tag{4.3d}$$

For CC,

$$\frac{\partial u_{\mathrm{CC}}}{\partial t} = D_{\mathrm{CC}}\frac{\partial^2 u_{\mathrm{CC}}}{\partial z^2} - k_{\mathrm{CC}}u_{\mathrm{CC}},\ z_{\mathrm{FL}} \le z \le z_{\mathrm{CC}}, \tag{4.4a}$$

$$u_{\mathrm{CC}}(z,t=0) = f_{\mathrm{CC}}(z), \tag{4.4b}$$

$$\frac{\partial u_{\mathrm{CC}}(z=z_{\mathrm{FL}},t)}{\partial z} = (D_{\mathrm{FL}}/D_{\mathrm{CC}})\frac{\partial u_{\mathrm{FL}}(z=z_{\mathrm{FL}},t)}{\partial z}, \tag{4.4c}$$

$$u_{\mathrm{CC}}(z=z_{\mathrm{CC}},t) = P_{\mathrm{CC\text{-}S}}(t). \tag{4.4d}$$

where $P_{\mathrm{CC\text{-}S}}$ is a prescribed function of t, typically a constant such as the O_2 concentration for normal breathing (see Fig. 4.2). Equations (4.2c), (4.3c), and (4.4c) express continuity of the O_2 flux across the interior interfaces.

4.2 MOL routines

Equations (4.1) to (4.4) constitute the complete O_2 transport model (without VEGF concentration and photoreceptor cell density, which will be considered subsequently). We now consider a set of MATLAB routines for the solution of these equations that include two test cases for the model equations and their computer implementation.

4.2.1 Main program

A main program, `pde_1_main`, is listed first.

```
%
% Four-section retinal O2 transport model equation
%
% Clear previous files
  clear all
```

```
  clc
%
% Model parameters shared with other routines
  global   nir      nor      nfl      ncc...
         zl_ir    zl_or    zl_fl    zl_cc...
         zg_ir    zg_or    zg_fl    zg_cc...
           Dir      Dor      Dfl      Dcc...
                 kir_or   kor_fl   kfl_cc...
           kir      kor      kfl      kcc...
         pir_s    pcc_s    ncall    ncase
%
% Select case
%
%   ncase = 1: metabolism rates = 0
%
%   ncase = 2: metabolism rates ne 0
  ncase=2;
%
% Number of grid points
  nir=11; nor=11; nfl=11; ncc=11;
%
% Lengths of four sections (microns)
  zl_ir=200; zl_or=200; zl_fl=200; zl_cc=200;
%
% Spatial grids;
  zg_ir=[0:zl_ir/10:zl_ir]'; zg_or=[0:zl_or/10:zl_or]';
  zg_fl=[0:zl_fl/10:zl_fl]'; zg_cc=[0:zl_cc/10:zl_cc]';
%
% Diffusivities (microns^2/s)
  Dir=1.0e+04; Dor=1.0e+04; Dfl=1.0e+04; Dcc=1.0e+04;
% Dir=0.1e+04; Dor=0.1e+04; Dfl=0.1e+04; Dcc=0.1e+04;
% Dir=0.5e+04; Dor=0.5e+04; Dfl=0.5e+04; Dcc=0.5e+04;
%
% Interface coefficients
  kir_or=1; kor_fl=1; kfl_cc=1;
%
% Metabolism rates
  if(ncase==1) kir=   0; kor=   0; kfl=   0; kcc=   0; end
  if(ncase==2) kir= 0.1; kor= 0.1; kfl= 0.1; kcc= 0.1; end
%
% Normal breathing O2 concentration (mm hg)
  pir_s=20;
  pcc_s=100;
%
% Independent variable t
  t0=0.0; tf=3.0e+01; tout=[t0:tf/6:tf]';
  nout=7;
%
% Initial condition
  u0=inital_1(t0);
%
```

```
% ODE integration
  mf=2;
  reltol=1.0e-06; abstol=1.0e-05;
  options=odeset('RelTol',reltol,'AbsTol',abstol);
%
% Explicit (nonstiff) integration
  if(mf==1)[t,u]=ode45(@pde_1,tout,u0,options); end
%
% Implicit (sparse stiff) integration
  if(mf==2)
    S=jpattern_num_1;
%   pause
    options=odeset(options,'JPattern',S)
    [t,u]=ode15s(@pde_1,tout,u0,options);
  end
%
% One vector to four vectors
  for it=1:nout
    for i=1:nir uir(it,i)=u(it,i);             end
    for i=1:nor uor(it,i)=u(it,i+nir);         end
    for i=1:nfl ufl(it,i)=u(it,i+nir+nor);     end
    for i=1:ncc ucc(it,i)=u(it,i+nir+nor+nfl); end
    if(it>=2)
        uir(it,1)  =pir_s;
        ucc(it,ncc)=pcc_s;
    end
  end
%
%   Display tabulated numerical solution
    for it=1:nout
      fprintf('\n    t     zg_ir    uir(z,t)\n')
      for i=1:nir
        fprintf('%5.2f%10.0f%12.2f\n',t(it),zg_ir(i),uir(it,i))
      end
      fprintf('\n    t     zg_or    uor(z,t)\n')
      for i=1:nor
        fprintf('%5.2f%10.0f%12.2f\n',t(it),zg_or(i),uor(it,i))
      end
      fprintf('\n    t     zg_fl    ufl(z,t)\n')
      for i=1:nfl
        fprintf('%5.2f%10.0f%12.2f\n',t(it),zg_fl(i),ufl(it,i))
      end
      fprintf('\n    t     zg_cc    ucc(z,t)\n')
      for i=1:ncc
        fprintf('%5.2f%10.0f%12.2f\n',t(it),zg_cc(i),ucc(it,i))
      end
%
%   Next t
    end
    fprintf('\n    ncall = %4d\n',ncall);
%
```

```
%    Four plots for uir, uor, ufl, ucc
     figure(2)
     subplot(2,2,1)
     plot(zg_ir,uir,'-')
     axis([0 200 0 100])
     xlabel('zg-ir, \mum'); ylabel('uir(z,t), mm hg O_2');
     title('Inner, t=0,5,...,30 s, D=1\times10^{4}\mum^2/s');
     subplot(2,2,2)
     plot(zg_or,uor,'-')
     axis([0 200 0 100])
     xlabel('zg-or, \mum'); ylabel('uor(z,t), mm hg O_2');
     title('Outer, t=0,10,...,30 s, D=1\times10^{4}\mum^2/s');
     subplot(2,2,3)
     plot(zg_fl,ufl,'-')
     axis([0 200 0 100])
     xlabel('zg-fl, \mum'); ylabel('ufl(z,t), mm hg O_2');
     title('Fluid, t=0,10,...,30 s, D=1\times10^{4}\mum^2/s');
     subplot(2,2,4)
     plot(zg_cc,ucc,'-')
     axis([0 200 0 100])
     xlabel('zg-cc, \mum'); ylabel('ucc(z,t), mm hg O_2');
     title('Choroid, t=0,10,...,30 s, D=1\times10^{4}\mum^2/s');
```

Listing 4.1 Main program pde_1_main for the MOL solution of eqs. (4.1) to (4.4)

We can note the following points about Listing 4.1.

- Previous files are cleared and selected variables and parameters are declared global so they can be shared with other routines.

```
%
% Four-section retinal O2 transport model equation
%
% Clear previous files
  clear all
  clc
%
% Model parameters shared with other routines
  global   nir      nor      nfl      ncc...
         zl_ir    zl_or    zl_fl    zl_cc...
         zg_ir    zg_or    zg_fl    zg_cc...
           Dir      Dor      Dfl      Dcc...
                 kir_or   kor_fl   kfl_cc...
           kir      kor      kfl      kcc...
         pir_s    pcc_s    ncall    ncase
```

- Two cases are programmed through ncase for zero and nonzero metabolism rate constants.

```
%
% Select case
%
%   ncase = 1: metabolism rates = 0
```

```
%
%   ncase = 2: metabolism rates ne 0
  ncase=2;
```

- Spatial grids are defined for the four sections of Fig. 4.1 (the resulting variables correspond to Fig. 4.2).

```
%
% Number of grid points
  nir=11; nor=11; nfl=11; ncc=11;
%
% Lengths of four sections (microns)
  zl_ir=200; zl_or=200; zl_fl=200; zl_cc=200;
%
% Spatial grids;
  zg_ir=[0:zl_ir/10:zl_ir]'; zg_or=[0:zl_or/10:zl_or]';
  zg_fl=[0:zl_fl/10:zl_fl]'; zg_cc=[0:zl_cc/10:zl_cc]';
```

Note that each section has 11 grid points (counting the two end points) and is divided into a grid with a spacing $200/10 = 20\,\mu$m (microns).

- The diffusivities of eqs. (4.1) to (4.4) are defined numerically.

```
%
% Diffusivities (microns^2/s)
  Dir=1.0e+04; Dor=1.0e+04; Dfl=1.0e+04; Dcc=1.0e+04;
% Dir=0.1e+04; Dor=0.1e+04; Dfl=0.1e+04; Dcc=0.1e+04;
% Dir=0.5e+04; Dor=0.5e+04; Dfl=0.5e+04; Dcc=0.5e+04;
```

Note that multiple sets of diffusivities are programmed. A particular set is selected by uncommenting the corresponding line. In this case, the first set is used, which serves as the base case for the model (the output for this case is discussed subsequently). The second and third sets correspond to a large reduction in O_2 transport, and a modest reduction, respectively, (the reader can easily activate these sets to observe the effect on the model, that is, the O_2 profiles in the four sections). This variation in the diffusivities demonstrates how a parameter can be investigated. If the parameter is sensitive as in the case of the diffusivities (has a large effect on the model output), further refinement of the numerical values is warranted.

- The interface coefficients in eqs. (4.1d), (4.2d), and (4.3d) are defined numerically.

```
%
% Interface coefficients
  kir_or=1; kor_fl=1; kfl_cc=1;
```

- The metabolism rate constants in eqs. (4.1a), (4.2a), (4.3a), and (4.4a) are defined numerically.

```
%
% Metabolism rates
  if(ncase==1) kir=   0; kor=   0; kfl=   0; kcc=   0; end
  if(ncase==2) kir= 0.1; kor= 0.1; kfl= 0.1; kcc= 0.1; end
```

Note that these constants are nonnegative, so the terms in which they appear are negative (owing to the minus sign) corresponding to a depletion (consumption) of O_2 as expected. Two cases are programmed (`ncase=1,2`) to demonstrate the effect of O_2 metabolism. This approach (by using a control variable such as `ncase`) illustrates a second approach to parametric variation (rather than activating statements as in the case of the diffusivities). Other approaches are commonplace such as a `for` loop, an `if`, a `while` or a `switch` statement.

- The BC O_2 concentrations are defined numerically at $z = z_L, z_{cc}$ (see Fig 4.2).

```
%
% Normal breathing O2 concentration (mm hg)
  pir_s=20;
  pcc_s=100;
```

These are the constants that drive the model response away from the zero ICs (specified subsequently). That is, if the boundary concentrations were zero, the solution of eqs. (4.1) to (4.4) would remain at the zero ICs.

- The interval in t is specified as $0 \le t \le 30$ s with output of the solution at $t = 0, 5, 10, ..., 30$ (seven outputs).

```
%
% Independent variable t
  t0=0.0; tf=3.0e+01; tout=[t0:tf/6:tf]';
  nout=7;
%
% Initial condition
  u0=inital_1(t0);
```

The ICs of eqs. (4.1b), (4.2b), (4.3b), and (4.4b) are set by a call to `inital_1` (discussed subsequently); recall that `t0=0`. Integration of the `nir+nor+nfl+ncc = 11 + 11 + 11 + 11 = 44` ODEs is by `ode15s` (see Section 1.2.3.3 for details about this ODE integrator).

- `ode15s` (with `mf=2`) is called after error tolerances for the numerical integration are specified.

```
%
% ODE integration
  mf=2;
  reltol=1.0e-06; abstol=1.0e-05;
  options=odeset('RelTol',reltol,'AbsTol',abstol);
%
% Explicit (nonstiff) integration
  if(mf==1)[t,u]=ode45(@pde_1,tout,u0,options); end
%
% Implicit (sparse stiff) integration
  if(mf==2)
    S=jpattern_num_1;
%   pause
    options=odeset(options,'JPattern',S)
    [t,u]=ode15s(@pde_1,tout,u0,options);
  end
```

For mf=1, the explicit (nonstiff) integrator ode45 is called. For ode15s, the sparse stiff option is used, which requires a routine jpattern_num_1 to define the ODE Jacobian matrix (discussed subsequently). In both cases (ode45, ode15s), the ODE routine is pde_1 (discussed subsequently). Also, the IC vector u0 passes along to ode45 or ode15s the size of the ODE problem (44 ODEs).

- The ODE solution vector returned by ode45 or ode15s, u, (a 44-vector) is placed in four vectors uir,uor,ufl,ucc corresponding to the dependent variables of eqs. (4.1a), (4.2a), (4.3a), and (4.4a), respectively, to facilitate the subsequent programming of the solution output.

```
%
% One vector to four vectors
  for it=1:nout
    for i=1:nir uir(it,i)=u(it,i);                 end
    for i=1:nor uor(it,i)=u(it,i+nir);             end
    for i=1:nfl ufl(it,i)=u(it,i+nir+nor);         end
    for i=1:ncc ucc(it,i)=u(it,i+nir+nor+nfl); end
    if(it>=2)
        uir(it,1)  =pir_s;
        ucc(it,ncc)=pcc_s;
    end
  end
```

Note that the boundary values $u_{IR}(z = z_L, t) = P_{IR\text{-}S}(t) =$ uir(it,1) and $u_{CC}(z = z_{CC}, t) = P_{CC\text{-}S}(t) =$ ucc(it,ncc) are not computed by the integration of ODEs in the ODE routine pde_1 and therefore are not returned in u. They therefore are set in two separate statements (for BCs (4.1c) and (4.4d)).

- The four vectors are displayed in tabular form.

```
%
%   Display tabulated numerical solution
    for it=1:nout
      fprintf('\n     t       zg_ir     uir(z,t)\n')
      for i=1:nir
        fprintf('%5.2f%10.0f%12.2f\n',t(it),zg_ir(i),uir(it,i))
      end
      fprintf('\n     t       zg_or     uor(z,t)\n')
      for i=1:nor
        fprintf('%5.2f%10.0f%12.2f\n',t(it),zg_or(i),uor(it,i))
      end
      fprintf('\n     t       zg_fl     ufl(z,t)\n')
      for i=1:nfl
        fprintf('%5.2f%10.0f%12.2f\n',t(it),zg_fl(i),ufl(it,i))
      end
      fprintf('\n     t       zg_cc     ucc(z,t)\n')
      for i=1:ncc
        fprintf('%5.2f%10.0f%12.2f\n',t(it),zg_cc(i),ucc(it,i))
      end
%
```

```
%   Next t
    end
    fprintf('\n    ncall = %4d\n',ncall);
```

This output includes the final value of the number of calls to pde_1, ncall, which is a measure of the computational effort required to produce the numerical ODE solution.

- The four dependent variables of eqs. (4.1a), (4.2a), (4.3a), and (4.4a) are displayed in a composite plot (using the subplot utility).

```
%
%   Four plots for uir, uor, ufl, ucc
    figure(2)
    subplot(2,2,1)
    plot(zg_ir,uir,'-')
    axis([0 200 0 100])
    xlabel('zg-ir, \mum'); ylabel('uir(z,t), mm hg O_2');
    title('Inner, t=0,5,...,30 s, D=1\times10^{4}\mum^2/s');
    subplot(2,2,2)
    plot(zg_or,uor,'-')
    axis([0 200 0 100])
    xlabel('zg-or, \mum'); ylabel('uor(z,t), mm hg O_2');
    title('Outer, t=0,10,...,30 s, D=1\times10^{4}\mum^2/s');
    subplot(2,2,3)
    plot(zg_fl,ufl,'-')
    axis([0 200 0 100])
    xlabel('zg-fl, \mum'); ylabel('ufl(z,t), mm hg O_2');
    title('Fluid, t=0,10,...,30 s, D=1\times10^{4}\mum^2/s');
    subplot(2,2,4)
    plot(zg_cc,ucc,'-')
    axis([0 200 0 100])
    xlabel('zg-cc, \mum'); ylabel('ucc(z,t), mm hg O_2');
    title('Choroid, t=0,10,...,30 s, D=1\times10^{4}\mum^2/s');
```

A title for each section subplot is programmed with the title utility.

4.2.2 ODE routine

The ODE routine pde_1 called by ode15s in Listing 4.1 is listed next.

```
  function ut=pde_1(t,u)
%
% Function pde_1 defines the ODEs in the MOL solution of the
% four-section retinal O2 transport model equations
%
% Model parameters
  global    nir      nor      nfl      ncc...
          zl_ir    zl_or    zl_fl    zl_cc...
          zg_ir    zg_or    zg_fl    zg_cc...
            Dir      Dor      Dfl      Dcc...
                   kir_or   kor_fl   kfl_cc...
```

```
        kir     kor     kfl     kcc...
      pir_s   pcc_s   ncall   ncase
%
% One vector to four vectors
  for i=1:nir uir(i)=u(i);                end
  for i=1:nor uor(i)=u(i+nir);            end
  for i=1:nfl ufl(i)=u(i+nir+nor);        end
  for i=1:ncc ucc(i)=u(i+nir+nor+nfl);  end
%
% First order spatial derivatives
  uir_z=dss004(0,zl_ir,nir,uir);
  uor_z=dss004(0,zl_or,nor,uor);
  ufl_z=dss004(0,zl_fl,nfl,ufl);
  ucc_z=dss004(0,zl_cc,ncc,ucc);
%
% BCs
%
%   Inner retina
    uir(1)=pir_s;
    uir(nir)=kir_or*uor(1);
%
%   Outer retina
    uor_z(1)=(Dir/Dor)*uir_z(nir);
    uor(nor)=kor_fl*ufl(1);
%
%   Fluid layer
    ufl_z(1)=(Dor/Dfl)*uor_z(nor);
    ufl(nfl)=kfl_cc*ucc(1);
%
%   Choriocapillaris
    ucc_z(1)=(Dfl/Dcc)*ufl_z(nfl);
    ucc(ncc)=pcc_s;
%
% Second order spatial derivatives
  nl=1; nu=1;
  uir_zz=dss044(0,zl_ir,nir,uir,uir_z,nl,nu);
  nl=2; nu=1;
  uor_zz=dss044(0,zl_or,nor,uor,uor_z,nl,nu);
  ufl_zz=dss044(0,zl_fl,nfl,ufl,ufl_z,nl,nu);
  ucc_zz=dss044(0,zl_cc,ncc,ucc,ucc_z,nl,nu);
%
% PDEs
  uir_t=Dir*uir_zz-kir*uir;
  uor_t=Dor*uor_zz-kor*uor;
  ufl_t=Dfl*ufl_zz-kfl*ufl;
  ucc_t=Dcc*ucc_zz-kcc*ucc;
  uir_t(1)  =0;
  ucc_t(ncc)=0;
%
% Four vectors to one vector
  for i=1:nir ut(i)            =uir_t(i); end
```

```
  for i=1:nor ut(i+nir)        =uor_t(i); end
  for i=1:nfl ut(i+nir+nor)    =ufl_t(i); end
  for i=1:ncc ut(i+nir+nor+nfl)=ucc_t(i); end
  ut=ut';
%
% Increment calls to pde_1
  ncall=ncall+1;
```

Listing 4.2 ODE routine `pde_1` for the MOL solution of eqs. (4.1) to (4.4)

We can note the following points about Listing 4.2.

- The function is defined and selected variables and parameters are declared as global.

```
  function ut=pde_1(t,u)
%
% Function pde_1 defines the ODEs in the MOL solution of the
% four-section retinal O2 transport model equations
%
% Model parameters
  global   nir     nor     nfl     ncc...
         zl_ir   zl_or   zl_fl   zl_cc...
         zg_ir   zg_or   zg_fl   zg_cc...
           Dir     Dor     Dfl     Dcc...
                kir_or  kor_fl  kfl_cc...
           kir     kor     kfl     kcc...
         pir_s   pcc_s   ncall   ncase
```

- The 44-vector u is redefined as four 11-vectors, the dependent variables of eqs. (4.1a), (4.2a), (4.3a), and (4.4a), as `uir,uor,ufl,ucc`.

```
%
% One vector to four vectors
  for i=1:nir uir(i)=u(i);              end
  for i=1:nor uor(i)=u(i+nir);          end
  for i=1:nfl ufl(i)=u(i+nir+nor);      end
  for i=1:ncc ucc(i)=u(i+nir+nor+nfl); end
```

- The first order spatial derivatives in z, $\partial u_{\text{IR}}/\partial z$ = `uir_z`, $\partial u_{\text{OR}}/\partial z$ = `uor_z`, $\partial u_{\text{FL}}/\partial z$ = `ufl_z`, and $\partial u_{\text{CC}}/\partial z$ = `ucc_z`, are computed by `dss004` (discussed in Section 1.2.1, particularly Listing 1.17).

```
%
% First order spatial derivatives
  uir_z=dss004(0,zl_ir,nir,uir);
  uor_z=dss004(0,zl_or,nor,uor);
  ufl_z=dss004(0,zl_fl,nfl,ufl);
  ucc_z=dss004(0,zl_cc,ncc,ucc);
```

- The BCs for eqs. (4.1a), (4.2a), (4.3a), and (4.4a) are programmed, starting with eqs. (4.1c) and (4.1d).

```
%
% BCs
%
%    Inner retina
     uir(1)=pir_s;
     uir(nir)=kir_or*uor(1);
```

$u_{IR}(z = z_L, t)$ = `uir(1)` of BC (4.1c) is programmed (a Dirichlet BC). Alternatively, a Neumann BC could be used, $D_{IR}(\partial u_{IR}(z = z_L, t)/\partial z) = r_{z_{L,IR}}$ where $r_{z_{L,IR}}$ is a prescribed flux for O_2 at the left end of the IR (according to Fourier's or Fick's first law), or a third type (Robin) BC could be used, $D_{IR}(\partial u_{IR}(z = z_L, t)/\partial z) = k_{z_{L,IR}}(P_{IR\text{-}S} - u_{IR}(z = z_L, t))$ where $k_{z_{L,IR}}$ is a prescribed mass transfer coefficient.

Also, $u_{IR}(z = z_{IR}, t) =$ `uir(nir)` of BC (4.1d) is programmed (a Dirichlet BC).

- BCs (4.2c) and (4.2d) are programmed, as a Neumann BC at the left end, $z = z_{IR}$, and a Dirichlet BC at the right end, $z = z_{OR}$.

```
%
%    Outer retina
     uor_z(1)=(Dir/Dor)*uir_z(nir);
     uor(nor)=kor_fl*ufl(1);
```

- Boundary conditions (4.3c) and (4.3d) are programmed as a Neumann BC at the left end, $z = z_{OR}$, and a Dirichlet BC at the right end, $z = z_{FL}$.

```
%
%    Fluid layer
     ufl_z(1)=(Dor/Dfl)*uor_z(nor);
     ufl(nfl)=kfl_cc*ucc(1);
```

- Boundary conditions (4.4c) and (4.4d) are programmed as a Neumann BC at the left end, $z = z_{FL}$, and a Dirichlet BC at the right end, $z = z_{CC}$.

```
%
%    Choriocapillaris
     ucc_z(1)=(Dfl/Dcc)*ufl_z(nfl);
     ucc(ncc)=pcc_s;
```

- The second order spatial derivatives in z, $\partial^2 u_{IR}/\partial z^2 =$ `uir_zz`, $\partial^2 u_{OR}/\partial z^2 =$ `uor_zz`, $\partial u_{FL}^2/\partial z =$ `ufl_zz` and $\partial^2 u_{CC}/\partial z^2 =$ `ucc_zz`, in eqs. (4.1a), (4.2a), (4.3a), and (4.4a), are computed by `dss044` (discussed in Section 1.3, particularly Listing 1.18). Note that for the inner retina, Dirichlet BCs are programmed at $z = z_L, z_{IR}$ (`nl=nu=1` for BCs (4.1c), (4.1d)). For the outer retina, fluid layer and choroid, a Neumann BC is declared at the left end (`nl=2` for BCs (4.2c), (4.3c), (4.3d)), and a Dirichlet BC is declared at the right end, (`nu=1` for BCs (4.2d), (4.3d), (4.4d)).

```
%
% Second order spatial derivatives
  nl=1; nu=1;
  uir_zz=dss044(0,zl_ir,nir,uir,uir_z,nl,nu);
  nl=2; nu=1;
  uor_zz=dss044(0,zl_or,nor,uor,uor_z,nl,nu);
```

```
  ufl_zz=dss044(0,zl_fl,nfl,ufl,ufl_z,nl,nu);
  ucc_zz=dss044(0,zl_cc,ncc,ucc,ucc_z,nl,nu);
```

- With these second derivatives available, PDEs (4.1a), (4.2a), (4.3a) and (4.4a) can be programmed. We can note the following details about the calculation of the second derivatives.
  - For IR, Dirichlet BCs are specified at $z = z_L$ and $z = z_{IR}$, that is `nl=1,nu=1`. This follows from BCs (4.1c) and (4.1d), for which u_{IR} is specified at both boundaries, $z = z_L$ and $z = z_{IR}$.
  - For OR, FL, and CC, a Neumann BC is specified at the left end (`nl=2`), and a Dirichlet BC is specified at the right end (`nu=1`). For example, for OR, BC (4.2c) is Neumann since $\partial u_{OR}(z = z_{IR}, t)/\partial z$ is specified and BC (4.2d) is Dirichlet since $u_{OR}(z = z_{OR}, t)$ is specified.

```
%
% PDEs
  uir_t=Dir*uir_zz-kir*uir;
  uor_t=Dor*uor_zz-kor*uor;
  ufl_t=Dfl*ufl_zz-kfl*ufl;
  ucc_t=Dcc*ucc_zz-kcc*ucc;
  uir_t(1)   =0;
  ucc_t(ncc)=0;
```

Note that the MATLAB vector utility has been used in computing the derivatives in t (the LHS of eqs. (4.1a), (4.2a), (4.3a), and (4.4a)). The PDEs could also be programmed within a `for` loop. Also, the terms for depletion of O_2 due to metabolism in eqs. (4.1a), (4.2a), (4.3a), and (4.4a), i.e., $-k_{IR}u_{IR}$, $-k_{OR}u_{IOR}$, $-k_{FL}u_{FL}$, and $-k_{CC}u_C$, have been included in the coding corresponding to $k_{IR} = k_{OR} = k_{FL} = k_{CC} = 0.1$ (for `ncase=2`). The final statements, `uir_t(1)=0, ucc_t(ncc)=0`, reflect BCs (4.1c) and (4.4d), i.e., the derivatives are set to zero so that the ODE integrator does not move the dependent variables $u_{IR}(z = z_L, t), u_{CC}(z = z_{CC}, t)$ away from the values prescribed by eqs. (4.1c) and (4.4d) (set previously as BCs, `uir(1)=pir_s, ucc(ncc)=pcc_s`).

- The 44 derivatives in t are placed in a single vector, `ut`, that is returned as the LHS output argument of `pde_1`.

```
%
% Four vectors to one vector
  for i=1:nir ut(i)            =uir_t(i); end
  for i=1:nor ut(i+nir)        =uor_t(i); end
  for i=1:nfl ut(i+nir+nor)    =ufl_t(i); end
  for i=1:ncc ut(i+nir+nor+nfl)=ucc_t(i); end
  ut=ut';
%
% Increment calls to pde_1
  ncall=ncall+1;
```

The transpose from a row to a column vector is required by `ode15s`. Finally, the counter for the number of calls to `pde_1` is incremented.

4.2.3 IC routine

The IC routine, inital_1, is listed next.

```
  function u=inital_1(t0)
%
% Function inital_1 is called by the main program to define the
% initial conditions of the four-section retinal O2 transport model
%
% Model parameters
  global   nir      nor      nfl      ncc...
         zl_ir   zl_or    zl_fl    zl_cc...
         zg_ir   zg_or    zg_fl    zg_cc...
           Dir      Dor      Dfl      Dcc...
                 kir_or   kor_fl   kfl_cc...
           kir      kor      kfl      kcc...
         pir_s   pcc_s    ncall    ncase
%
% Initial conditions
%
%    Inner retina
     for i=1:nir
      uir(i)=0;
        u(i)=uir(i);
     end
%
%    Outer retina
     for i=1:nor
       uor(i)=0;
       u(i+nir)=uor(i);
     end
%
%    Fluid layer
     for i=1:nfl
       ufl(i)=0;
       u(i+nir+nor)=ufl(i);
     end
%
%    Choriocapillaris
     for i=1:ncc
       ucc(i)=0;
       u(i+nir+nor+nfl)=ucc(i);
     end
%
% Initialize calls to pde_1
  ncall=0;
```

Listing 4.3 IC routine inital_1 for eqs. (4.1b), (4.2b), (4.3b), and (4.4b)

We can note the following points about Listing 4.3.

- The function is defined and selected variables and parameters are declared global.

```
  function u=inital_1(t0)
%
% Function inital_1 is called by the main program to define the
% initial conditions of the four-section retinal O2 transport model
%
% Model parameters
  global   nir      nor      nfl      ncc...
         zl_ir    zl_or    zl_fl    zl_cc...
         zg_ir    zg_or    zg_fl    zg_cc...
           Dir      Dor      Dfl      Dcc...
                 kir_or   kor_fl   kfl_cc...
           kir      kor      kfl      kcc...
         pir_s    pcc_s    ncall    ncase
```

The RHS argument is the current value of t from `pde_1_main`, which is `t0=0` for the ICs. The LHS is the 44-vector of initial values, u, for eqs. (4.1b), (4.2b), (4.3b), and (4.4b).

- The ICs are programmed as a series of `for` loops. For example, eq. (4.1b) is programmed as

```
%
% Initial conditions
%
%    Inner retina
     for i=1:nir
      uir(i)=0;
        u(i)=uir(i);
     end
```

The MATLAB vector utility could have been used in place of the `for` loop. Also, the initial value is zero (initially the O_2 concentration in the IR is zero), but this could be set to any initial distribution in z according to $f_{IR}(z)$ of eq. (4.1b).

- Similarly, the ICs for OR, FL, and CC are programmed as

```
%
%    Outer retina
     for i=1:nor
       uor(i)=0;
       u(i+nir)=uor(i);
     end
%
%    Fluid layer
     for i=1:nfl
       ufl(i)=0;
       u(i+nir+nor)=ufl(i);
     end
%
%    Choriocapillaris
     for i=1:ncc
       ucc(i)=0;
       u(i+nir+nor+nfl)=ucc(i);
     end
```

```
%
% Initialize calls to pde_1
  ncall=0;
```

Again, all of the initial O_2 concentrations are zero, but the functions $f_{OR}(z), f_{FL}(z)$, and $f_{IR}(z)$ in eqs. (4.2b), (4.3b), and (4.4b) could have been generalized to any initial distributions in z. Finally, the counter for the calls to `pde_1` is initialized.

This discussion suggests some additional points about ICs and related modeling details:

- Initial conditions are required for time-dependent PDEs such as eqs. (4.1a), (4.2a), (4.3a), (4.4a) (because of the derivatives in t). In physical applications, a realistic IC may not be apparent. For example, in the case of eqs. (4.1a), (4.2a), (4.3a), (4.4a), homogeneous (zero) ICs (4.1b), (4.2b), (4.3b), (4.4b) were selected, which is probably not realistic physically; that is, the O_2 concentration is unlikely to be zero throughout the four sections. However, we need to use some ICs to fill the requirement for eqs. (4.1a), (4.2a), (4.3a), (4.4a).
- Starting with the homogeneous ICs of eqs. (4.1b), (4.2b), (4.3b), (4.4b), we can observe how the solution evolves to a steady-state or equilibrium condition that could be realistic physically. This steady-state solution could be considered a normal condition for O_2 diffusion; then we could impose a change, e.g., in the boundary O_2 concentration, $P_{CC\text{-}S}$, at $z = z_{cc}$ of BC (4.4d) and observe how the solution responds to the change (departs from the steady state). Physically, a change in $P_{CC\text{-}S}$ might represent an abnormal condition, such as a reduction in the blood supply. We would then observe the effect of this nonnormal condition on the O_2 spatial distributions throughout the four sections ($P_{IR}, P_{OR}, P_{FL}, P_{CC}$ as a function of x and t).
- The BCs, eqs. (4.1c) and (4.4d), can be considered as forcing functions that move the four section concentrations away from their nominal (normal) steady-state values. For example, after integrating the PDE system to a steady state corresponding to BC (4.4d) $P_{CC\text{-}S} = 100$, this boundary value could be changed to $P_{CC\text{-}S} = 50$, (a 50% reduction in choroidal O_2 supply) and the effect on the solution could be observed. Alternatively, the O_2 concentrations of BCs (4.1c) and (4.4d) could be reduced simultaneously to observe the combined effect of these changes. This discussion gives some idea of the numerical experiments that can easily be carried out once the PDE model is running numerically.
- Integration in t is an open-ended process over the interval (for example) $0 \le t < \infty$. This is basically why t is termed an initial value variable (it starts at $t = 0$ and proceeds indefinitely for $t > 0$).
- Practically, we can integrate the PDEs forward in t for any period of time (seconds, minutes, hours, days, etc.) as long as the numerical solution remains stable and reasonably accurate.
- The numerical solution will be computed as a function of t (and z) where time has the units corresponding to the parameters (constants) in the model equations. For

example, in the main program of Listing 4.1, the diffusivities have the time units of seconds (s),

```
%
% Diffusivities (microns^2/s)
  Dir=1.0e+04; Dor=1.0e+04; Dfl=1.0e+04; Dcc=1.0e+04;
% Dir=0.1e+04; Dor=0.1e+04; Dfl=0.1e+04; Dcc=0.1e+04;
% Dir=0.5e+04; Dor=0.5e+04; Dfl=0.5e+04; Dcc=0.5e+04;
```

and therefore the solution will be in seconds. This presupposes that all of the parameters will be in seconds, including the rate constants

```
%
% Metabolism rates
  if(ncase==1) kir=   0; kor=   0; kfl=   0; kcc=   0; end
  if(ncase==2) kir= 0.1; kor= 0.1; kfl= 0.1; kcc= 0.1; end
```

If the parameters are not all consistent with respect to units, e.g., s for t, μm (microns for z), the computed solution will be meaningless (incorrect).

- The ICs of eqs. (4.1b) and (4.4b), and the BCs of eqs. (4.1c) and (4.4d) might be inconsistent. For example, for the ICs

$$P_{\mathrm{IR}}(z=z_{\mathrm{L}},t=0)=0;\ P_{\mathrm{CC}}(z=z_{\mathrm{CC}},t=0)=0,$$

while for the BCs

$$P_{\mathrm{IR}}(z=z_{\mathrm{L}},t>0)=20;\ P_{\mathrm{CC}}(z=z_{\mathrm{CC}},t>0)=100.$$

In other words, there is a discontinuous change (step, discontinuity) in the O_2 concentration at the boundaries. This step may cause a problem numerically (e.g., the numerical solution might exhibit unrealistic oscillations). Whether this happens depends mainly on the form of the PDEs. In the case of eqs. (4.1a) to (4.1d), a discontinuity at the boundaries does not cause a problem since these PDEs are parabolic (first order in t and second order in z). Physically, parabolic equations model diffusion, which tends to smooth (diffuse away) discontinuities (in contrast with hyperbolic PDEs, which tend to propagate discontinuities and the associated numerical distortions).

- The time scale was selected in the main program of Listing 4.1 as

```
%
% Independent variable t
  t0=0.0; tf=3.0e+01; tout=[t0:tf/6:tf]';
  nout=7;
```

that is, $0 \le t \le 30$ s with solution output at $t = 0, 5, ..., 30$. This time scale was selected to demonstrate how the numerical solution moves to a steady-state condition (no further changes in t). If the t scale is selected much shorter than over 30 s, the solution will appear to remain at the IC. If the t scale is selected much greater than over 30 s, the solution will appear to move instantaneously from the IC to the final equilibrium solution. Thus, some judgement (possibly by trial and error) is required in selecting the time scale according to the rate of response of the solution.

– As a related item, the scale in z is defined by

```
%
% Lengths of four sections (microns)
  zl_ir=200; zl_or=200; zl_fl=200; zl_cc=200;
%
% Spatial grids;
  zg_ir=[0:zl_ir/10:zl_ir]'; zg_or=[0:zl_or/10:zl_or]';
  zg_fl=[0:zl_fl/10:zl_fl]'; zg_cc=[0:zl_cc/10:zl_cc]';
```

The use of 11 grid points in each of the four sections is a compromise between reasonable accuracy in z (setting a lower limit on the number of points) and reasonable computational effort (setting an upper limit on the number of points). Fortunately, because eqs. (4.1a), (4.2a), (4.3a), and (4.4a) are parabolic, they tend to smooth the solutions and a modest number of grid points (11) is sufficient for each section. This smoothness is apparent in the plotted solutions discussed subsequently.

These additional considerations indicate that the formulation of a PDE model requires attention to details such as time and space scales, with units defined by the parameters of the PDE model.

4.2.4 Sparse matrix routine

A portion of the ODE sparsity routine, `jpattern_num_1`, is given in Listing 4.4.

```
  function S=jpattern_num_1
%
  global   nir     nor     nfl     ncc
%
        .                    .
        .                    .
        .                    .
  for i=1:nir+nor+nfl+ncc
    ybase(i)=0.5;
  end
        .                    .
        .                    .
        .                    .
   ytbase=pde_1(tbase,ybase);
  fac=[];
  thresh=1e-16;
  vectorized='on';
  [Jac,fac]=numjac(@pde_1,tbase,ybase,ytbase,thresh,fac,vectorized);
        .                    .
        .                    .
        .                    .
```

Listing 4.4 Sparsity routine `jpattern_num_1` called by `ode15s` in `pde_1_main`

We can note the following details about this code.

- A `for` loop is programmed with an upper limit `nir+nor+nfl+ncc`, corresponding to the 44 ODEs used in the MOL approximation of eqs. (4.1) to (4.4)

```
for i=1:nir+nor+nfl+ncc
```

- The ODE routine, `pde_1`, is called in two places.

These are the details in `jpattern_num_1` pertaining specifically to eqs. (4.1) to (4.4). Execution of `jpattern_num_1` produces the Jacobian map discussed subsequently (Fig. 4.3).

This completes the programming of eqs. (4.1), (4.2), (4.3), and (4.4). We now consider the numerical and graphical output produced by the routines of Listings 4.1, 4.2, 4.3, and 4.4. Selected numerical output is given in Table 4.2.

4.3 Base case output

The output from the routines in Listings 4.1 to 4.4 is now discussed for `ncase=2`. We will consider this as a base case since extensions to the model will be considered subsequently. Abbreviated numerical output follows in Table 4.2.
We can note the following details about the solution in Table 4.2.

- The list of features of the ODE Jacobian (from `jpattern_num_1`) indicates a 44×44 matrix as expected for the 44 ODEs. Also, the error tolerances for the ODE integrator are `reltol = ` 10^{-6}, `abstol = ` 10^{-5} (set in `pde_1_main`). These tolerances were set by trial and error to be small enough that further reductions did not change the solution appreciably, but not so small that the computational effort becomes excessive (because the integration interval is excessively small to meet the more stringent tolerances).
- The homogeneous (zero) ICs set in `inital_1` of Listing 4.3 are correct (always a good check).
- The O_2 from the zero ICs redistributes at subsequent t. This entire process is driven by $P_{\text{IR-S}}(t) = 20, P_{\text{CC-S}}(t) = 100$ set as BCs (4.1c) and (4.4d) in `pde_1`. As a check on the coding, if the homogeneous (zero) BCs $P_{\text{IR-S}}(t) = 0, P_{\text{CC-S}}(t) = 0$ are used, all 44 values of the O_2 concentration remain at zero. While this may seem like a trivial check, it is worth making; if any of the concentrations depart from zero, we would know that an error in the programming must be corrected (which would most probably be in `pde_1`, where an error can easily be made).
- The computational effort is modest (`ncall = 304`), which reflects the computational efficiency of `ode15s`.

The graphical output appears in Figs. 4.3 and 4.4. The Jacobian map in Fig. 4.3 reflects the four sections of the model.

- Only 11.983% of the elements are nonzero, indicating that the sparse utility of `ode15s` is used to good advantage (and this number would be smaller (greater sparsity) if more grid points in z are used (>44) to improve the accuracy of the numerical solution).

- The nonzero elements of the Jacobian matrix appear down a diagonal of the map. In particular, the four sections of the PDE model are evident.
- Within each section, a row typically has five nonzero elements (a pentadiagonal structure). This appearance of five elements results from the five point finite difference (FD) approximations used in dss044 called by pde_1 of Listing 4.2. Specifically,

Table 4.2. Abbreviated output from the routines of Listings 4.1 to 4.4 for ncase=2

```
options =

              AbsTol: 1.0000e-005
                 BDF: []
              Events: []
         InitialStep: []
            Jacobian: []
           JConstant: []
            JPattern: [44x44 double]
                Mass: []
        MassConstant: []
        MassSingular: []
            MaxOrder: []
             MaxStep: []
         NonNegative: []
         NormControl: []
           OutputFcn: []
           OutputSel: []
              Refine: []
              RelTol: 1.0000e-006
               Stats: []
          Vectorized: []
    MStateDependence: []
           MvPattern: []
        InitialSlope: []


     t      zg_ir    uir(z,t)
  0.00          0        0.00
  0.00         20        0.00
  0.00         40        0.00
  0.00         60        0.00
  0.00         80        0.00
  0.00        100        0.00
  0.00        120        0.00
  0.00        140        0.00
  0.00        160        0.00
  0.00        180        0.00
  0.00        200        0.00
```

```
     t      zg_or    uor(z,t)
  0.00          0        0.00
  0.00         20        0.00
  0.00         40        0.00
  0.00         60        0.00
  0.00         80        0.00
  0.00        100        0.00
  0.00        120        0.00
  0.00        140        0.00
  0.00        160        0.00
  0.00        180        0.00
  0.00        200        0.00

     t      zg_fl    ufl(z,t)
  0.00          0        0.00
  0.00         20        0.00
  0.00         40        0.00
  0.00         60        0.00
  0.00         80        0.00
  0.00        100        0.00
  0.00        120        0.00
  0.00        140        0.00
  0.00        160        0.00
  0.00        180        0.00
  0.00        200        0.00

     t      zg_cc    ucc(z,t)
  0.00          0        0.00
  0.00         20        0.00
  0.00         40        0.00
  0.00         60        0.00
  0.00         80        0.00
  0.00        100        0.00
  0.00        120        0.00
  0.00        140        0.00
  0.00        160        0.00
  0.00        180        0.00
  0.00        200        0.00
            .          .
            .          .
            .          .
  Output for t = 5,10,15,20,25
           removed
            .          .
            .          .
            .          .
     t      zg_ir    uir(z,t)
 30.00          0       20.00
 30.00         20       19.78
 30.00         40       19.63
 30.00         60       19.56
```

```
   30.00          80          19.57
   30.00         100          19.66
   30.00         120          19.83
   30.00         140          20.08
   30.00         160          20.41
   30.00         180          20.82
   30.00         200          21.31

       t       zg_or       uor(z,t)
   30.00           0          21.32
   30.00          20          21.89
   30.00          40          22.55
   30.00          60          23.31
   30.00          80          24.16
   30.00         100          25.10
   30.00         120          26.14
   30.00         140          27.29
   30.00         160          28.55
   30.00         180          29.93
   30.00         200          31.42

       t       zg_fl       ufl(z,t)
   30.00           0          31.42
   30.00          20          33.03
   30.00          40          34.78
   30.00          60          36.67
   30.00          80          38.70
   30.00         100          40.89
   30.00         120          43.24
   30.00         140          45.77
   30.00         160          48.48
   30.00         180          51.38
   30.00         200          54.48

       t       zg_cc       ucc(z,t)
   30.00           0          54.49
   30.00          20          57.80
   30.00          40          61.35
   30.00          60          65.15
   30.00          80          69.20
   30.00         100          73.53
   30.00         120          78.16
   30.00         140          83.10
   30.00         160          88.37
   30.00         180          94.00
   30.00         200         100.00

       ncall =   304
```

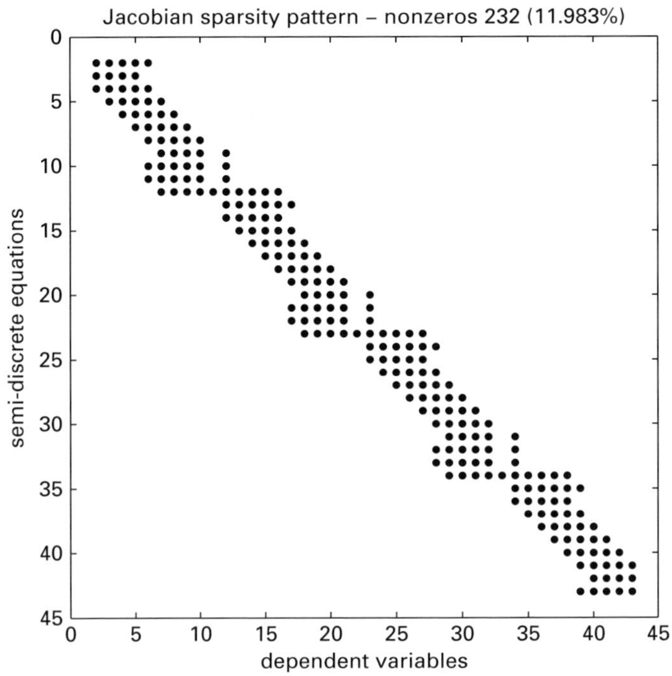

Figure 4.3 Map of the 44-ODE system for `ncase=2`

the second order, spatial derivatives in z of eqs. (4.1a), (4.2a), (4.3a), and (4.4a) are approximated with five point FD approximations.

We can note the following details of the Jacobian map.

- To elaborate a bit further, any given row in the map of Fig. 4.3 corresponds to one of the 44 ODEs integrated by `ode15s` (note the vertical axis has an index running from 1 to 44; the 0 and 45 end values result from the plotting software and have no relevance to the map or ODE system). The nonzero elements in a row indicate the RHS of the corresponding ODE is a function of the dependent variables identified along the horizontal axis (that is, 44 dependent variables, $u_1, u_2, ..., u_{44}$). For example, the first row (top left corner, Fig. 4.3) indicates an ODE of the form

$$\frac{\mathrm{d}u_2}{\mathrm{d}t} = f_2(u_2, u_3, u_4, u_5, u_6).$$

This example indicates that generally an ODE derivative (e.g., $\mathrm{d}u_2/\mathrm{d}t$) depends on only a relatively small number of dependent variables, (e.g., u_2, u_3, u_4, u_5, u_6) and not the full set of 44 dependent variables. This dependency on a small number of dependent variables is the reason for the banded structure in Fig. 4.3 and the relatively large number of zero elements.

Note also that the ODE for $\mathrm{d}u_1/\mathrm{d}t$ does not appear in the map since u_1 is set as a constant ($u(z = z_L, t) = P_{\text{IR-S}} = 20$) according to BC (4.1c) and is therefore not set by an ODE.

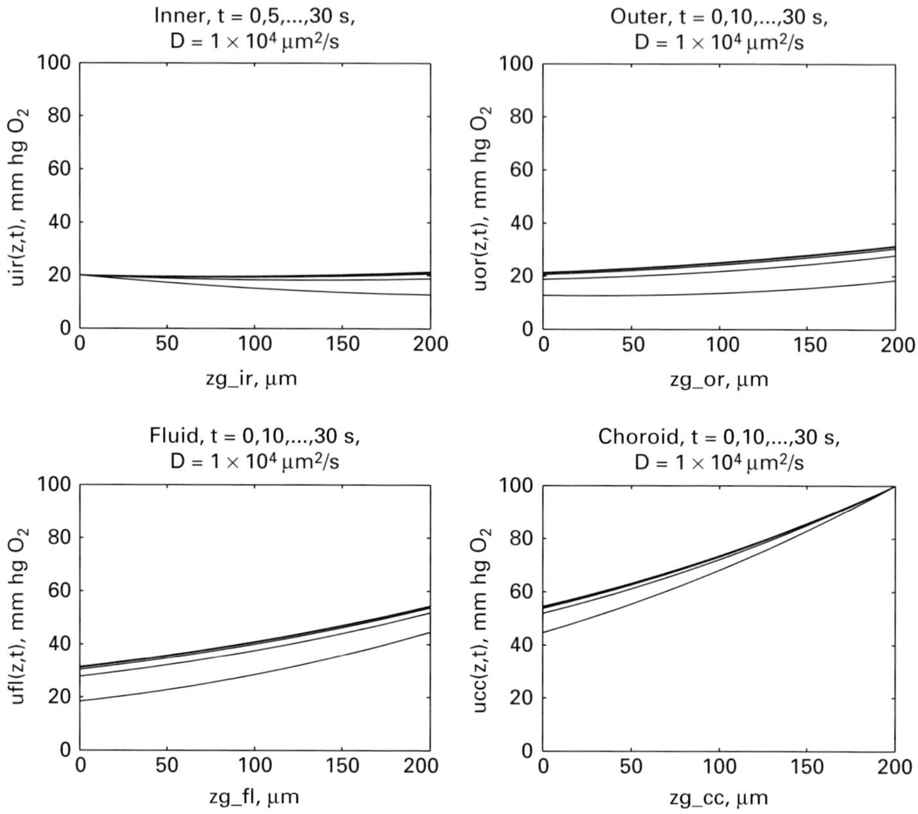

Figure 4.4 O_2 z distribution in IC, OC, FL, CC, `ncase` = 2, t=0,5,...,30 s (bottom to top)

As another example, the fifth row corresponds to an ODE of the form

$$\frac{du_5}{dt} = f_5(u_3, u_4, u_5, u_6, u_7).$$

In this case, the FD approximation of the second derivative in z, ($\partial^2 U_{IR}/\partial z^2$ in eq. (4.1a)) is centered about the value u_5.

- The situation at the interfaces between the four sections is somewhat more complicated (as programmed in `pde_1`). This additional detail results from the FD approximations of the PDEs at the interfaces in combination with the associated BCs (eqs. (4.1d), (4.2c), (4.2d), (4.3c), (4.3d), (4.4c)).

In summary, the ODE Jacobian map gives a picture of the overall structure of the MOL approximation of the PDE system.

The redistribution O_2 with increasing t can be appreciated by consideration of Fig. 4.4. We can note the following details about Fig. 4.4.

- The O_2 concentration starts at zero at $t = 0$ as expected (programmed in `inital_1` of Listing 4.3).

- $P_{\text{IR-S}}(t) = 20, P_{\text{CC-S}}(t) = 100$ set as BCs (4.1c),(4.4d) at $z = z_L, z = z_{CC}$ is clear.
- The O_2 profiles in IR, OR, FL, CC approach a steady state by $t = 30$ s (no further change with increasing t).
- The solutions "connect" from one section to the two adjacent sections as a consequence of BCs (4.1d), (4.2d), (4.3d) with unit interface coefficients, that is, $k_{\text{IR-OR}} = k_{\text{OR-FL}} = k_{\text{FL-CC}} = 1$. Also, the slopes at these interfaces are the same as a consequence of BCs (4.2c), (4.3c), and (4.4c) with unit values of the ratios of the diffusivities, that is, $D_{IR}/D_{OR} = D_{OR}/D_{FL} = D_{FL}/D_{CC} = 1$.

The effect of metabolism (normal O_2 consumption) could be investigated by comparing the solutions for `ncase=1` and `ncase=2`. We will not consider these two cases further, but rather, we now consider the extension of the basic model by adding PDEs.

4.4 Model including photoreceptor cell density

The preceding model of eqs. (4.1) to (4.4), and the associated MATLAB routines of Listings 4.1 to 4.4, can be considered as a base case starting point for further investigations. We will now illustrate the use of this base case to investigate hypotheses (concepts, scenarios) that might be proposed concerning the modeled system, in this case, the four-section system of Fig. 4.1. As a first example, we hypothesize that if the O_2 concentration falls below a critical value, the photoreceptor cells (rods and cones) in the outer segment will begin to fail (as a result of insufficient O_2 or hypoxia).

To model this situation we add a PDE for the photoreceptor cell density in the outer retina, designated as $u_{2,OR}$.

$$\frac{\partial u_{2,OR}}{\partial t} = 0, \; u_{1,OR} \geq u_{1,ORt}, \; z_{IR} \leq z \leq z_{OR}, \tag{4.5a}$$

$$\frac{\partial u_{2,OR}}{\partial t} = -k_{2,OR}(u_{1,ORt} - u_{1,OR}), \; u_{1,OR} < u_{1,ORt}, \; z_{IR} \leq z \leq z_{OR}, \tag{4.5b}$$

$$u_{2,OR}(z, t = 0) = u_{2,ORn}. \tag{4.5c}$$

Equations (4.5) require some additional explanation.

- Cell density is designated with a subscript 2, $u_{2,OR}$, since it is a second PDE-dependent variable. The first dependent variable is the O_2 concentration in eqs. (4.1) to (4.4), which will now be changed from u to u_1 (with an additional designation of the section, so that, for example, u_{OR} becomes $u_{1,OR}$). This procedure illustrates the naming required as dependent variables, and their associated PDEs, are added. By convention, we use u to designate a PDE-dependent variable, with an associated number, e.g., u_1.
- The PDE is stated in two parts, eqs. (4.5a) and (4.5b). For eq. (4.5a), the OR O_2 concentration $u_{1,OR}$ is at or above a critical or threshold value, $u_{1,ORt}$, so the cell density does not change (sufficient O_2 is available to maintain the photoreceptor cells). For eq. (4.5b), the OR O_2 concentration $u_{1,OR}$ is below the critical value, $u_{1,ORt}$, so the cell

Table 4.3. Variables and parameters of eqs. (4.5)

Variable	Interpretation and units
$u_{1,OR}$	OR O_2 concentration (mm Hg)
$u_{2,OR}$	OR photoreceptor cell density (cells/cm^2)
z	position in OR (μm)
t	time (s)
$u_{1,ORn}$	OR O_2 IC concentration (mm Hg)
$k_{2,OR}$	rate constant for OR photoreceptor cell density (cells/cm^2 s mm Hg)
$u_{2,ORt}$	threshold OR O_2 concentration (mm Hg)

density decreases as photoreceptor cells begin to fail (insufficient O_2 is available to maintain the photoreceptor cells). The switch between eqs. (4.5a) and (4.5b) is easily accomplished numerically in the ODE routine pde_1 discussed subsequently.

- Equation (4.5b) does not have a diffusion term (the photoreceptor cells are considered as fixed in space z (in the outer retina, OR), but a diffusion term to model their movement could be included as in eq. (4.2a)). Therefore, BCs are not required for eq. (4.5b). This step suggests that as a hypothesis or concept is considered mathematically, assumptions are inherently part of the process, in this case, no cell movement. In other words, mathematical models are based on a set of assumptions that should be kept in mind when the model is used, and the output is interpreted.
- The IC of eq. (4.5c) is required for the derivative $\partial u_{2,OR}/\partial t$ of eqs. (4.5a) and (4.5b). $u_{2,ORn}$ is a normal cell density, which is taken as 10^6 cells/cm^2. Note that this is an area density (based on cm^2); it could just as well be a volume density with units cells/cm^3.
- The rate of change of the cell density, $\partial u_{2,OR}/\partial t$, from eqs. (4.5a) and (4.5b) equals $-k_{2,OR}(u_{1,ORt} - u_{1,OR})$, where $k_{2,OR}$ is a rate constant for u_2 and $u_{1,ORt}$ is the threshold value of $u_{1,OR}$, as mentioned. Note that $k_{2,OR} \geq 0$ but the minus in the RHS of eq. (4.5b) ensures a decrease in cell density when $u_{1,OR} < u_{1,ORt}$. $k_{2,OR}$ and $u_{1,ORt}$ are important parameters that can be varied in the MATLAB main program to elucidate their effects.

The variables and parameters in eqs. (4.5) are further reiterated in Table 4.3.

Note that the units of these variables and parameters are consistent with those of eqs. (4.1) to (4.4).

4.4.1 ODE routine

The ODE routine is a straightforward extension of pde_1 in Listing 4.2.

```
  function ut=pde_1(t,u)
%
% Function pde_1 defines the ODEs in the MOL solution of the
% four-section retinal O2 transport model equations
%
% Model parameters
```

```
  global  nir     nor     nfl     ncc...
         zl_ir   zl_or   zl_fl   zl_cc...
         zg_ir   zg_or   zg_fl   zg_cc...
          D1ir    D1or    D1fl    D1cc...
               k1ir_or k1or_fl k1fl_cc...
          k1ir    k1or    k1fl    k1cc...
         u1ort    k2or                ...
         pir_s   pcc_s   ncall   ncase      nt
%
% One vector to five vectors
%
%   u1
    for i=1:nir u1ir(i)=u(i);                 end
    for i=1:nor u1or(i)=u(i+nir);             end
    for i=1:nfl u1fl(i)=u(i+nir+nor);         end
    for i=1:ncc u1cc(i)=u(i+nir+nor+nfl);     end
%
%   u2
    for i=1:nor u2or(i)=u(nt+i);              end
%
% First order spatial derivatives, u1
  u1ir_z=dss004(0,zl_ir,nir,u1ir);
  u1or_z=dss004(0,zl_or,nor,u1or);
  u1fl_z=dss004(0,zl_fl,nfl,u1fl);
  u1cc_z=dss004(0,zl_cc,ncc,u1cc);
%
% BCs, u1
%
%   Inner retina
    u1ir(1)=pir_s;
    u1ir(nir)=k1ir_or*u1or(1);
%
%   Outer retina
    u1or_z(1)=(D1ir/D1or)*u1ir_z(nir);
    u1or(nor)=k1or_fl*u1fl(1);
%
%   Fluid layer
    u1fl_z(1)=(D1or/D1fl)*u1or_z(nor);
    u1fl(nfl)=k1fl_cc*u1cc(1);
%
%   Choriocapillaris
    u1cc_z(1)=(D1fl/D1cc)*u1fl_z(nfl);
    if(ncase==1)u1cc(ncc)=pcc_s;    end
    if(ncase==2)u1cc(ncc)=0.1*pcc_s;end
%
% Second order spatial derivatives, u1
  nl1=1; nu1=1;
  u1ir_zz=dss044(0,zl_ir,nir,u1ir,u1ir_z,nl1,nu1);
  nl1=2; nu1=1;
  u1or_zz=dss044(0,zl_or,nor,u1or,u1or_z,nl1,nu1);
  u1fl_zz=dss044(0,zl_fl,nfl,u1fl,u1fl_z,nl1,nu1);
```

```
  u1cc_zz=dss044(0,zl_cc,ncc,u1cc,u1cc_z,nl1,nu1);
%
% PDEs
%
%   u1
    u1ir_t=D1ir*u1ir_zz-k1ir*u1ir;
    u1or_t=D1or*u1or_zz-k1or*u1or;
    u1fl_t=D1fl*u1fl_zz-k1fl*u1fl;
    u1cc_t=D1cc*u1cc_zz-k1cc*u1cc;
    u1ir_t(1)  =0;
    u1cc_t(ncc)=0;
%
%   u2
    for i=1:nor
      if(u1or(i)>=u1ort)
        u2or_t(i)=0;
      else
        u2or_t(i)=-k2or*(u1ort-u1or(i));
      end
    end
%
% Five vectors to one vector
%
%   u1
    for i=1:nir ut(i)                =u1ir_t(i); end
    for i=1:nor ut(i+nir)            =u1or_t(i); end
    for i=1:nfl ut(i+nir+nor)        =u1fl_t(i); end
    for i=1:ncc ut(i+nir+nor+nfl)    =u1cc_t(i); end
%
%   u2
    for i=1:nor ut(nt+i)             =u2or_t(i); end
  ut=ut';
%
% Increment calls to pde_1
  ncall=ncall+1;
```

Listing 4.5 ODE routine pde_1 for the MOL solution of eqs. (4.1) to (4.5) including photoreceptor cell density

We can note the following points about Listing 4.5, primarily as departures from Listing 4.2.

- The function pde_1 is defined and selected variables and parameters are declared as global. Again nt=nio+nor+nfl+ncc=11+11+11+11=44 is set in the main program discussed subsequently.
- Equations (4.5a) and (4.5b) are added to the previous PDEs, eqs. (4.1a) to (4.4a) (u_2 is added to u_1).

```
%
% One vector to five vectors
%
```

```
%    u1
     for i=1:nir u1ir(i)=u(i);                  end
     for i=1:nor u1or(i)=u(i+nir);              end
     for i=1:nfl u1fl(i)=u(i+nir+nor);          end
     for i=1:ncc u1cc(i)=u(i+nir+nor+nfl);      end
%
%    u2
     for i=1:nor u2or(i)=u(nt+i);               end
```

Note that eqs. (4.5a) and (4.5b) with dependent variable u2or are defined only in the OR since we assume photoreceptor cells are only in the OR. Thus, the total number of ODEs is nt+nor =44+11=55.

- The first and second derivatives of u_1 in z with BCs are handled the same way as in Listing 4.2 (eqs. (4.5a) and (4.5b) do not require these calculations since they do not have a second derivative in z for diffusion).

```
%
% First order spatial derivatives, u1
  u1ir_z=dss004(0,zl_ir,nir,u1ir);
  u1or_z=dss004(0,zl_or,nor,u1or);
  u1fl_z=dss004(0,zl_fl,nfl,u1fl);
  u1cc_z=dss004(0,zl_cc,ncc,u1cc);
%
% BCs, u1
%
%    Inner retina
     u1ir(1)=pir_s;
     u1ir(nir)=k1ir_or*u1or(1);
%
%    Outer retina
     u1or_z(1)=(D1ir/D1or)*u1ir_z(nir);
     u1or(nor)=k1or_fl*u1fl(1);
%
%    Fluid layer
     u1fl_z(1)=(D1or/D1fl)*u1or_z(nor);
     u1fl(nfl)=k1fl_cc*u1cc(1);
%
%    Choriocapillaris
     u1cc_z(1)=(D1fl/D1cc)*u1fl_z(nfl);
     if(ncase==1)u1cc(ncc)=pcc_s;     end
     if(ncase==2)u1cc(ncc)=0.1*pcc_s;end
%
% Second order spatial derivatives, u1
  nl1=1; nu1=1;
  u1ir_zz=dss044(0,zl_ir,nir,u1ir,u1ir_z,nl1,nu1);
  nl1=2; nu1=1;
  u1or_zz=dss044(0,zl_or,nor,u1or,u1or_z,nl1,nu1);
  u1fl_zz=dss044(0,zl_fl,nfl,u1fl,u1fl_z,nl1,nu1);
  u1cc_zz=dss044(0,zl_cc,ncc,u1cc,u1cc_z,nl1,nu1);
```

In the CC, two cases are programmed.

– ncase=1 corresponds to a normal condition in which the CC right boundary ($z = z_{CC}$) is at O_2 concentration $u_{1,CC} = P_{CC\text{-}S} = 100$.
– ncase=2 corresponds to an abnormal condition in which the CC right boundary ($z = z_{CC}$) is at O_2 concentration $u_{1,CC} = 0.1P_{CC\text{-}S} = (0.1)(100) = 10$. This could represent a condition of seriously interrupted blood supply.

- The five PDEs, eqs. (4.1a) to (4.5a), are programmed.

```
%
% PDEs
%
%   u1
    u1ir_t=D1ir*u1ir_zz-k1ir*u1ir;
    u1or_t=D1or*u1or_zz-k1or*u1or;
    u1fl_t=D1fl*u1fl_zz-k1fl*u1fl;
    u1cc_t=D1cc*u1cc_zz-k1cc*u1cc;
    u1ir_t(1)  =0;
    u1cc_t(ncc)=0;
%
%   u2
    for i=1:nor
      if(u1or(i)>=u1ort)
        u2or_t(i)=0;
      else
        u2or_t(i)=-k2or*(u1ort-u1or(i));
      end
    end
```

The O_2 depletion is included as the second RHS terms in eqs. (4.1a) to (4.4a) (based on the rate constants `k1ir,k1or,k1fl,k1cc`). The programming for `u2` as eqs. (4.5a) and (4.5b) is done with an `if`. Again, the total number of ODEs, with derivatives in t and denoted with `_t` in the LHS variable names, is now `nir+2nor+nfl+ncc = 11+(2)(11)+11+11=55` (11 additional ODEs in OR for u_2).

- The five derivative vectors in t are placed in a single vector `ut` of length `nt + nor = 55`.

```
%
% Five vectors to one vector
%
%   u1
    for i=1:nir ut(i)               =u1ir_t(i); end
    for i=1:nor ut(i+nir)           =u1or_t(i); end
    for i=1:nfl ut(i+nir+nor)       =u1fl_t(i); end
    for i=1:ncc ut(i+nir+nor+nfl)   =u1cc_t(i); end
%
%   u2
    for i=1:nor ut(nt+i)            =u2or_t(i); end
  ut=ut';
%
% Increment calls to pde_1
  ncall=ncall+1;
```

The usual transpose (required for ode15s to receive a column vector of derivatives) and incrementing of the number of calls to pde_1 conclude pde_1.

In summary, the pde_1 of Listing 4.5 demonstrates the use of simultaneous or coupled PDEs (in u1 and u2); this is an important concept in developing PDE models. Also, we have demonstrated how a PDE is added to just one section (rather than all four).

4.4.2 Main program

The main program of Listing 4.6 is a straightforward extension of pde_1_main in Listing 4.1.

```
%
% Four-section retinal O2 transport model equation
%
% Clear previous files
  clear all
  clc
%
% Model parameters shared with other routines
%
% Model parameters
  global    nir      nor      nfl      ncc...
          zl_ir    zl_or    zl_fl    zl_cc...
          zg_ir    zg_or    zg_fl    zg_cc...
           D1ir     D1or     D1fl     D1cc...
                k1ir_or k1or_fl k1fl_cc...
           k1ir     k1or     k1fl     k1cc...
          u1ort     k2or                ...
          pir_s    pcc_s    ncall    ncase       nt
%
% Select case
%
%   ncase = 1: Normal O2 at z=z_cc
%
%   ncase = 2: Reduced O2 at z=z_cc
  ncase=2;
%
% Number of grid points
  nir=11; nor=11; nfl=11; ncc=11;
  nt=nir+nor+nfl+ncc;
%
% Lengths of four sections (microns)
  zl_ir=200; zl_or=200; zl_fl=200; zl_cc=200;
%
% Spatial grids;
  zg_ir=[0:zl_ir/10:zl_ir]'; zg_or=[0:zl_or/10:zl_or]';
  zg_fl=[0:zl_fl/10:zl_fl]'; zg_cc=[0:zl_cc/10:zl_cc]';
%
% Diffusivities (microns^2/s)
  D1ir=1.0e+04; D1or=1.0e+04; D1fl=1.0e+04; D1cc=1.0e+04;
```

```
%
% Interface coefficients
  kb_ir=1; k1ir_or=1; k1or_fl=1; k1fl_cc=1;
%
% Metabolism rates
  k1ir=0.1; k1or=0.1; k1fl=0.1; k1cc=0.1;
%
% Photoreceptor rate
  k2or=2.0e+01;
%
% Normal breathing O2 concentration (mm hg)
  pir_s= 20;
  pcc_s=100;
%
% Photoreceptor threshold
  u1ort=20;
%
% Independent variable t
  t0=0.0; tf=7200; tout=[t0:tf/6:tf]';
  nout=7;
%
% Initial condition
  u0=inital_1(t0);
%
% ODE integration
  mf=2;
  reltol=1.0e-06; abstol=1.0e-05;
  options=odeset('RelTol',reltol,'AbsTol',abstol);
%
% Explicit (nonstiff) integration
  if(mf==1)[t,u]=ode45(@pde_1,tout,u0,options); end
%
% Implicit (sparse stiff) integration
  if(mf==2)
    S=jpattern_num_1;
%   pause
    options=odeset(options,'JPattern',S)
    [t,u]=ode15s(@pde_1,tout,u0,options);
  end
%
% One vector to five vectors
%
% u1
    for it=1:nout
      for i=1:nir u1ir(it,i)=u(it,i);                end
      for i=1:nor u1or(it,i)=u(it,i+nir);            end
      for i=1:nfl u1fl(it,i)=u(it,i+nir+nor);        end
      for i=1:ncc u1cc(it,i)=u(it,i+nir+nor+nfl);    end
      if(it>=2)
        u1ir(it,1)  =pir_s;
        if(ncase==1)u1cc(it,ncc)=pcc_s;     end
```

```
      if(ncase==2)u1cc(it,ncc)=0.1*pcc_s; end
    end
  end
%
% u2
  for it=1:nout
    for i=1:nor u2or(it,i)=u(it,nt+i);              end
  end
%
% Display tabulated numerical solution
%
% Inner retina
  for it=1:nout
    fprintf('\n    t     zg_ir   u1ir(z,t)')
    for i=1:nir
      fprintf('%5.0f%10.0f%12.2f\n'  ,t(it)/60,zg_ir(i),u1ir(it,i))
    end
%
%   Outer retina
    fprintf('\n    t     zg_or   u1or(z,t)')
    fprintf('\n    t     zg_or   u2or(z,t)\n')
    for i=1:nor
      fprintf('%5.0f%10.0f%12.2f\n'  ,t(it)/60,zg_or(i),u1or(it,i))
      fprintf('%5.0f%10.0f%12.0f\n\n',t(it)/60,zg_or(i),u2or(it,i))
    end
%
%   Fluid layer
    fprintf('\n    t     zg_fl   u1fl(z,t)\n')
    for i=1:nfl
      fprintf('%5.0f%10.0f%12.2f\n'  ,t(it)/60,zg_fl(i),u1fl(it,i))
    end
%
%   Choriocapillaris
    fprintf('\n    t     zg_cc   u1cc(z,t)\n')
    for i=1:ncc
      fprintf('%5.0f%10.0f%12.2f\n'  ,t(it)/60,zg_cc(i),u1cc(it,i))
    end
%
% Next t
  end
  fprintf('\n    ncall = %4d\n',ncall);
%
% Four plots for u1ir, u1or, u1fl, u1cc
  figure(2)
  subplot(2,2,1)
  plot(zg_ir,u1ir,'-')
  axis([0 200 0 100])
  xlabel('zg-ir, \mum'); ylabel('u1ir(z,t), mm hg O_2');
  title('Inner retina O_2, t=0,20,...,120 min');
  subplot(2,2,2)
  plot(zg_or,u1or,'-')
```

```
    axis([0 200 0 100])
    xlabel('zg-or, \mum'); ylabel('u1or(z,t), mm hg O_2');
    title('Outer retina O_2, t=0,20,...,120 min');
    subplot(2,2,3)
    plot(zg_fl,u1fl,'-')
    axis([0 200 0 100])
    xlabel('zg-fl, \mum'); ylabel('u1fl(z,t), mm hg O_2');
    title('Fluid layer O_2, t=0,20,...,120 min');
    subplot(2,2,4)
    plot(zg_cc,u1cc,'-')
    axis([0 200 0 100])
    xlabel('zg-cc, \mum'); ylabel('u1cc(z,t), mm hg O_2');
    title('Choriocapillaris O_2, t=0,20,...,120 min');
%
%   One plot for u2or
    figure(3)
    plot(zg_or,u2or,'-')
    axis([0 200 0 1.0e+07])
    xlabel('zg-or, \mum'); ylabel('u2or(z,t), cells/cm^2');
    title('Outer retina photoreceptors, t=0,20,...,120 min');
```

Listing 4.6 Main program pde_1_main for the MOL solution of eqs. (4.1) to (4.5)

Here we comment primarily on the extensions of Listing 4.1.

- Previous files are cleared and selected variables and parameters are declared global. Then two cases are established, as explained subsequently.

```
%
% Select case
%
%   ncase = 1: Normal O2 at z=z_cc
%
%   ncase = 2: Reduced O2 at z=z_cc
  ncase=2;
```

- The grid in z for the four sections is defined.

```
%
% Number of grid points
  nir=11; nor=11; nfl=11; ncc=11;
  nt=nir+nor+nfl+ncc;
%
% Lengths of four sections (microns)
  zl_ir=200; zl_or=200; zl_fl=200; zl_cc=200;
%
% Spatial grids;
  zg_ir=[0:zl_ir/10:zl_ir]'; zg_or=[0:zl_or/10:zl_or]';
  zg_fl=[0:zl_fl/10:zl_fl]'; zg_cc=[0:zl_cc/10:zl_cc]';
```

- Parameters such as the diffusivities and interface coefficients are defined numerically for each of the four sections. Then the depletion rate constants in eqs. (4.1a) to (4.4a), $k_{IR}, k_{OR}, k_{FL}, k_{CC}$, the photoreceptor rate constant in eq. (4.5b), $k_{2,IR}$, the O_2 normal breathing concentrations in BCs (4.1c) and (4.4d), $P_{\text{IR-S}}, P_{\text{CC-S}}$, and the O_2 threshold, below which photoreceptor cells fails, $u_{1,\text{ORt}}$, are defined numerically.

```
%
% Diffusivities (microns^2/s)
  D1ir=1.0e+04; D1or=1.0e+04; D1fl=1.0e+04; D1cc=1.0e+04;
%
% Interface coefficients
  k1ir_or=1; k1or_fl=1; k1fl_cc=1;
%
% Metabolism rates
  k1ir=0.1; k1or=0.1; k1fl=0.1; k1cc=0.1;
%
% Photoreceptor rate
  k2or=2.0e+01;
%
% Normal breathing O2 concentration (mm hg)
  pir_s= 20;
  pcc_s=100;
%
% Photoreceptor threshold
  u1ort=20;
```

- The total interval in t for the solution, $0 \le t \le 7200$, and the output interval 1200 are specified for seven output points (including the IC $t = 0$). The ICs of eqs. (4.1b), (4.2b), (4.3b), (4.4b), and (4.5c) are then set by a call to `inital_1` (discussed subsequently).

```
%
% Independent variable t
  t0=0.0; tf=7200; tout=[t0:tf/6:tf]';
  nout=7;
%
% Initial condition
  u0=inital_1(t0);
```

The final $t = 7200$ s was selected to establish a significant variation in the numerical solution with t.

- The integration of the 55 ODEs by `ode15s` is the same as in Listing 4.1. The single solution vector from `ode15s`, `u`, is placed in separate arrays for the five PDEs, eqs. (4.1a) to (4.4a), (4.5a), and (4.5b), to facilitate subsequent programming.

```
%
% One vector to five vectors
%
% u1
    for it=1:nout
      for i=1:nir u1ir(it,i)=u(it,i);             end
      for i=1:nor u1or(it,i)=u(it,i+nir);         end
      for i=1:nfl u1fl(it,i)=u(it,i+nir+nor);     end
      for i=1:ncc u1cc(it,i)=u(it,i+nir+nor+nfl); end
      if(it>=2)
        u1ir(it,1)  =pir_s;
```

```
        if(ncase==1)u1cc(it,ncc)=pcc_s;     end
        if(ncase==2)u1cc(it,ncc)=0.1*pcc_s; end
      end
    end
%
%   u2
    for it=1:nout
      for i=1:nor u2or(it,i)=u(it,nt+i);              end
    end
```

The five vectors correspond to the series of seven values in t specified by the index it.

- The numerical output is the same as in Listing 4.1 except that u2 (from eqs. (4.5a), (4.5b)) is added to the output for the OR.

```
%
%     Outer retina
      fprintf('\n    t     zg_or    u1or(z,t)')
      fprintf('\n    t     zg_or    u2or(z,t)\n')
      for i=1:nor
        fprintf('%5.0f%10.0f%12.2f\n'  ,t(it)/60,zg_or(i),u1or(it,i))
        fprintf('%5.0f%10.0f%12.0f\n\n ,t(it)/60,zg_or(i),u2or(it,i))
      end
```

The division by 60 was used to convert the output from s to min (e.g., 7200 s = 120 min).

- The graphical output for eqs. (4.1a) to (4.4a) is essentially the same as in Listing 4.1. A second plot was added for eqs. (4.5a) and (4.5b).

```
%
%   One plot for u2or
    figure(3)
    plot(zg_or,u2or,'-')
    axis([0 200 0 1.0e+07])
    xlabel('zg-or, \mum'); ylabel('u2or(z,t), cells/cm^2');
    title('Outer retina photoreceptors, t=0,20,...,120 min');
```

4.4.3 IC routine

The IC routine inital_1 (Listing 4.7) is similar to that of Listing 4.3.

```
  function u=inital_1(t0)
%
% Function inital_1 is called by the main program to define the
% initial conditions of the four-section retinal O2 transport model
%
% Model parameters
  global   nir      nor      nfl      ncc...
         zl_ir    zl_or    zl_fl    zl_cc...
         zg_ir    zg_or    zg_fl    zg_cc...
          D1ir     D1or     D1fl     D1cc...
               k1ir_or k1or_fl k1fl_cc...
```

```
          k1ir    k1or    k1fl    k1cc...
          u1ort   k2or            ...
          pir_s   pcc_s   ncall   ncase    nt
%
% Initial conditions
%
%   Inner retina
    for i=1:nir
     u1ir(i)=pir_s;
     u(i)=u1ir(i);
    end
%
%   Outer retina
    for i=1:nor
      u1or(i)=pir_s;
      u2or(i)=1.0e+07;
      u(i+nir)=u1or(i);
      u(nt+i) =u2or(i);
    end
%
%   Fluid layer
    for i=1:nfl
      u1fl(i)=pir_s;
      u(i+nir+nor)=u1fl(i);
    end
%
%   Choriocapillaris
    for i=1:ncc
      u1cc(i)=pir_s;
      u(i+nir+nor+nfl)=u1cc(i);
    end
%
% Initialize calls to pde_1
  ncall=0;
```

Listing 4.7 IC routine inital_1 for eqs. (4.1b), (4.2b), (4.3b), (4.4b), and (4.5c)

Note in particular the programming of IC (4.5c).

```
u2ir(i)=1.0e+07;
```

where N_0 in eq. (4.5c) is given the value 10^7 cells/cm^2. inital_1 defines the 55 ICs required for the MOL solution of eqs. (4.1) to (4.5) in composite array u for use by ode15s (the LHS argument of inital_1). Also, the counter for the calls to pde_1 is initialized.

4.4.4 Sparse matrix routine

A change in jpattern_num_1 of Listing 4.4 reflects the addition of eqs. (4.5a) and (4.5b).

```
for i=1:nt+nor
  ybase(i)=0.5;
end
```

That is, the number of ODEs is now `nt+nor`$= 44 + 11 = 55$ rather than `nt` in Listing 4.4.

4.4.5 Model output

The tabulated numerical output is not discussed to conserve space. The graphical output is in Figs. 4.5, 4.6, and 4.7.

The reduction in the photoreceptor cell density due to O_2 deficiency is clear in Fig. 4.5.

Figure 4.5 suggests an impairment of vision from the loss of photoreceptor (rod, cone) cells due to O_2 deficiency. This deficiency might be due to an injury or a retinal detachment. This could be studied further, for example, by reducing one or more of the diffusivities to simulate reduced O_2 transport (see the variation in diffusivities programmed in `pde_1_main` of Listing 4.6) or by reducing the normal breathing O_2 concentrations, $P_{\text{IR-S}}, P_{\text{CC-S}}$ at the boundaries $z = z_L, z_{CC}$ as a function of t (since t is available as an input argument of `pde_1` of Listing 4.5). This reduction in the boundary O_2 could therefore take place at a value of t after the steady-state profile is established for normal O_2.

Also, the photoreceptor cell density `u2` would continue to drop indefinitely (in Fig. 4.5)) once `u1` drops below the threshold `u1ort` since there is nothing in eqs. (4.5) to limit a reduction in `u2`.

The redistribution of O_2 with increasing t can be appreciated by consideration of Fig. 4.6.

Note that the plots approach a steady state generally below 20 mm Hg (due to the BC `u1cc(it,ncc)=0.1*pcc_s=10` in `pde_1`).

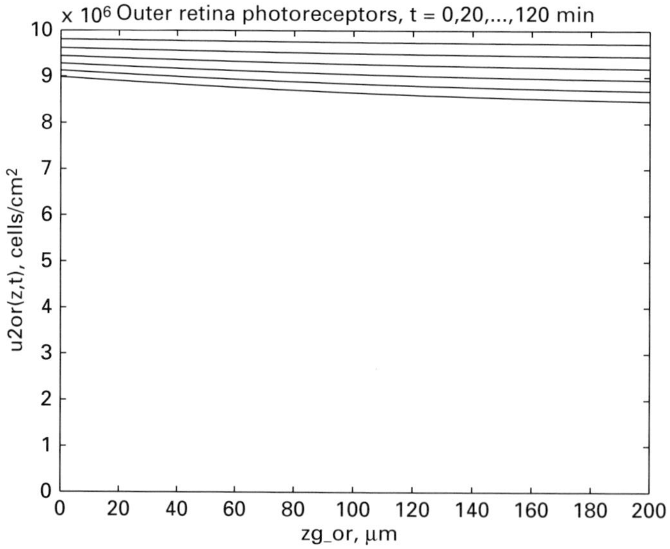

Figure 4.5 Photoreceptor cell density from eqs. (4.5a), (4.5b), `ncase=2`, t=0,20,...,120 min (top to bottom)

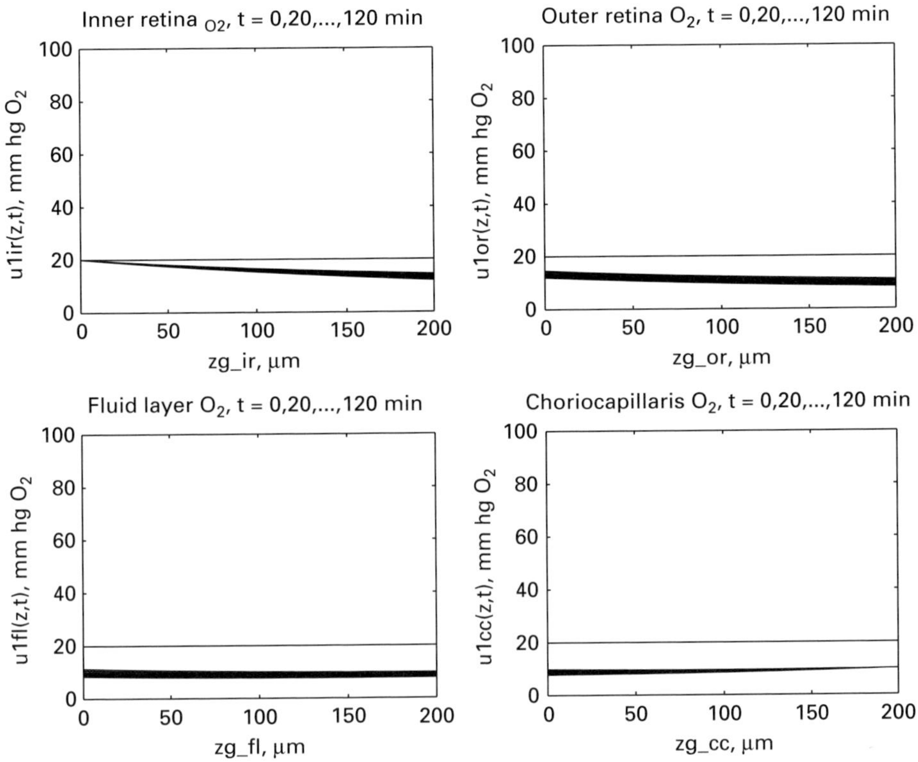

Figure 4.6 O_2 z distribution in IC, OC, FL, CC, `ncase=2`, t=0,20,...,120 min (top to bottom)

The decline in the photoreceptor cell density illustrated in Fig. 4.6 indicates a reduction in vision that warrants further study with the model. This loss of vision is due to an impairment of O_2 transport through the four sections considered in the model. Possible causes for reduced O_2 transport can be studied with the model, including the effect of model parameters such as the O_2 diffusivities and depletion rate constants. This parameter sensitivity in turn suggests experimental measurements that can provide more reliable parameter values for use in the model. This interplay between experiment and theory is an important guide to continuing research and is a primary justification for computer-based modeling.

The ODE Jacobian map is in Fig. 4.7.

The addition of eqs. (4.5a) and (4.5b) produces a second diagonal in the lower left corner of this map. This diagonal has only one entry for each ODE (denoted as ODEs 45 to 55 along the vertical axis) since eq. (4.5b) does not have a diffusion term. Also, the RHS of eq. (4.5b) is a function of u_1 (the O_2 concentration) and not u_2 (the photoreceptor cell density), which is why the diagonal appears in the lower left corner. In other words, the horizontal axis of Fig. 4.7 has only ODE-dependent variables 1 to 44 since none of the five PDEs has RHS terms that depend on ODE-dependent variables 45 to 55 from the solution of eq. (4.5b).

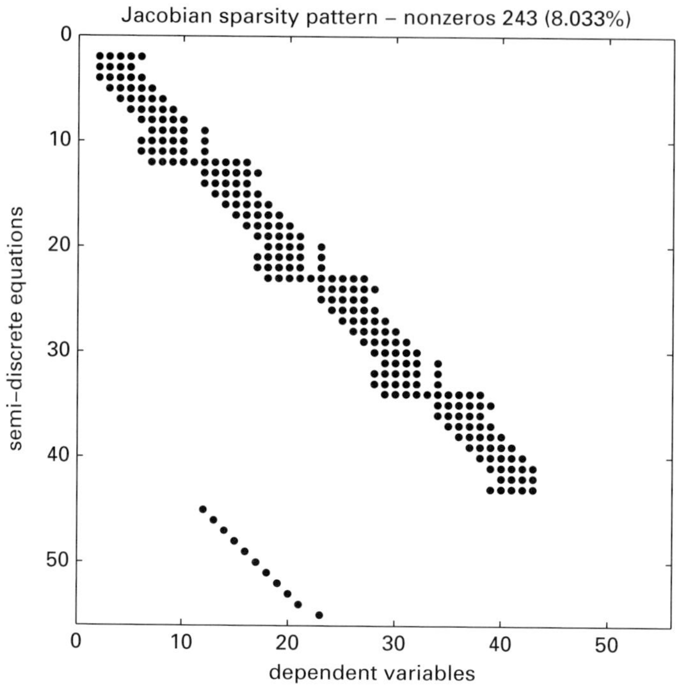

Figure 4.7 Map of the 55-ODE system for `ncase=2`

The preceding model can be extended to include the production of vascular endothelial growth factor (VEGF) leading to neovascularization (angiogenesis). Such an extension could be achieved in two ways:

- Reduction of the diffusivities (due to neovascularization) as an explicit function of t. This could be done by programming the diffusivities as a function for t in the ODE routine `pde_1`.
- Addition of a PDE for VEGF production, possibly with diffusion, to one or more of the four sections. This approach is now discussed.

4.5 Model including VEGF production

We now consider an extension of the base case model of eqs. (4.1) to (4.4) by adding a PDE to each of the four sections for VEGF production. These additional four PDEs follow (with dependent variable u_2 for VEGF concentration). For the IR, we have

$$\frac{\partial u_{2,\mathrm{IR}}}{\partial t} = D_{2,\mathrm{IR}} \frac{\partial^2 u_{2,\mathrm{IR}}}{\partial z^2}, \; u_{1,\mathrm{IR}} \geq u_{1,\mathrm{IRt}}, \; z_{\mathrm{L}} \leq z \leq z_{\mathrm{IR}}, \tag{4.6a}$$

$$\frac{\partial u_{2,\text{IR}}}{\partial t} = D_{2,\text{IR}} \frac{\partial^2 u_{2,\text{IR}}}{\partial z^2} + k_{2,\text{IR}}(u_{1,\text{IRt}} - u_{1,\text{IR}}), \; u_{1,\text{IR}} < u_{1,\text{IRt}}, \; z_L \le z \le z_{\text{IR}}, \tag{4.6b}$$

$$u_{2,\text{IR}}(z, t = 0) = u_{2,\text{IRn}}, \tag{4.6c}$$

$$\frac{\partial u_{2,\text{IR}}(z = z_L, t)}{\partial z} = 0, \tag{4.6d}$$

$$u_{2,\text{IR}}(z = z_{\text{IR}}, t) = k_{\text{IR-OR}} u_{2,\text{OR}}(z = z_{\text{IR}}, t). \tag{4.6e}$$

We can note the following details about eqs. (4.6).

- The VEGF concentration is designated with a subscript 2, $u_{2,\text{IR}}$, since it is a second PDE-dependent variable. Again, the first dependent variable is the O_2 concentration in eqs. (4.1) to (4.4), which will be changed from u to u_1 (with an additional designation of the section, so that, for example, u_{IR} becomes $u_{1,\text{IR}}$).
- The PDE is stated in two parts, eqs. (4.6a) and (4.6b). For eq. (4.6a), the IR O_2 concentration $u_{1,\text{IR}}$ is at or above a critical or threshold value, $u_{1,\text{IRt}}$, so VEGF is not produced (sufficient O_2 is available to exclude VEGF production). For eq. (4.6b), the IR O_2 concentration $u_{1,\text{IR}}$ is below the critical value, $u_{1,\text{IRt}}$, so that VEGF is produced (insufficient O_2 is available to avoid VEGF production). The switch between eqs. (4.6a) and (4.6b) is easily accomplished numerically in routine `pde_1` discussed subsequently.
- Equations (4.6a) and (4.6b) have a diffusion term $D_{2,\text{IR}}(\partial^2 u_{2,\text{IR}}/\partial z^2)$ (VEGF can move throughout the IR by diffusion), i.e., these equations are based on Fourier's or Fick's second law. Therefore, BCs are required for eqs. (4.6a) and (4.6b). Boundary condition (4.6d) specifies a zero-flux condition at the left end of the IR ($z = z_L$). In other words, VEGF does not leave the IR at the left end. Boundary condition (4.6e) is the usual equilibrium condition at the IR-OR interface ($z = z_{\text{IR}}$), where $k_{\text{IR-OR}}$ is an equilibrium constant.
- The rate of change of the VEGF concentration, $\partial u_{2,\text{IR}}/\partial t$, from eq. (4.6b) consists of two parts.
  - Diffusion, with the diffusivity $D_{2,\text{IR}}$, which designates u_2 (VEGF) in the IR. In other words, the diffusivity can be specific to the section, in this case IR.
  - Generation of VEGF modeled as $k_{2,\text{IR}}(u_{1,\text{IRt}} - u_{1,\text{IR}})$, where $k_{2,\text{IR}}$ is a rate constant for u_2 and $u_{1,\text{IRt}}$ is the threshold value of $u_{1,\text{IR}}$ discussed already. Note that $k_{2,\text{IR}} \ge 0$ so the RHS of eq. (4.5b) ensures an increase in VEGF concentration when $u_{1,\text{IR}} < u_{1,\text{IRt}}$. $k_{2,\text{IR}}$ and $u_{1,\text{IRt}}$ are important parameters that can be varied in the MATLAB main program to elucidate their effects.
- The IC of eq. (4.6c) is required for the derivative $\partial u_{2,\text{IR}}/\partial t$ of eqs. (4.6a) and (4.6b). $u_{2,\text{IRn}}$ is an initial VEGF concentration (taken as zero).

The VEGF PDEs for OR, FL, and CC are similar to eqs. (4.6). For OR,

$$\frac{\partial u_{2,\text{OR}}}{\partial t} = D_{2,\text{OR}} \frac{\partial^2 u_{2,\text{OR}}}{\partial z^2}, \; u_{1,\text{OR}} \ge u_{1,\text{OR}t}, \; z_{\text{IR}} \le z \le z_{\text{OR}}, \tag{4.7a}$$

$$\frac{\partial u_{2,\mathrm{OR}}}{\partial t} = D_{2,\mathrm{OR}}\frac{\partial^2 u_{2,\mathrm{OR}}}{\partial z^2} + k_{2,\mathrm{OR}}(u_{1,\mathrm{OR}t} - u_{1,\mathrm{OR}}),\ u_{1,\mathrm{OR}} < u_{1,\mathrm{OR}t},\ z_{\mathrm{IR}} \le z \le z_{\mathrm{OR}}, \tag{4.7b}$$

$$u_{2,\mathrm{OR}}(z, t = 0) = u_{2,\mathrm{ORn}}, \tag{4.7c}$$

$$\frac{\partial u_{2,\mathrm{OR}}(z = z_{\mathrm{IR}}, t)}{\partial z} = (D_{2,\mathrm{IR}}/D_{2,\mathrm{OR}})\frac{\partial u_{2,\mathrm{IR}}(z = z_{\mathrm{IR}}, t)}{\partial z}, \tag{4.7d}$$

$$u_{2,\mathrm{OR}}(z = z_{\mathrm{OR}}, t) = k_{\mathrm{OR\text{-}FL}} u_{2,FL}(z = z_{\mathrm{OR}}, t). \tag{4.7e}$$

Note that BC (4.7d) specifies the usual continuity in the fluxes at $z = z_{\mathrm{IR}}$ (at the IR–OR interface), while BC (4.7e) specifies the usual equilibrium at $z = z_{\mathrm{OR}}$ (the OR–FL interface).

The PDE for FL are

$$\frac{\partial u_{2,\mathrm{FL}}}{\partial t} = D_{2,\mathrm{FL}}\frac{\partial^2 u_{2,\mathrm{FL}}}{\partial z^2},\ u_{1,\mathrm{FL}} \ge u_{1,\mathrm{FLt}},\ z_{\mathrm{OR}} \le z \le z_{\mathrm{FL}}, \tag{4.8a}$$

$$\frac{\partial u_{2,\mathrm{FL}}}{\partial t} = D_{2,\mathrm{FL}}\frac{\partial^2 u_{2,\mathrm{FL}}}{\partial z^2} + k_{2,\mathrm{FL}}(u_{1,\mathrm{FLt}} - u_{1,\mathrm{FL}}),\ u_{1,\mathrm{FL}} < u_{1,\mathrm{FLt}},\ z_{\mathrm{OR}} \le z \le z_{\mathrm{FL}}, \tag{4.8b}$$

$$u_{2,\mathrm{FL}}(z, t = 0) = u_{2,\mathrm{FLn}}, \tag{4.8c}$$

$$\frac{\partial u_{2,\mathrm{FL}}(z = z_{\mathrm{OR}}, t)}{\partial z} = (D_{2,\mathrm{OR}}/D_{2,\mathrm{FL}})\frac{\partial u_{2,\mathrm{OR}}(z = z_{\mathrm{OR}}, t)}{\partial z}, \tag{4.8d}$$

$$u_{2,\mathrm{FL}}(z = z_{\mathrm{FL}}, t) = k_{\mathrm{FL-CC}} u_{2,\mathrm{CC}}(z = z_{\mathrm{FL}}, t). \tag{4.8e}$$

The PDEs for CC are

$$\frac{\partial u_{2,\mathrm{CC}}}{\partial t} = D_{2,\mathrm{CC}}\frac{\partial^2 u_{2,\mathrm{CC}}}{\partial z^2},\ u_{1,\mathrm{CC}} \ge u_{1,\mathrm{CCt}},\ z_{\mathrm{FL}} \le z \le z_{\mathrm{CC}}, \tag{4.9a}$$

$$\frac{\partial u_{2,\mathrm{CC}}}{\partial t} = D_{2,\mathrm{CC}}\frac{\partial^2 u_{2,\mathrm{CC}}}{\partial z^2} + k_{2,\mathrm{CC}}(u_{1,\mathrm{CCt}} - u_{1,\mathrm{CC}}),\ u_{1,\mathrm{CC}} < u_{1,\mathrm{CCt}},\ z_{\mathrm{FL}} \le z \le z_{\mathrm{CC}}, \tag{4.9b}$$

$$u_{2,\mathrm{CC}}(z, t = 0) = u_{2,\mathrm{CCn}}, \tag{4.9c}$$

$$\frac{\partial u_{2,\mathrm{CC}(z=z_{\mathrm{FL}},t)}}{\partial z} = (D_{2,\mathrm{FL}}/D_{2,\mathrm{CC}})\frac{\partial u_{2,\mathrm{FL}}(z = z_{\mathrm{FL}}, t)}{\partial z}, \tag{4.9d}$$

$$\frac{\partial u_{2,\mathrm{CC}}(z = z_{\mathrm{CC}}, t)}{\partial z} = 0. \tag{4.9e}$$

Note that eq. (4.9e) specifies a zero flux (homogeneous Neumann) BC for VEGF, so that VEGF does not leave the right end of the CC.

4.5.1 ODE routine

The ODE routine for eqs. (4.1) to (4.4), and (4.6) to (4.9) is in Listing 4.8.

```
  function ut=pde_1(t,u)
%
% Function pde_1 defines the ODEs in the MOL solution of the
% four-section retinal O2 transport model equations
%
% Model parameters
  global   nir      nor      nfl      ncc...
         zl_ir    zl_or    zl_fl    zl_cc...
         zg_ir    zg_or    zg_fl    zg_cc...
          D1ir     D1or     D1fl     D1cc...
          D2ir     D2or     D2fl     D2cc...
               k1ir_or k1or_fl k1fl_cc...
               k2ir_or k2or_fl k2fl_cc...
          k1ir     k1or     k1fl     k1cc...
          k2ir     k2or     k2fl     k2cc...
         u1irt    u1ort    u1flt    u1cct...
         pir_s    pcc_s    ncall      nt
%
% One vector to eight vectors
%
%   u1
    for i=1:nir u1ir(i)=u(i);                end
    for i=1:nor u1or(i)=u(i+nir);            end
    for i=1:nfl u1fl(i)=u(i+nir+nor);        end
    for i=1:ncc u1cc(i)=u(i+nir+nor+nfl);    end
%
%   u2
    for i=1:nir u2ir(i)=u(nt+i);             end
    for i=1:nor u2or(i)=u(nt+i+nir);         end
    for i=1:nfl u2fl(i)=u(nt+i+nir+nor);     end
    for i=1:ncc u2cc(i)=u(nt+i+nir+nor+nfl); end
%
% First order spatial derivatives, u1
  u1ir_z=dss004(0,zl_ir,nir,u1ir);
  u1or_z=dss004(0,zl_or,nor,u1or);
  u1fl_z=dss004(0,zl_fl,nfl,u1fl);
  u1cc_z=dss004(0,zl_cc,ncc,u1cc);
%
% BCs, u1
%
%   Inner retina
    u1ir(1)=pir_s;
    u1ir(nir)=k1ir_or*u1or(1);
%
%   Outer retina
    u1or_z(1)=(D1ir/D1or)*u1ir_z(nir);
    u1or(nor)=k1or_fl*u1fl(1);
%
%   Fluid layer
    u1fl_z(1)=(D1or/D1fl)*u1or_z(nor);
    u1fl(nfl)=k1fl_cc*u1cc(1);
```

```
%
%   Choriocapillaris
    u1cc_z(1)=(D1fl/D1cc)*u1fl_z(nfl);
    u1cc(ncc)=pcc_s;
%
% Second order spatial derivatives, u1
  nl1=1; nu1=1;
  u1ir_zz=dss044(0,zl_ir,nir,u1ir,u1ir_z,nl1,nu1);
  nl1=2; nu1=1;
  u1or_zz=dss044(0,zl_or,nor,u1or,u1or_z,nl1,nu1);
  u1fl_zz=dss044(0,zl_fl,nfl,u1fl,u1fl_z,nl1,nu1);
  u1cc_zz=dss044(0,zl_cc,ncc,u1cc,u1cc_z,nl1,nu1);
%
% First order spatial derivatives, u2
  u2ir_z=dss004(0,zl_ir,nir,u2ir);
  u2or_z=dss004(0,zl_or,nor,u2or);
  u2fl_z=dss004(0,zl_fl,nfl,u2fl);
  u2cc_z=dss004(0,zl_cc,ncc,u2cc);
%
% BCs, u2
%
%   Inner retina
    u2ir_z(1)=0;
    u2ir(nir)=k2ir_or*u2or(1);
%
%   Outer retina
    u2or_z(1)=(D2ir/D2or)*u2ir_z(nir);
    u2or(nor)=k2or_fl*u2fl(1);
%
%   Fluid layer
    u2fl_z(1)=(D2or/D2fl)*u2or_z(nor);
    u2fl(nfl)=k2fl_cc*u2cc(1);
%
%   Choriocapillaris
    u2cc_z(1)=(D2fl/D2cc)*u2fl_z(nfl);
    u2cc_z(ncc)=0;
%
% Second order spatial derivatives, u2
  nl2=2; nu2=1;
  u2ir_zz=dss044(0,zl_ir,nir,u2ir,u2ir_z,nl2,nu2);
  u2or_zz=dss044(0,zl_or,nor,u2or,u2or_z,nl2,nu2);
  u2fl_zz=dss044(0,zl_fl,nfl,u2fl,u2fl_z,nl2,nu2);
  nl2=2; nu2=2;
  u2cc_zz=dss044(0,zl_cc,ncc,u2cc,u2cc_z,nl2,nu2);
%
% PDEs
%
%   u1
    u1ir_t=D1ir*u1ir_zz-k1ir*u1ir;
    u1or_t=D1or*u1or_zz-k1or*u1or;
    u1fl_t=D1fl*u1fl_zz-k1fl*u1fl;
```

```
    u1cc_t=D1cc*u1cc_zz-k1cc*u1cc;
    u1ir_t(1)  =0;
    u1cc_t(ncc)=0;
%
%   u2
    for i=1:nir
      if(u1ir(i)>=u1irt)
        u2ir_t(i)=D2ir*u2ir_zz(i);
      else
        u2ir_t(i)=D2ir*u2ir_zz(i)...
                  +k2ir*(u1irt-u1ir(i));
      end
    end
    for i=1:nor
      if(u1or(i)>=u1ort)
        u2or_t(i)=D2or*u2or_zz(i);
      else
        u2or_t(i)=D2or*u2or_zz(i)...
                  +k2or*(u1ort-u1or(i));
      end
    end
    for i=1:nfl
      if(u1fl(i)>=u1flt)
        u2fl_t(i)=D2fl*u2fl_zz(i);
      else
        u2fl_t(i)=D2fl*u2fl_zz(i)...
                  +k2fl*(u1flt-u1fl(i));
      end
    end
    for i=1:ncc
      if(u1cc(i)>=u1cct)
        u2cc_t(i)=D2cc*u2cc_zz(i);
      else
        u2cc_t(i)=D2cc*u2cc_zz(i)...
                  +k2cc*(u1cct-u1cc(i));
      end
    end
%
% Eight vectors to one vector
%
%   u1
    for i=1:nir ut(i)                =u1ir_t(i); end
    for i=1:nor ut(i+nir)            =u1or_t(i); end
    for i=1:nfl ut(i+nir+nor)        =u1fl_t(i); end
    for i=1:ncc ut(i+nir+nor+nfl)    =u1cc_t(i); end
%
%   u2
    for i=1:nir ut(nt+i)             =u2ir_t(i); end
    for i=1:nor ut(nt+i+nir)         =u2or_t(i); end
    for i=1:nfl ut(nt+i+nir+nor)     =u2fl_t(i); end
    for i=1:ncc ut(nt+i+nir+nor+nfl)=u2cc_t(i); end
```

```
  ut=ut';
%
% Increment calls to pde_1
  ncall=ncall+1;
```

Listing 4.8 ODE routine pde_1 for the MOL solution of eqs. (4.1) to (4.4), (4.6) to (4.9), including VEGF concentration

We can note the following details about pde_1.

- The function pde_1 is defined and selected variables and parameters are declared global.
- The model of eqs. (4.1) to (4.4) and (4.6) to (4.9) has eight PDEs. To facilitate the programming in pde_1, the composite solution vector u (an input or RHS argument to pde_1) is placed in eight vectors, u1ir to u2cc.

```
%
% One vector to eight vectors
%
%   u1
    for i=1:nir u1ir(i)=u(i);                  end
    for i=1:nor u1or(i)=u(i+nir);              end
    for i=1:nfl u1fl(i)=u(i+nir+nor);          end
    for i=1:ncc u1cc(i)=u(i+nir+nor+nfl);      end
%
%   u2
    for i=1:nir u2ir(i)=u(nt+i);               end
    for i=1:nor u2or(i)=u(nt+i+nir);           end
    for i=1:nfl u2fl(i)=u(nt+i+nir+nor);       end
    for i=1:ncc u2cc(i)=u(nt+i+nir+nor+nfl);   end
```

  u_1 (O_2 concentration) is placed in arrays u1ir to u1cc and u_2 (VEGF concentration) is placed in arrays u2ir to u2cc. Again, nt=nir+nor+nfl+ncc (set in the main program, discussed subsequently).

- Equations (4.1) to (4.4) for u_1 are programmed first, starting with the first derivatives in z computed by the library routine dss004.

```
%
% First order spatial derivatives, u1
  u1ir_z=dss004(0,zl_ir,nir,u1ir);
  u1or_z=dss004(0,zl_or,nor,u1or);
  u1fl_z=dss004(0,zl_fl,nfl,u1fl);
  u1cc_z=dss004(0,zl_cc,ncc,u1cc);
```

  The resulting first derivatives, u1ir_z to u1cc_z, are then available for use in the u_1 BCs.

- The BCs (4.1c) and (4.1d) for the IR, Boundary conditions (4.2c) and (4.2d) for the OR, Boundary conditions (4.3c) and (4.3d) for the FL, and Boundary conditions (4.4c) and (4.4d) for the CC are programmed. Since this programming was discussed previously for Listing 4.2, it is not considered further here.

```
%
% BCs, u1
%
%    Inner retina
     u1ir(1)=pir_s;
     u1ir(nir)=k1ir_or*u1or(1);
%
%    Outer retina
     u1or_z(1)=(D1ir/D1or)*u1ir_z(nir);
     u1or(nor)=k1or_fl*u1fl(1);
%
%    Fluid layer
     u1fl_z(1)=(D1or/D1fl)*u1or_z(nor);
     u1fl(nfl)=k1fl_cc*u1cc(1);
%
%    Choriocapillaris
     u1cc_z(1)=(D1fl/D1cc)*u1fl_z(nfl);
     u1cc(ncc)=pcc_s;
```

- The second derivatives in eq. (4.1) to (4.4) are computed by a call to `dss044`. The designation of the types of BCs through `nl1,nu1` was discussed previously (for Listing 4.2) and will therefore not be considered further here.

```
%
% Second order spatial derivatives, u1
  nl1=1; nu1=1;
  u1ir_zz=dss044(0,zl_ir,nir,u1ir,u1ir_z,nl1,nu1);
  nl1=2; nu1=1;
  u1or_zz=dss044(0,zl_or,nor,u1or,u1or_z,nl1,nu1);
  u1fl_zz=dss044(0,zl_fl,nfl,u1fl,u1fl_z,nl1,nu1);
  u1cc_zz=dss044(0,zl_cc,ncc,u1cc,u1cc_z,nl1,nu1);
```

- The first derivatives for u_2 are computed in the same way as for u_1.

```
%
% First order spatial derivatives, u2
  u2ir_z=dss004(0,zl_ir,nir,u2ir);
  u2or_z=dss004(0,zl_or,nor,u2or);

  u2fl_z=dss004(0,zl_fl,nfl,u2fl);
  u2cc_z=dss004(0,zl_cc,ncc,u2cc);
```

- The BCs for u_2, eqs. (4.6d) and (4.6e) for IR, eqs. (4.7d) and (4.7e) for OR, eqs. (4.8d) and (4.8e) for FL, and eqs. (4.9d) and (4.9e) for CC, are programmed in the same way as for u_1 (above). There are two essential differences. Boundary condition (4.6d) is programmed as a Neumann BC, `u2ir_z(1)=0`. Similarly, BC (4.9e) is programmed as a Neumann BC, `u2cc_z(ncc)=0`.

```
%
% BCs, u2
%
%    Inner retina
     u2ir_z(1)=0;
```

```
      u2ir(nir)=k2ir_or*u2or(1);
%
%     Outer retina
      u2or_z(1)=(D2ir/D2or)*u2ir_z(nir);
      u2or(nor)=k2or_fl*u2fl(1);
%
%     Fluid layer
      u2fl_z(1)=(D2or/D2fl)*u2or_z(nor);
      u2fl(nfl)=k2fl_cc*u2cc(1);
%
%     Choriocapillaris
      u2cc_z(1)=(D2fl/D2cc)*u2fl_z(nfl);
      u2cc_z(ncc)=0;
```

- All of the second derivatives in z are now available so the PDEs can be programmed. For u_1, the MATLAB vector utility is used so that subscripting (in a `for` loop) is not required.

```
%
% PDEs
%
%     u1
      u1ir_t=D1ir*u1ir_zz-k1ir*u1ir;
      u1or_t=D1or*u1or_zz-k1or*u1or;
      u1fl_t=D1fl*u1fl_zz-k1fl*u1fl;
      u1cc_t=D1cc*u1cc_zz-k1cc*u1cc;
      u1ir_t(1)  =0;
      u1cc_t(ncc)=0;
```

This programming is the same as in Listing 4.2.

- The programming for u_2 reflects the two parts for each PDE, e.g., eqs. (4.6a) and (4.6b) for the IR. Note that for the second part of each PDE, the VEGF production is included.

```
%
%     u2
      for i=1:nir
        if(u1ir(i)>=u1irt)
          u2ir_t(i)=D2ir*u2ir_zz(i);
        else
          u2ir_t(i)=D2ir*u2ir_zz(i)...
                    +k2ir*(u1irt-u1ir(i));
        end
      end
      for i=1:nor
        if(u1or(i)>=u1ort)
          u2or_t(i)=D2or*u2or_zz(i);
        else
          u2or_t(i)=D2or*u2or_zz(i)...
                    +k2or*(u1ort-u1or(i));
        end
      end
```

```
    for i=1:nfl
      if(u1fl(i)>=u1flt)
        u2fl_t(i)=D2fl*u2fl_zz(i);
      else
        u2fl_t(i)=D2fl*u2fl_zz(i)...
                  +k2fl*(u1flt-u1fl(i));
      end
    end
    for i=1:ncc
      if(u1cc(i)>=u1cct)
        u2cc_t(i)=D2cc*u2cc_zz(i);
      else
        u2cc_t(i)=D2cc*u2cc_zz(i)...
                  +k2cc*(u1cct-u1cc(i));
      end
    end
```

All 88 derivatives in t are now computed (44 for u_1 from eqs. (4.1) to (4.4), 44 for u_2 from eqs. (4.6) to (4.9)).

- The 88 derivatives in t are now placed in a single vector, `ut`, to be returned as a LHS output argument of `pde_1`.

```
%
% Eight vectors to one vector
%
%   u1
    for i=1:nir ut(i)                 =u1ir_t(i); end
    for i=1:nor ut(i+nir)             =u1or_t(i); end
    for i=1:nfl ut(i+nir+nor)         =u1fl_t(i); end
    for i=1:ncc ut(i+nir+nor+nfl)     =u1cc_t(i); end
%
%   u2
    for i=1:nir ut(nt+i)              =u2ir_t(i); end
    for i=1:nor ut(nt+i+nir)          =u2or_t(i); end
    for i=1:nfl ut(nt+i+nir+nor)      =u2fl_t(i); end
    for i=1:ncc ut(nt+i+nir+nor+nfl)=u2cc_t(i); end
  ut=ut';
%
% Increment calls to pde_1
  ncall=ncall+1;
```

`pde_1` concludes with the usual transpose required by `ode15s` and incrementing of the counter for the calls to `pde_1`.

4.5.2 Main program

The main program that calls `pde_1` through `ode15s` is in Listing 4.9.

```
%
% Four-section retinal O2 transport model equation
%
```

```
% Clear previous files
  clear all
  clc
%
% Model parameters shared with other routines
%
% Model parameters
  global   nir      nor      nfl      ncc...
         zl_ir    zl_or    zl_fl    zl_cc...
         zg_ir    zg_or    zg_fl    zg_cc...
          D1ir     D1or     D1fl     D1cc...
          D2ir     D2or     D2fl     D2cc...
               k1ir_or k1or_fl k1fl_cc...
               k2ir_or k2or_fl k2fl_cc...
          k1ir     k1or     k1fl     k1cc...
          k2ir     k2or     k2fl     k2cc...
         u1irt    u1ort    u1flt    u1cct...
         pir_s    pcc_s    ncall      nt
%
% Number of grid points
  nir=11; nor=11; nfl=11; ncc=11;
  nt=nir+nor+nfl+ncc;
%
% Lengths of four sections (microns)
  zl_ir=200; zl_or=200; zl_fl=200; zl_cc=200;
%
% Spatial grids;
  zg_ir=[0:zl_ir/10:zl_ir]'; zg_or=[0:zl_or/10:zl_or]';
  zg_fl=[0:zl_fl/10:zl_fl]'; zg_cc=[0:zl_cc/10:zl_cc]';
%
% Diffusivities (microns^2/s)
  D1ir=1.0e+04; D1or=1.0e+04; D1fl=1.0e+04; D1cc=1.0e+04;
  D2ir=1.0e+03; D2or=1.0e+03; D2fl=1.0e+03; D2cc=1.0e+03;
%
% Interface coefficients
  k1ir_or=1; k1or_fl=1; k1fl_cc=1;
  k2ir_or=1; k2or_fl=1; k2fl_cc=1;
%
% Metabolism rates
  k1ir=0.1; k1or=0.1; k1fl=0.1; k1cc=0.1;
%
% VEGF rates
  k2ir=1.0e-05; k2or=1.0e-05; k2fl=1.0e-05; k2cc=1.0e-05;
%
% Normal breathing O2 concentration (mm hg)
  pir_s= 20;
  pcc_s=100;
  pcc_s=  0;
%
% O2 thresholds
  u1irt=10; u1ort=10; u1flt=10; u1cct=10;
```

```
%
% Independent variable t
  t0=0.0; tf=7200; tout=[t0:tf/6:tf]';
  nout=7;
%
% Initial condition
  u0=inital_1(t0);
%
% ODE integration
  mf=2;
  reltol=1.0e-06; abstol=1.0e-05;
  options=odeset('RelTol',reltol,'AbsTol',abstol);
%
% Explicit (nonstiff) integration
  if(mf==1)[t,u]=ode45(@pde_1,tout,u0,options); end
%
% Implicit (sparse stiff) integration
  if(mf==2)
    S=jpattern_num_1;
    options=odeset(options,'JPattern',S)
    [t,u]=ode15s(@pde_1,tout,u0,options);
  end
%
% One vector to eight vectors
%
% u1
    for it=1:nout
      for i=1:nir u1ir(it,i)=u(it,i);                  end
      for i=1:nor u1or(it,i)=u(it,i+nir);              end
      for i=1:nfl u1fl(it,i)=u(it,i+nir+nor);          end
      for i=1:ncc u1cc(it,i)=u(it,i+nir+nor+nfl);      end
      if(it>=2)
        u1ir(it,1)  =pir_s;
        u1cc(it,ncc)=pcc_s;
      end
    end
%
% u2
    for it=1:nout
      for i=1:nir u2ir(it,i)=u(it,nt+i);               end
      for i=1:nor u2or(it,i)=u(it,nt+i+nir);           end
      for i=1:nfl u2fl(it,i)=u(it,nt+i+nir+nor);       end
      for i=1:ncc u2cc(it,i)=u(it,nt+i+nir+nor+nfl); end
    end
%
%   Display tabulated numerical solution
%
%   Inner retina
    for it=1:nout
      fprintf('\n    t     zg_ir   u1ir(z,t)')
      fprintf('\n    t     zg_ir   u2ir(z,t)\n')
```

```
      for i=1:nir
        fprintf('%5.0f%10.0f%12.2f\n'  ,t(it)/60,zg_ir(i),u1ir(it,i))
        fprintf('%5.0f%10.0f%12.2f\n\n',t(it)/60,zg_ir(i),u2ir(it,i))
      end
%
%     Outer retina
      fprintf('\n    t     zg_or   u1or(z,t)')
      fprintf('\n    t     zg_or   u2or(z,t)\n')
      for i=1:nor
        fprintf('%5.0f%10.0f%12.2f\n'  ,t(it)/60,zg_or(i),u1or(it,i))
        fprintf('%5.0f%10.0f%12.2f\n\n',t(it)/60,zg_or(i),u2or(it,i))
      end
%
%     Fluid layer
      fprintf('\n    t     zg_fl   u1fl(z,t)\n')
      fprintf('\n    t     zg_or   u2fl(z,t)\n')
      for i=1:nfl
        fprintf('%5.0f%10.0f%12.2f\n'  ,t(it)/60,zg_fl(i),u1fl(it,i))
        fprintf('%5.0f%10.2f%12.2f\n\n',t(it)/60,zg_fl(i),u2fl(it,i))
      end
%
%     Choriocapillaris
      fprintf('\n    t     zg_cc   u1cc(z,t)\n')
      for i=1:ncc
        fprintf('%5.0f%10.0f%12.2f\n'  ,t(it)/60,zg_cc(i),u1cc(it,i))
        fprintf('%5.0f%10.2f%12.2f\n\n',t(it)/60,zg_cc(i),u2cc(it,i))
      end
%
%   Next t
    end
    fprintf('\n    ncall = %4d\n',ncall);
%
%   Four plots for u1ir, u1or, u1fl, u1cc
    figure(2)
    subplot(2,2,1)
    plot(zg_ir,u1ir,'-')
    axis([0 200 0 100])
    xlabel('zg-ir, \mum'); ylabel('u1ir(z,t), mm hg O_2');
    title('Inner retina O_2, t=0,20,...,120 min');
    subplot(2,2,2)
    plot(zg_or,u1or,'-')
    axis([0 200 0 100])
    xlabel('zg-or, \mum'); ylabel('u1or(z,t), mm hg O_2');
    title('Outer retina O_2, t=0,20,...,120 min');
    subplot(2,2,3)
    plot(zg_fl,u1fl,'-')
    axis([0 200 0 100])
    xlabel('zg-fl, \mum'); ylabel('u1fl(z,t), mm hg O_2');
    title('Fluid layer O_2, t=0,20,...,120 min');
    subplot(2,2,4)
    plot(zg_cc,u1cc,'-')
```

```
      axis([0 200 0 100])
      xlabel('zg-cc, \mum'); ylabel('u1cc(z,t), mm hg O_2');
      title('Choriocapillaris O_2, t=0,20,...,120 min');
%
%     Four plots for u2ir, u2or, u2fl, u2cc
      figure(3)
      subplot(2,2,1)
      plot(zg_ir,u2ir,'-')
      axis([0 200 0 1])
      xlabel('zg-ir, \mum'); ylabel('u2ir(z,t), ng/ml');
      title('Inner retina VEGF, t=0,20,...,120 min');
      subplot(2,2,2)
      plot(zg_or,u2or,'-')
      axis([0 200 0 1])
      xlabel('zg-or, \mum'); ylabel('u2or(z,t), ng/ml');
      title('Outer retina VEGF, t=0,20,...,120 min');
      subplot(2,2,3)
      plot(zg_fl,u2fl,'-')
      axis([0 200 0 1])
      xlabel('zg-fl, \mum'); ylabel('u2fl(z,t), ng/ml');
      title('Fluid layer VEGF, t=0,20,...,120 min');
      subplot(2,2,4)
      plot(zg_cc,u2cc,'-')
      axis([0 200 0 1])
      xlabel('zg-cc, \mum'); ylabel('u2cc(z,t), ng/ml');
      title('Choriocapillaris VEGF, t=0,20,...,120 min');
```

Listing 4.8 Main program pde_1_main for the MOL solution of eqs. (4.1) to (4.4), (4.6) to (4.9)

pde_1_main of Listing 4.9 is similar to the main programs in Listings 4.1 and 4.6 so only the essential differences are discussed next. We can note the following points about pde_1_main.

- Previous files are cleared and selected variables and parameters are declared as global.
- The grids in z for u_1 and u_2 are defined as in Listing 4.6.
- The model parameters are defined numerically.

```
%
% Diffusivities (microns^2/s)
  D1ir=1.0e+04; D1or=1.0e+04; D1fl=1.0e+04; D1cc=1.0e+04;
  D2ir=1.0e+03; D2or=1.0e+03; D2fl=1.0e+03; D2cc=1.0e+03;
%
% Interface coefficients
  k1ir_or=1; k1or_fl=1; k1fl_cc=1;
  k2ir_or=1; k2or_fl=1; k2fl_cc=1;
%
% Metabolism rates
  k1ir=0.1; k1or=0.1; k1fl=0.1; k1cc=0.1;
%
% VEGF rates
  k2ir=1.0e-05; k2or=1.0e-05; k2fl=1.0e-05; k2cc=1.0e-05;
```

```
%
% Normal breathing O2 concentration (mm hg)
  pir_s= 20;
  pcc_s=100;
  pcc_s=  0;
%
% O2 thresholds
  u1irt=10; u1ort=10; u1flt=10; u1cct=10;
```

Note in particular:

- Diffusivities for VEGF are defined (and used in pde_1 of Listing 4.8).

```
D2ir=1.0e+03; D2or=1.0e+03; D2fl=1.0e+03; D2cc=1.0e+03;
```

  These diffusivities are in $\mu m^2/s$ and are a factor of ten smaller than those for O_2, since VEGF has a much higher molecular weight than O_2.
- The VEGF interface coefficients are defined (and used in pde_1 of Listing 4.8).

```
k2ir_or=1; k2or_fl=1; k2fl_cc=1;
```

- The VEGF production rates are defined (and used in pde_1 of Listing 4.8).

```
%
% VEGF rates
  k2ir=1.0e-05; k2or=1.0e-05; k2fl=1.0e-05; k2cc=1.0e-05;
```

  These rates were selected by trial and error to give a significant level of VEGF production, as indicated in the output discussed subsequently.
- The boundary O_2 concentrations are set. Note that pcc_s=0 is used, corresponding to the elimination of the O_2 supply at the boundary $z = z_{CC}$. If this statement is deactivated as a comment, the normal O_2 concentration pcc_s=100 is used. Thus, a comparison of the model output for these two cases gives an indication of the effect of O_2 failure at $z = z_L$.

```
%
% Normal breathing O2 concentration (mm hg)
  pir_s= 20;
  pcc_s=100;
  pcc_s=  0;
```

- The time scale is again $0 \leq t \leq 7200$ (total of 120 min), with seven outputs at $t = 0, 1200, ..., 7200$ s or $t = 0, 20, ..., 120$ min.

```
%
% Independent variable t
  t0=0.0; tf=7200; tout=[t0:tf/6:tf]';
  nout=7;
%
% Initial condition
  u0=inital_1(t0);
```

Function inital_1 is then called to set the ICs of the eight PDEs (discussed subsequently).

- The 88 ODEs are integrated by a call to ode15s as in Listings 4.1 and 4.6.
- The solution vector u returned by ode15s is placed in eight vectors for u_1, u_2 of eqs. (4.1) to (4.4) and (4.6) to (4.9).

```
%
% One vector to eight vectors
%
% u1
    for it=1:nout
      for i=1:nir u1ir(it,i)=u(it,i);                  end
      for i=1:nor u1or(it,i)=u(it,i+nir);              end
      for i=1:nfl u1fl(it,i)=u(it,i+nir+nor);          end
      for i=1:ncc u1cc(it,i)=u(it,i+nir+nor+nfl);      end
      if(it>=2)
        u1ir(it,1)   =pir_s;
        u1cc(it,ncc)=pcc_s;
      end
    end
%
% u2
    for it=1:nout
      for i=1:nir u2ir(it,i)=u(it,nt+i);               end
      for i=1:nor u2or(it,i)=u(it,nt+i+nir);           end
      for i=1:nfl u2fl(it,i)=u(it,nt+i+nir+nor);       end
      for i=1:ncc u2cc(it,i)=u(it,nt+i+nir+nor+nfl); end
```

The eight vectors correspond to the series of seven values in t specified by the index it.

- Two composite plots (figure(2), figure(3)) are produced for eqs. (4.1) to (4.4) and eqs. (4.6) to (4.9), respectively.

```
%
%   Four plots for u1ir, u1or, u1fl, u1cc
    figure(2)
    subplot(2,2,1)
    plot(zg_ir,u1ir,'-')
    axis([0 200 0 100])
    xlabel('zg-ir, \mum'); ylabel('u1ir(z,t), mm hg O_2');
    title('Inner retina O_2, t=0,20,...,120 min');
    subplot(2,2,2)
    plot(zg_or,u1or,'-')
    axis([0 200 0 100])
    xlabel('zg-or, \mum'); ylabel('u1or(z,t), mm hg O_2');
    title('Outer retina O_2, t=0,20,...,120 min');
    subplot(2,2,3)
    plot(zg_fl,u1fl,'-')
    axis([0 200 0 100])
    xlabel('zg-fl, \mum'); ylabel('u1fl(z,t), mm hg O_2');
    title('Fluid layer O_2, t=0,20,...,120 min');
    subplot(2,2,4)
    plot(zg_cc,u1cc,'-')
    axis([0 200 0 100])
```

```
    xlabel('zg-cc, \mum'); ylabel('u1cc(z,t), mm hg O_2');
    title('Choriocapillaris O_2, t=0,20,...,120 min');
%
%   Four plots for u2ir, u2or, u2fl, u2cc
    figure(3)
    subplot(2,2,1)
    plot(zg_ir,u2ir,'-')
    axis([0 200 0 1])
    xlabel('zg-ir, \mum'); ylabel('u2ir(z,t), ng/ml');
    title('Inner retina VEGF, t=0,20,...,120 min');
    subplot(2,2,2)
    plot(zg_or,u2or,'-')
    axis([0 200 0 1])
    xlabel('zg-or, \mum'); ylabel('u2or(z,t), ng/ml');
    title('Outer retina VEGF, t=0,20,...,120 min');
    subplot(2,2,3)
    plot(zg_fl,u2fl,'-')
    axis([0 200 0 1])
    xlabel('zg-fl, \mum'); ylabel('u2fl(z,t), ng/ml');
    title('Fluid layer VEGF, t=0,20,...,120 min');
    subplot(2,2,4)
    plot(zg_cc,u2cc,'-')
    axis([0 200 0 1])
    xlabel('zg-cc, \mum'); ylabel('u2cc(z,t), ng/ml');
    title('Choriocapillaris VEGF, t=0,20,...,120 min');
```

4.5.3 IC routine

The IC routine, inital_1, is in Listing 4.10.

```
  function u=inital_1(t0)
%
% Function inital_1 is called by the main program to define the
% initial conditions of the four-section retinal O2 transport model
%
% Model parameters
  global  nir     nor     nfl     ncc...
        zl_ir   zl_or   zl_fl   zl_cc...
        zg_ir   zg_or   zg_fl   zg_cc...
         D1ir    D1or    D1fl    D1cc...
         D2ir    D2or    D2fl    D2cc...
              k1ir_or k1or_fl k1fl_cc...
              k2ir_or k2or_fl k2fl_cc...
         k1ir    k1or    k1fl    k1cc...
         k2ir    k2or    k2fl    k2cc...
        u1irt   u1ort   u1flt   u1cct...
        pir_s   pcc_s   ncall      nt
%
% Initial conditions
%
%    Inner retina
```

```
      for i=1:nir
       u1ir(i)=pir_s;
       u2ir(i)=0;
         u(i)    =u1ir(i);
         u(nt+i)=u2ir(i);
      end
%
%     Outer retina
      for i=1:nor
        u1or(i)=pir_s;
        u2or(i)=0;
        u(i+nir)    =u1or(i);
        u(nt+i+nir)=u2or(i);
      end
%
%     Fluid layer
      for i=1:nfl
        u1fl(i)=pir_s;
        u2fl(i)=0;
        u(i+nir+nor)    =u1fl(i);
        u(nt+i+nir+nor)=u2fl(i);
      end
%
%     Choriocapillaris
      for i=1:ncc
        u1cc(i)=pir_s;
        u2cc(i)=0;
        u(i+nir+nor+nfl)    =u1cc(i);
        u(nt+i+nir+nor+nfl)=u2cc(i);
      end
%
% Initialize calls to pde_1
  ncall=0;
```

Listing 4.10 IC routine `inital_1` for (a) eqs. (4.1b), (4.2b), (4.3b), (4.4b) and (b) eqs. (4.6b), (4.7b), (4.8b), (4.9b)

Note that the initial value of u_1 (O_2) is `pir_s` (set in `pde_1_main`) while the initial value of u_2 (VEGF) is zero. `inital_1` defines the 88 ICs required for the MOL solution of eqs. (4.1) to (4.4) and (4.6) to (4.9) returned in the composite array `u` for use by `ode15s` (the LHS argument of `inital_1`). Also, the counter for the calls to `pde_1` is initialized.

4.5.4 Sparse matrix routine

A change in `jpattern_num_1` of Listing 4.4 reflects the addition of eqs. (4.6) to (4.9).

```
for i=1:2*nt
  ybase(i)=0.5;
end
```

That is, the number of ODEs is now `2*nt`$= (2)(44) = 88$ rather than `nt` in Listing 4.4.

4.5.5 Model output

The production of VEGF due to O_2 deficiency is clear in Fig. 4.8.

Figure 4.8 indicates flat VEGF profiles in each of the four sections (IR,OR,FL,CC), owing to essentially uniform VEGF production in the four sections (from nearly uniform O_2 profiles in Fig. 4.9), and dispersion of the VEGF by diffusion to level whatever VEGF variation may occur in z. These effects could be studied further, e.g., by reducing the u_2 (VEGF) diffusivities (or setting them to zero). Also, an important comparison could be made by returning to normal O_2 supply (using `pcc_s=100` in place of `pcc_s=0` in `pde_1_main` of Listing 4.9) so that no VEGF production takes place (prevented by sufficient O_2).

The redistribution of O_2 with increasing t is clear Fig. 4.9. Note that the plots approach a steady state generally below 20 mm Hg.

The ODE Jacobian map is in Fig. 4.10.

The main diagonal includes all of the ODEs (1 to 88 on the vertical axis) since all eight PDEs have diffusion terms (and therefore the main diagonal is essentially pentadiagonal through the use of the five point FDs in `dss044` called in `pde_1`). The addition of eqs. (4.6) to (4.9) also produces a second diagonal in the lower left corner of the map (resulting from the test on u_1 for O_2 above or below a threshold value). The Jacobian map has

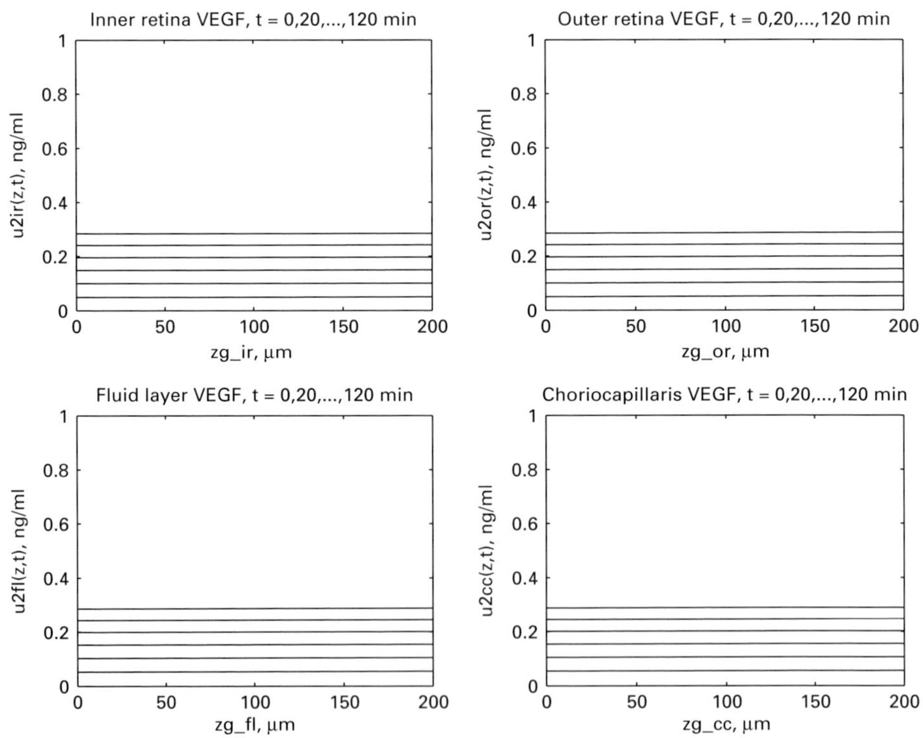

Figure 4.8 VEGF concentration from eqs. (4.6), (4.7), (4.8), (4.9), t=0,20,...,120 min (bottom to top)

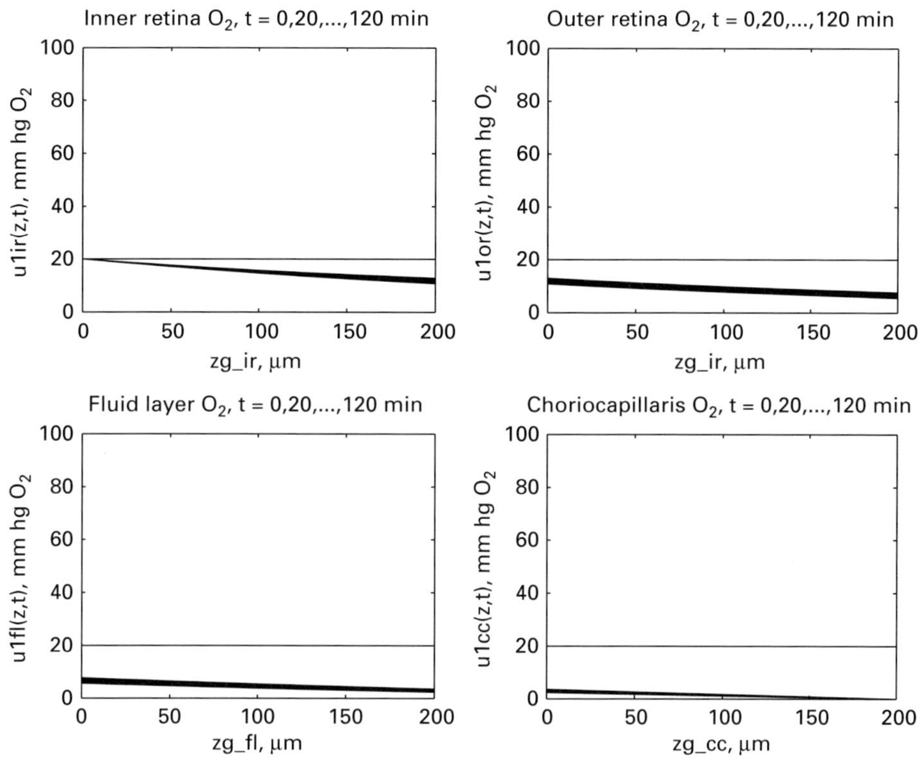

Figure 4.9 O_2 z distribution in IC, OC, FL, CC, t=0,20,...,120 min (top to bottom)

increased complexity (compared with Fig. 4.7) since the model now has eight PDEs (rather than five as in Fig 4.7).

This completes the discussion of the O_2 transport model. The basic version of eqs. (4.1) to (4.4) has been extended to include the photoreceptor cell density to illustrate the addition of another PDE to the base case model, that is, eqs. (4.5). The basic model has also been extended to include VEGF production to illustrate the addition of four PDEs to the base case model, eqs. (4.6) to (4.9). The intention is to demonstrate how models can be assembled and then extended to investigate various hypotheses and concepts. Numerical experiments with the models are also demonstrated, such as the occurrence of O_2 deficiency.

The scale in t could be extended to months, or even a few years (since t is an initial value variable that has no inherent upper limit) to reflect the observed slower changes in the retina. This raises the basic question of what determines the time scale for any particular implementation of a PDE-based model. The general answer is that anything that appears on the RHS of the PDEs, which in turn defines the LHS derivatives in t, will influence the time scale, e.g., the LHS derivatives in t of eqs. (4.6) to (4.9). For example, if the diffusivities or VEGF rates are reduced, the time response of the model will be slowed (lengthened); i.e., the derivatives in t will be reduced, thereby producing a slower model response in t.

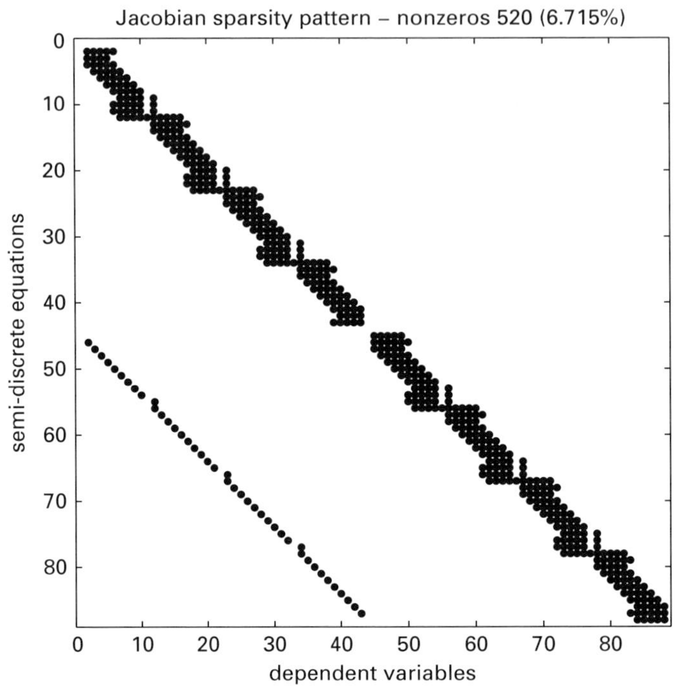

Figure 4.10 Map of the 88-ODE system from eqs. (4.1) to (4.4), (4.6) to (4.9)

As a related detail, the units of the time scale for the solution are the same as the units of the LHS derivatives in t. For example, if the LHS derivatives have the units s^{-1}, the time scale of the solution will be in s; of course, another time scale can be defined for the solution by a simple multiplication with a unit conversion factor, e.g., the use of the conversion factor $1/60$ as in Listing 4.9 to convert from s to min. This highlights another important, and perhaps obvious, detail. For a system of simultaneous or coupled PDEs, the units for t must be the same for all of the PDEs.

We conclude this discussion of the O_2 transport model, first with a few comments about the accuracy of the numerical solution, and second, a final interpretation of the model. The solution accuracy has two aspects:

- The accuracy of the ODE integration in t is determined by:
  - The length of the specified integration step in t, such as h in the Euler, modified and RK4 methods discussed in Chapter 1. Variation of h to investigate the accuracy of the integration in t is termed h-refinement.
  - The error tolerances for a variable step ODE integrator, such as `reltol=1.0e-06; abstol=1.0e-05;` for `ode15s` in Listing 4.9. In other words, variation in h (h-refinement) is automatic, as in `ode15s`, in an attempt to meet the specified error tolerances.

- The accuracy of the spatial approximations in z, for example, for the second derivatives in eqs. (4.1) to (4.4) and (4.6) to (4.9). This accuracy can be viewed in two ways:
  - The spatial finite difference interval, Δz, can be varied; the accuracy of the derivatives in z would vary as $O(\Delta z^p)$ ($p = 4$ for `dss004,dss044`). Variation of Δz is a form of h-refinement. For eqs. (4.1) to (4.4) and (4.6) to (4.9), this form of error analysis could be accomplished by increasing the number of grid points in each section (above 11 as defined in Listing 4.9) and observing the effect on the numerical solution.
  - The order of the approximation can be varied and the effect on the solution observed. For example, the second derivatives in eqs. (4.1) to (4.4) and (4.6) to (4.9) could be calculated with `dss006,dss0046` which are $O(\Delta z^6)$ and the solution compared with the solution from `dss004,dss044`. This variation in order p is termed p refinement.

Generally, the error in the initial value integration (in t) and the boundary value integration (in z) should be investigated by an error analysis, such as through h and p refinement, to estimate the accuracy of the numerical solution (specifically, to balance the initial and boundary value errors). This can generally be done numerically and does not require an analytical solution (which usually will not be available).

As a brief interpretation of the solution in Figs. 4.8 to 4.10, the increase in the VEGF concentration illustrated in Fig. 4.8 could lead to a possible retinal neovascularization and then a reduction in vision. This loss of vision is ultimately due to an impairment of O_2 transport through the four sections considered in the model, for example, from a retinal detachment or age-related macular degeneration (AMD). Possible causes for reduced O_2 transport can be studied with the model, including the effect of model parameters such as: (a) reduction in the O_2 and VEGF diffusivities, (b) increases in the VEGF production rate constants, and (c) choroidal reduction in O_2 at $z = z_L$ and $z = z_{CC}$. This parameter sensitivity in turn suggests experimental measurements that can provide more reliable parameter values for use in the model. This interplay between experiment and theory is an important guide to continuing research and is a primary justification for computer-based modeling.

Acknowledgements

The interest and suggestions of Dr. Robert Weber, Dr. Robert Linsenmeier, and Dr. Mark Pavilack are gratefully acknowledged.

References

[1] Linsenmeier, R. A. and Padnick-Silver, L. (2000), Metabolic dependence of photoreceptors on the choroid in the normal and detached retina, *Invest. Ophth. Vis. Sci.*, **41**, 3117–3123

[2] Stefánsson, E., Geirsdóttir, Á., and Sigurdsson, H. (2011), Metabolic physiology in age related macular degeneration, *Prog. Retin. Eye Res.*, **30**, 72–80

5 Hemodialyzer dynamics

When the kidneys fail to remove sufficient impurities from the blood, a device for removing the impurities is used, which is termed a hemodialyzer or just a dialyzer. Basically it transfers the impurities from the blood to another fluid termed the dialyzate by mass transfer through a membrane. A schematic diagram of a dialyzer is given in Fig. 5.1.

We now consider the derivation of a PDE model based on mass conservation.

5.1 1D PDE model

The configuration of a 1D hemodialyzer model is explained in Fig. 5.1, primarily with words.

We can note the following details about the model represented in Fig. 5.1:

- The model is one dimensional (1D) with distance along the dialyzer, z, as the spatial (boundary value) independent variable. Time t is an initial value independent variable.
- Two PDE-dependent variables, $u_1(z,t), u_2(z,t)$, represent the impurity concentrations in the blood and dialyzate, respectively. The PDEs that define these dependent variables are derived subsequently.
- Blood enters the left end at concentration $u_{1L}(t)$. This BC is not designated as $u_1(z = 0,t)$ because of a header volume at the left end (explained next).
- Similarly, the exiting blood concentration at the right end is designated as $u_{1R}(t)$ rather than $u_1(z = z_L,t)$ (again, because of a header volume).
- The entering and exiting dialyzate concentrations are $u_2(z = z_L,t)$ and $u_2(z = 0,t)$, respectively.
- The overall objective in formulating the model and computing numerical solutions is to determine $u_1(z,t), u_2(z,t)$, and in particular, how effective the dialyzer is in reducing the exiting (outflow) blood concentration $u_{1R}(t)$ below its entering value $u_{1L}(t)$.

A mass balance on the blood gives

$$\epsilon A \Delta z \frac{\partial u_1}{\partial t} = \epsilon A v_1 u_1|_z - \epsilon A v_1 u_1|_{z+\Delta z} + A_M \Delta z k_M (u_2 - u_1), \tag{5.1}$$

with variables and parameters explained in Table 5.1.

Table 5.1. Variables and parameters of eq. (5.1)

Variable	Interpretation
u_1	concentration of impurities in blood
u_2	concentration of impurities in dialyzate
t	time
z	axial position along the dialyzer
A	cross sectional area of dialyzer (transverse to z)
ϵ	fraction of A for blood flow
v_1	superficial velocity of blood flow
A_M	area for mass transfer per unit length in z
k_M	membrane mass transfer coefficient

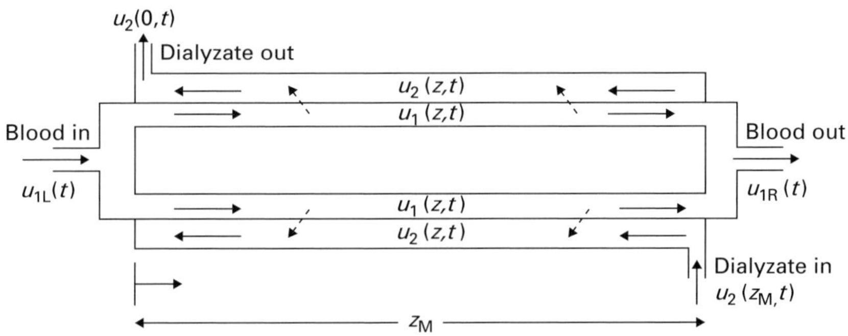

Figure 5.1 Diagram of a countercurrent hemodialyzer

Equation (5.1) is a mass conservation balance for blood with the terms explained further in the following comments.

LHS-1: $\epsilon A \Delta z(\partial u_1/\partial t)$ – Accumulation of impurities in an incremental volume $\epsilon A \Delta z$. The units of this term are (cm^2)(cm)(gmol/cm^3)(1/s) = gmol/s, that is, the accumulation of impurities per second (or the depletion of impurities if the derivative in t is negative).

RHS-1: $\epsilon A v_1 u_1|_z$ – Flow (by convection) of impurities into the incremental volume at z. The units of this term are (cm^2)(cm/s)(gmol/cm^3) = gmol/s, that is, the flow of impurities per second into the incremental volume.

RHS-2: $-\epsilon A v_1 u_1|_{z+\Delta z}$ – Flow (by convection) of impurities out of the incremental volume at $z + \Delta z$. Again, the units of this term are (cm^2)(cm/s)(gmol/cm^3) = gmol/s, that is, the flow of impurities per second out of the incremental volume.

RHS-3: $+A_M \Delta z k_M(u_2 - u_1)$ – Mass transfer of impurities between blood and dialyzate into or out of the incremental volume at z. The units of this term are (cm^2/cm)(cm)(cm/s)(gmol/cm^3) = gmol/s, that is, the transfer of impurities per second into or out of the incremental volume. Three additional points about this term can be observed.

- The transfer of impurities will be from blood to dialyzate if $u_1 > u_2$, which causes the derivative in t (the LHS of eq. (3.1)) to become more negative, as expected, that is, for u_1 to decrease with t. This should be the usual case since the purpose of the dialyzer is to purify the blood. This may seem like an obvious detail, but it emphasizes the importance of using the correct sign for this term.
- The mass transfer coefficient k_m has the units of cm/s. Of course, this coefficient is key to the performance of the dialyzer and therefore its evaluation (estimation) is quite important. We would expect that for a final design, experimental values of k_m would be measured. But for preliminary designs based on the use of the model, a reliable estimate of this coefficient is desirable; alternatively a preliminary analysis based on a range of values of k_m could be used as a guide for a further feasibility study and an experimental program.
- This mass transfer term presupposes that essentially only impurities pass through the membrane and that the principal components of blood remain in the blood stream. That is, the membrane is selective for the impurities. This is a basis of the operation of the dialyzer, and the development of an effective (efficient) membrane is the key step in the production of the dialyzer. A detailed analysis of membrane performance is given in [1, 2].

If eq. (5.1) is divided by $\epsilon A\Delta z$,

$$\frac{\partial u_1}{\partial t} = -\frac{v_1 u_1|_{z+\Delta z} - v_1 u_1|_z}{\Delta z} + \frac{A_M k_M}{\epsilon A}(u_2 - u_1),$$

or for $\Delta z \to 0$,

$$\frac{\partial u_1}{\partial t} = -\frac{\partial (v_1 u_1)}{\partial z} + \frac{A_M k_M}{\epsilon A}(u_2 - u_1). \tag{5.2}$$

Equation (5.2) is the PDE for the calculation of $u_1(z,t)$. For the subsequent analysis and programming, we will take v_1 as independent of z so that it can be taken outside the derivative in z (even though the transfer of impurities could affect v_1, but this will be neglected). Also, v_1 as a function of t is an interesting case that could be investigated through the use of eq. (5.2).

A PDE for u_2 follows from an analogous mass balance for the dialyzate. The starting point is

$$(1-\epsilon)A\Delta z\frac{\partial u_2}{\partial t} = (1-\epsilon)Av_2u_2|_z - (1-\epsilon)Av_2u_2|_{z+\Delta z} + A_M\Delta z k_M(u_2 - u_1).$$

Division by $(1-\epsilon)A\Delta z$ followed by $\Delta z \to 0$ gives

$$\frac{\partial u_2}{\partial t} = -\frac{\partial (v_2 u_2)}{\partial z} + \frac{A_M k_M}{(1-\epsilon)A}(u_1 - u_2). \tag{5.3}$$

Note that the convective terms in eqs. (5.2) and (5.3) have the same sign, even though the flow in Fig. 5.1 is countercurrent. But as presented in Fig. 5.1, $v_1 > 0, v_2 < 0$ (the numerical values for these velocities are positive and negative, respectively). Note also that the mass transfer terms in eqs. (5.2) and (5.3) are opposite in sign,

Table 5.2. Variables and parameters of eqs. (5.5)

Variable	Interpretation
V_{1L}	left volume
q_1	blood volumetric flow
u_{1L}	entering blood concentration
u_{10}	initial value of $u_1(z=0,t)$ (for $t=0$)

indicating that the impurities that leave the blood equal the impurities that enter the dialyzate.

Equations (5.2) and (5.3) are first order in t and z (they are termed first order, hyperbolic PDEs). Therefore, each requires an initial condition (IC) and a boundary condition (BC). The ICs are

$$u_1(z,t=0)=f_1(z);\ u_2(z,t=0)=f_2(z). \tag{5.4a,b}$$

The BCs are somewhat more complicated because of the entering and exiting volumes for the blood as illustrated in Fig. 5.1 (these header volumes are a result of the design of the dialyzer). In each of these volumes, we assume perfect or complete mixing. Therefore, the blood concentration in each volume is described by an ordinary differential equation (ODE) in t (variations in z do not occur through the perfect mixing assumption). The ODE for the left header is

$$\frac{V_{1L}\mathrm{d}u_1(z=0,t)}{\mathrm{d}t}=q_1(u_{1L}(t)-u_1(z=0,t));\ u_1(z=0,t=0)=u_{10}, \tag{5.5a,b}$$

as explained in Table 5.2.

Note that the solution to eq. (5.5a) produces $u_1(z=0,t)$, that is, the entering value of u_1 for the blood and therefore eq. (5.2) has eq. (5.5a) as a BC. ($u_{1L}(t)$ is a prescribed function of t).

Also, the right hand header volume is described by the ODE

$$\frac{V_{1R}\mathrm{d}u_{1R}(t)}{\mathrm{d}t}=q_1(u_1(z=z_L,t)-u_{1R}(t));\ u_{1R}(t=0)=u_{1R0}, \tag{5.6a,b}$$

which gives the exiting blood concentration $u_{1R}(t)$. Note that the input to eq. (5.6a) is the exiting blood concentration $u_1(z=z_L,t)$ (from eq. (5.2)); z_L is the length of the membrane. Equation (5.6a) is an ODE in addition to the PDEs, eqs. (5.2) and (5.3). Also, $q_1=v_1\epsilon A$ which relates the blood volumetric and linear flow rates.

The BC for eq. (5.3) is

$$u_2(z=z_L,t)=g_2(t), \tag{5.7}$$

where $g_2(t)$ is a prescribed function.

Equations (5.2) to (5.7) constitute the model for the dialyzer. They are also summarized in Fig. 5.2. The coding of the model equations is considered next.

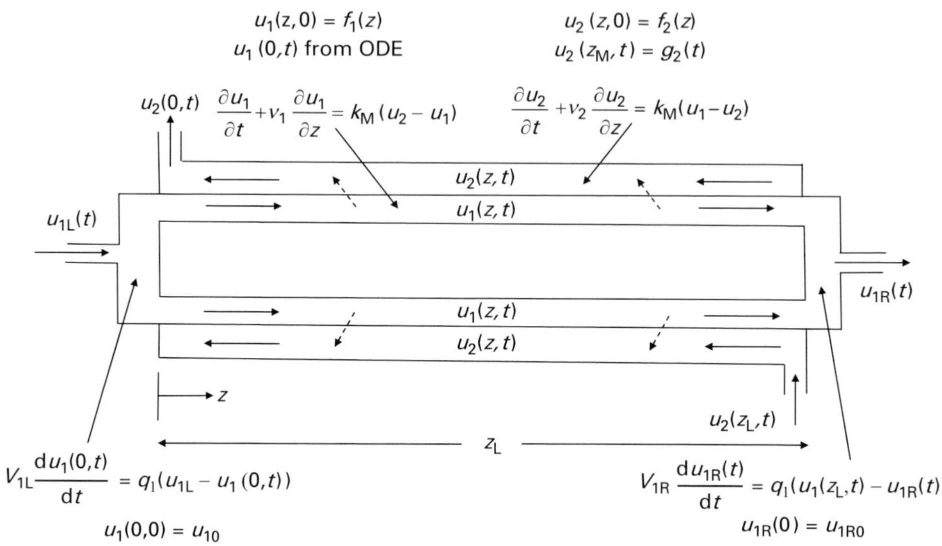

Figure 5.2 Diagram of a countercurrent hemodialyzer with model equations

5.2 MOL routines

The method of lines (MOL) format discussed in Chapter 1 is used here to compute a numerical solution to eqs. (5.2) to (5.7). The discussion of the routines starts with the main program.

5.2.1 Main program

The listing of the main program, pde_1_main, follows.

```
  clc
  clear all
%
%   1D dialyzer model
%
%   The ODE/PDE system is
%
%   u1_t = -v1*u1_z + kM1*(u2 - u1)                    (PDE)(1a)
%
%   u2_t = -v2*u2_z + kM2*(u1 - u2)                    (PDE)(1b)
%
%   V1L*u1_t(z=0,t) = q1*(u1L - u1(z=0,t))             (ODE)(1c)
%
%   V1R*u1R_t(t) = q1*(u1(z=zL,t) - u1R(t))            (ODE)(1d)
%
%   For the countercurrent case (v1 > 0, v2 < 0).
%
```

```
%   The primary outputs are u1R(t), u2(z=0,t) as a function t.
%
%   The method of lines (MOL) solution for eqs. (1) is coded
%   below.  Specifically, the spatial derivatives in the fluid
%   balances, u1_z, u2_z, are replaced by one of six approximations
%   as selected by the  variable ifd.
%
%   The following cases are programmed:
%
%   ncase = 1: kM = 0 (no mass transfer)
%
%   ncase = 2: kM = 0.001 (blood to dialysate mass transfer)
%
  global zL q1 q2 v1 v2 V1L V1R kM1 kM2 u1L u2zL u1 u2 ifd n...
         ncase ncall
%
% Step through cases
  for ncase=1:2
%
%   Model parameters
    D=5; A=pi*D^2/4; AM=A; q1=0.25; q2=0.25; eps=0.5;
    v1=q1/(eps*A); v2=-q2/((1-eps)*A); u1L=1;
    V1L=A; V1R=A; u10=0; u20=0; zL=50; n=21;
%
%   Set parameters for each case
    if(ncase==1) kM=0;      u2zL=1; end
    if(ncase==2) kM=0.001;  u2zL=0; end
    kM1=AM*kM/(A*eps);
    kM2=AM*kM/(A*(1-eps));
%
%   Display parameter summary
    fprintf(...
    '\n\n D = %3.1f  A = %4.1f  q1 = %4.2f  q2 = %4.2f
    eps = %4.2f\n',D,A,q1,q2,eps);
    fprintf(...
    '\n v1 = %5.3f  v2 = %5.3f  u1L = %5.3f  u2zL = %4.2f
    kM = %5.3f\n', v1,v2,u1L,u2zL,kM);
    fprintf(...
    '\n u10 = %4.2f  u20 = %4.2f  zL = %4.1f  n = %3d\n',...
    u10,u20,zL,n);
%
% Select an approximation for the convective derivatives
% u1z, u2z
%
%   ifd = 1: Two point upwind approximation
%
%   ifd = 2: Centered approximation
%
%   ifd = 3: Five point, biased upwind approximation
%
%   ifd = 4: van Leer flux limiter
```

```
%
%   ifd = 5: Superbee flux limiter
%
%   ifd = 6: Smart flux limiter
%
  ifd=1;
%
% Level of output
%
%   Detailed output - ip = 1
%
%   Brief (IC) output - ip = 2
%
  ip=1;
%
% Parameters for fourth order Runge Kutta integration
  nsteps=10;
  h=14.4;
%
% Initial condition
  for i=1:n
      u(i)=u10;
    u(i+n)=u20;
  end
  u(2*n+1)=u10;
  t=0;
%
% Display ifd, ncase, h, CFL
  fprintf('\n ifd = %2d   ncase = %2d   h = %10.3e
          CFL = %4.2f\n\n',ifd,ncase,h,v1*h/(zL/(n-1)));
%
% Display heading
  fprintf('    t    u1R(t)   u2(0,t)\n');
%
% Display numerical solution at t = 0
  fprintf('%5.2f%10.4f%10.4f\n',t/3600,u(2*n+1),u(n+1));
%
% Store solution for plotting
   u1plot(1)=u(2*n+1);
   u2plot(1)=u(n+1);
   tplot(1)=t;
%
% nout output points
  nout=51;
  ncall=0;
  for iout=2:nout
%
%   Fourth order Runge Kutta integration
    u0=u; t0=t;
    [u,t]=rk4(u0,t0,h,nsteps);
%
```

```
%   Numerical solutions
    if(ip==1)
      fprintf('%5.2f%10.4f%10.4f\n',t/3600,u(2*n+1),u(n+1));
    end
%
%   Store solution for plotting
     u1plot(iout)=u(2*n+1);
     u2plot(iout)=u(n+1);
     tplot(iout)=t/3600;
%
% Next output
  end
%
% Plots for u1R(t), u2(z=0,t)
  figure(ncase);
  plot(tplot,u1plot,'-o');
  axis([0 2 -0.1 1.1]);
  ylabel('u1R(t),u2(0,t)');xlabel('t');
  if(ncase==1) title('ncase = 1; u1 - o; u2 - x'); end
  if(ncase==2) title('ncase = 2; u1 - o; u2 - x'); end
  hold on
  plot(tplot,u2plot,'-x');
%
% Next case
  end
```

Listing 5.1 Main program pde_1_main for eqs. (5.2) to (5.7)

We can note the following details about pde_1_main.

- Previous files are cleared and selected variables and parameters are declared global so that they can be shared with other routines.

```
  clc
  clear all
%
%   1D dialyzer model
%
    (some documentation comments deleted to conserve space)
%
%   The following cases are programmed:
%
%   ncase = 1: kM = 0 (no mass transfer)
%
%   ncase = 2: kM = 0.001 (blood to dialysate mass transfer)
%
  global zL q1 q2 v1 v2 V1L V1R kM1 kM2 u1L u2zL u1 u2 ifd n...
         ncase ncall
%
% Step through cases
  for ncase=1:2
```

Two cases are indicated, with k_M in eqs. (5.2) and (5.3) set to zero for `ncase=1` to investigate the expected behavior of the model with no mass transfer.

- The model parameters are defined numerically.

```
%
%   Model parameters
    D=5; A=pi*D^2/4; AM=A; q1=0.25; q2=0.25; eps=0.5;
    v1=q1/(eps*A); v2=-q2/((1-eps)*A); u1L=1;
    V1L=A; V1R=A; u10=0; u20=0; zL=50; n=21;
```

These numerical values are explained briefly next.

- **D**: Diameter of the dialyzer, cm.
- **A**: Cross sectional area of the dialyzer, cm^2; used in eqs. (5.2) and (5.3).
- **AM**: Mass transfer area per unit length of the dialyzer, cm^2/cm; used in eqs. (5.2) and (5.3). `AM` can be assigned any reasonable value; here we use the value `AM=A` just for the purpose of the program execution.
- **q1, q2**: Volumetric flow rates of blood and dialyzate, respectively, cm^3/s
- **eps**: Fraction of `A` available for blood flow, $0 \le \epsilon \le 1$, dimensionless; thus, `1 - eps` is the fraction of `A` available for dialyzate flow.
- **v1, v2**: Linear flow velocity for blood and dialyzate, respectively, cm/s; used in eqs. (5.2) and (5.3). Note that `v1 > 0, v2 < 0` for countercurrent flow.
- **u1L**: Normalized entering blood concentration (at $z = 0$), dimensionless.
- **v1L, v2R**: Header volumes for u_1 at $z = 0, z_L$, cm^3; for the values stated, the length of the header volumes is 1 cm (`V1L=1*A`), but these volumes can be any positive values (not zero because of the division by the volume in the numerical integration of ODEs (5.5a) and (5.6a)). Also, as these volumes become smaller, the ODE/PDE model becomes stiffer; that is, eqs. (5.5a) and (5.6a) become faster or stiffer.
- **u10, u20**: ICs for eqs. (5.2), (5.3), dimensionless (in eqs. (5.4), $u_1(z,t=0) = f_1(z) = u_{10}$; $u_2(z,t=0) = f_2(z) = u_{20}$).
- **zL**: Dialyzer length, cm.
- **n**: Number of grid points in z.

- The mass transfer coefficient, k_M, is set for `ncase=1,2`. Note that for `ncase=1`, mass transfer between the blood and dialyzate does not take place; this special case provides a test of the numerical solution as explained subsequently.

```
%
%   Set parameters for each case
    if(ncase==1) kM=0;      u2zL=1; end
    if(ncase==2) kM=0.001;  u2zL=0; end
    kM1=AM*kM/(A*eps);
    kM2=AM*kM/(A*(1-eps));
```

The coefficients in eqs. (5.2) and (5.3), k_{M1}, k_{M2}, are then computed.

- The parameters are displayed.

```
%
%   Display parameter summary
```

```
fprintf(...
'\n\n D = %3.1f   A = %4.1f   q1 = %4.2f   q2 = %4.2f
eps = %4.2f\n',D,A,q1,q2,eps);
fprintf(...
'\n v1 = %5.3f   v2 = %5.3f   u1L = %5.3f   u2zL = %4.2f
kM = %5.3f\n', v1,v2,u1L,u2zL,kM);
fprintf(...
'\n u10 = %4.2f   u20 = %4.2f   zL = %4.1f   n = %3d\n',...
u10,u20,zL,n);
```

- An approximation for the derivatives in z in eqs. (5.2) and (5.3) is selected with `ifd` as in Section 1.2.4.

```
%
% Select an approximation for the convective derivatives u1z, u2z
%
%   ifd = 1: Two point upwind approximation
%
%   ifd = 2: Centered approximation
%
%   ifd = 3: Five point, biased upwind approximation
%
%   ifd = 4: van Leer flux limiter
%
%   ifd = 5: Superbee flux limiter
%
%   ifd = 6: Smart flux limiter
%
  ifd=1;
```

- A level of tabulated numerical output is specified with `ip`.

```
%
% Level of output
%
%   Detailed output - ip = 1
%
%   Brief (IC) output - ip = 2
%
  ip=1;
```

- The parameters for the Runge Kutta integration in `rk4` (Listing 1.5) provide ten RK steps each of length 14.4 s or $(10)(14.4) = 144$ s for each output; 144 was selected since it is evenly divisable by 3600 ($144/3600 = 0.04$) in a subsequent conversion from s to h.

```
%
% Parameters for fourth order Runge Kutta integration
  nsteps=10;
  h=14.4;
```

- The ICs of eqs. (5.4) are defined in a `for` loop (for `t=0`).

```
%
% Initial condition
  for i=1:n
      u(i)=u10;
    u(i+n)=u20;
  end
  u(2*n+1)=u10;
  t=0;
```

The IC `u(2*n+1)=u10` is for eq. (5.6b), $u_{1R}(t=0)=u_{1R0}=u_{10}$. In other words, u_1 from eq. (5.2) corresponds to dependent variables `u(1)` to `u(21)` (recall `n=21`), u_2 of eq. (5.3) corresponds to `u(22)` to `u(42)`, and u_{1R} from eq. (5.6a) corresponds to `u(43)` (since $2n+1=2(21)+1=43$).

- Additional parameters are displayed.

```
%
% Display ifd, ncase, h, CFL
  fprintf('\n ifd = %2d   ncase = %2d   h = %10.3e
          CFL = %4.2f\n\n',ifd,ncase,h,v1*h/(zL/(n-1)));
```

In particular, the dimensionless Courant–Friedrichs–Lewy number $= v_1 h/\Delta z$, `CFL`, is computed and displayed. This number is an indication of the stability of the numerical MOL solution of eqs. (5.2) and (5.3). If h is increased, eventually the numerical solution will become unstable.

- A heading for the numerical solution is displayed and the values $u_{1R}(t=0)$ from eq. (5.6a) and $u_2(z=0,t=0)$ from eq. (5.3) are placed under the heading.

```
%
% Display heading
  fprintf('    t    u1R(t)   u2(0,t)\n');
%
% Display numerical solution at t = 0
  fprintf('%5.2f%10.4f%10.4f\n',t/3600,u(2*n+1),u(n+1));
%
% Store solution for plotting
   u1plot(1)=u(2*n+1);
   u2plot(1)=u(n+1);
   tplot(1)=t;
```

Also, $u_{1R}(t=0)$ from eq. (5.6a) and $u_2(z=0,t=0)$ from eq. (5.3) are stored for subsequent plotting (note the LHS subscript `1` for the first points in the plots). The factor 3600 converts t from s to h (the model solution is in terms of s since v_1, v_2 are in cm/s).

- The solution to eqs. (5.2) to (5.7) is computed by `rk4` (Listing 1.5) with output at `nout=51` points in t (`iout` starts at 2 because of the previous use of `1` for the IC).

```
%
% nout output points
  nout=51;
  ncall=0;
  for iout=2:nout
```

```
%
%   Fourth order Runge Kutta integration
    u0=u; t0=t;
    [u,t]=rk4(u0,t0,h,nsteps);
```

The ODE routine pde_1 discussed next is called from rk4 (Listing 1.5).

- The solution is displayed and stored for subsequent plotting (a continuation of the previous output at $t = 0$).

```
%
%   Numerical solutions
    if(ip==1)
      fprintf('%5.2f%10.4f%10.4f\n',t/3600,u(2*n+1),u(n+1));
    end
%
%   Store solution for plotting
     u1plot(iout)=u(2*n+1);
     u2plot(iout)=u(n+1);
     tplot(iout)=t/3600;
%
% Next output
  end
```

The end concludes the for loop in iout.

- The terminal (exiting) blood and dialyzate concentrations are plotted against t in h.

```
%
% Plots for u1R(t), u2(z=0,t)
  figure(ncase);
  plot(tplot,u1plot,'-o');
  axis([0 2 -0.1 1.1]);
  ylabel('u1R(t),u2(0,t)');xlabel('t');
  if(ncase==1) title('ncase = 1; u1 - o; u2 - x'); end
  if(ncase==2) title('ncase = 2; u1 - o; u2 - x'); end
  hold on
  plot(tplot,u2plot,'-x');
%
% Next case
  end
```

The end terminates the for loop in ncase.

5.2.2 ODE routine

The ODE routine pde_1 called by rk4 (Listing 1.5) is in Listing 5.2.

```
  function ut=pde_1(u,t)
%
% Function pde_1 computes the t derivative vector of the u
% vector
%
  global zL q1 q2 v1 v2 V1L V1R kM1 kM2 u1L u2zL u1 u2 ifd n...
```

```
  ncase ncall
%
% One vector to two PDEs, one ODE
  for i=1:n
    u1(i)=u(i);
    u2(i)=u(i+n);
  end
  u1R=u(2*n+1);
%
% Boundary condition
  u2(n)=u2zL;
%
% First order spatial derivative
%
%   ifd = 1: Two point upwind finite difference (2pu)
    if(ifd==1) [u1z]=dss012(0.0,zL,n,u1,v1); end
    if(ifd==1) [u2z]=dss012(0.0,zL,n,u2,v2); end
%
%   ifd = 2: Three point center finite difference (3pc)
    if(ifd==2) [u1z]=dss002(0.0,zL,n,u1); end
    if(ifd==2) [u2z]=dss002(0.0,zL,n,u2); end
%
%   ifd = 3: Five point biased upwind approximation (5pbu)
    if(ifd==3) [u1z]=dss020(0.0,zL,n,u1,v1); end
    if(ifd==3) [u2z]=dss020(0.0,zL,n,u2,v2); end
%
%   ifd = 4: van Leer flux limiter
    if(ifd==4) [u1z]=vanl(0.0,zL,n,u1,v1); end
    if(ifd==4) [u2z]=vanl(0.0,zL,n,u2,v2); end
%
%   ifd = 5: Superbee flux limiter
    if(ifd==5) [u1z]=super(0.0,zL,n,u1,v1); end
    if(ifd==5) [u2z]=super(0.0,zL,n,u2,v2); end
%
%   ifd = 6: Smart flux limiter
    if(ifd==6) [u1z]=smart(0.0,zL,n,u1,v1); end
    if(ifd==6) [u2z]=smart(0.0,zL,n,u2,v2); end
%
% Temporal derivatives
%
%    u1t
     u1t(1)=(1/V1L)*q1*(u1L-u1(1));
     for i=2:n
       u1t(i)=-v1*u1z(i)+kM1*(u2(i)-u1(i));
     end
     u1Rt=(1/V1R)*q1*(u1(n)-u1R);
%
%    u2t
     u2t(n)=0.0;
     for i=1:n-1
       u2t(i)=-v2*u2z(i)+kM2*(u1(i)-u2(i));
```

```
    end
%
% Two PDEs, one ODE to one vector
  for i=1:n
      ut(i)=u1t(i);
    ut(i+n)=u2t(i);
  end
  ut(2*n+1)=u1Rt;
%
% Increment calls to pde_1
  ncall=ncall+1;
```

Listing 5.2 ODE routine pde_1 for eqs. (5.2) to (5.7)

We can note the following points about pde_1.

- The function is defined and selected variables and parameters are declared global so that they can be shared with the main program of Listing 5.1.

```
  function ut=pde_1(u,t)
%
% Function pde_1 computes the t derivative vector of the u
% vector
%
  global zL q1 q2 v1 v2 V1L V1R kM1 kM2 u1L u2zL u1 u2 ifd n...
  ncase ncall
```

- The single vector u that is an input (RHS argument) to pde_1 is placed in two vectors, u1 for eq. (5.2) and u2 for eq. (5.3), and one ODE dependent variable, u1R for eq. (5.6a).

```
%
% One vector to two PDEs, one ODE
  for i=1:n
    u1(i)=u(i);
    u2(i)=u(i+n);
  end
  u1R=u(2*n+1);
```

- The BC for eqs. (5.3) and (5.7) with $u_2(z = z_L, t) = g_2(t) =$ u2zL=1 (a normalized dialyzate entering concentration) is specified (for u2(n)).

```
%
% Boundary condition
  u2(n)=u2zL;
```

- The first derivatives in z in eqs. (5.2) and (5.3), $(\partial u_1/\partial z)$ and $(\partial u_2/\partial z)$, are computed by one of six spatial differentiators (discussed in Section 1.2.4).

```
%
% First order spatial derivative
%
%   ifd = 1: Two point upwind finite difference (2pu)
    if(ifd==1) [u1z]=dss012(0.0,zL,n,u1,v1); end
```

```
      if(ifd==1) [u2z]=dss012(0.0,zL,n,u2,v2); end
%
%     ifd = 2: Three point center finite difference (3pc)
      if(ifd==2) [u1z]=dss002(0.0,zL,n,u1); end
      if(ifd==2) [u2z]=dss002(0.0,zL,n,u2); end
%
%     ifd = 3: Five point biased upwind approximation (5pbu)
      if(ifd==3) [u1z]=dss020(0.0,zL,n,u1,v1); end
      if(ifd==3) [u2z]=dss020(0.0,zL,n,u2,v2); end
%
%     ifd = 4: van Leer flux limiter
      if(ifd==4) [u1z]=vanl(0.0,zL,n,u1,v1); end
      if(ifd==4) [u2z]=vanl(0.0,zL,n,u2,v2); end
%
%     ifd = 5: Superbee flux limiter
      if(ifd==5) [u1z]=super(0.0,zL,n,u1,v1); end
      if(ifd==5) [u2z]=super(0.0,zL,n,u2,v2); end
%
%     ifd = 6: Smart flux limiter
      if(ifd==6) [u1z]=smart(0.0,zL,n,u1,v1); end
      if(ifd==6) [u2z]=smart(0.0,zL,n,u2,v2); end
```

- The programming of PDE (5.2) and ODE (5.6a) follows directly from these two equations.

```
%
% Temporal derivatives
%
%     u1t
      u1t(1)=(1/V1L)*q1*(u1L-u1(1));
      for i=2:n
        u1t(i)=-v1*u1z(i)+kM1*(u2(i)-u1(i));
      end
      u1Rt=(1/V1R)*q1*(u1(n)-u1R);
```

We note two steps in this programming.

- The MOL ODE for the entering header at $z = 0$ (see Figs. 5.1 and 5.2) gives the derivative $(du_1(z=0,t)/dt) =$ `u1t(1)`. Note the division by `V1L` so this volume cannot be set to zero to eliminate the header. Rather, `u1t(1)` would be included in the `for` loop (for `i=1`). Also, as this volume is reduced, the header equation would become faster (stiffer) which could cause a problem with the use of `rk4` (called in `pde_1_main` in Listing 5.1) since this is a nonstiff integrator.
- Equation (5.6a) for exiting header gives the derivative $(du_{1R}/dt) =$ `u1RT`. Again, the division by `V1R` precludes setting the exiting header volume to zero.

- Equation (5.3) is programmed, including the use of eq. (5.7) with $(du_2(z=z_L,t)/dt) =$ `u2t(n) = 0`.

```
%
%     u2t
      u2t(n)=0.0;
```

```
    for i=1:n-1
      u2t(i)=-v2*u2z(i)+kM2*(u1(i)-u2(i));
    end
```

- $21+21+1=43$ derivatives in t are now programmed and can be transferred to a single derivative vector `ut` to be returned from `pde_1`.

```
%
% Two PDEs, one ODE to one vector
  for i=1:n
      ut(i)=u1t(i);
    ut(i+n)=u2t(i);
  end
  ut(2*n+1)=u1Rt;
%
% Increment calls to pde_1
  ncall=ncall+1;
```

A transpose to a column vector is not required by `rk4` (as for `ode15s`). Finally, the counter for the calls to `pde_1` is incremented.

This completes the programming of eqs. (5.2) to (5.7). Now the output from the routines in Listings 5.1 and 5.2 is considered, starting with abbreviated tabular numerical output in Table 5.3.

5.3 Model output

Abbreviated output from the routines of Section 5.2 follows.

Table 5.3. Selected numerical output for eqs. (5.2) to (5.7) from `pde_1_main` and `pde_1` for `ncase=1,2`

```
D = 5.0  A = 19.6  q1 = 0.25  q2 = 0.25  eps = 0.50

v1 = 0.025  v2 = -0.025  u1L = 1.000  u2zL = 1.00  kM = 0.000

u10 = 0.00  u20 = 0.00  zL = 50.0  n =  21

ifd =  1   ncase =  1   h = 1.440e+001  CFL = 0.15

   t     u1R(t)   u2(0,t)
0.00    0.0000    0.0000
0.04    0.0000    0.0000
0.08    0.0000    0.0000
0.12    0.0000    0.0000
0.16    0.0000    0.0000
0.20    0.0000    0.0001
0.24    0.0002    0.0008
0.28    0.0012    0.0046
0.32    0.0059    0.0173
```

```
0.36    0.0198    0.0484
0.40    0.0516    0.1071
0.44    0.1093    0.1973
0.48    0.1964    0.3142
0.52    0.3086    0.4456
0.56    0.4352    0.5765
0.60    0.5627    0.6941
0.64    0.6790    0.7906
0.68    0.7762    0.8637
0.72    0.8514    0.9154
0.76    0.9059    0.9498
0.80    0.9429    0.9714
0.84    0.9667    0.9843
0.88    0.9813    0.9917
0.92    0.9899    0.9958
0.96    0.9947    0.9979
1.00    0.9973    0.9990
1.04    0.9987    0.9995
1.08    0.9994    0.9998
1.12    0.9997    0.9999
1.16    0.9999    1.0000
1.20    0.9999    1.0000
1.24    1.0000    1.0000
1.28    1.0000    1.0000
  .                 .
  .                 .
  .                 .
(output for t = 1.32 to
     1.92 deleted)
  .                 .
  .                 .
  .                 .
1.96    1.0000    1.0000
2.00    1.0000    1.0000

ncall = 2000

D = 5.0  A = 19.6  q1 = 0.25  q2 = 0.25  eps = 0.50

v1 = 0.025  v2 = -0.025  u1L = 1.000  u2zL = 0.00  kM = 0.001

u10 = 0.00  u20 = 0.00  zL = 50.0  n =  21

ifd =  1   ncase =  2   h = 1.440e+001  CFL = 0.15

   t     u1R(t)   u2(0,t)
0.00    0.0000    0.0000
0.04    0.0000    0.1007
0.08    0.0000    0.2117
0.12    0.0000    0.2976
0.16    0.0000    0.3646
```

```
0.20     0.0000     0.4179
0.24     0.0000     0.4612
0.28     0.0003     0.4969
0.32     0.0010     0.5269
0.36     0.0030     0.5523
0.40     0.0068     0.5743
  .                   .
  .                   .
  .                   .
(output for t = 0.44 to
     1.76 deleted)
  .                   .
  .                   .
  .                   .
1.80     0.1867     0.7815
1.84     0.1879     0.7826
1.88     0.1890     0.7836
1.92     0.1900     0.7846
1.96     0.1909     0.7855
2.00     0.1918     0.7863

ncall = 2000
```

We can note the following details about Table 5.3.

- The grid in z is $0 \leq z \leq 50$ with 21 points (zL=50, n=21).
- The approximation of the derivatives in z in eqs. (5.2) and (5.3) is based on two point upwinding ifd=1 set in pde_1_main of Listing 5.1.
- The volumetric flow rates for blood and dialyzate are q1 = q2 = 0.25 cm^3/s.
- The blood and dialyzate linear velocities (computed from q1,q2 in pde_1_main) are v1=0.025,v2=-0.025 cm/s (opposite in sign for countercurrent flow).
- The output is at intervals of 0.04 hr. For the integration step in t, h = 14.4 s, 10 steps for the output interval, (14.4)(10)/3600 = 0.04 hr.
- The mass transfer coefficient is ncase=1, kM=0 (no mass transfer), ncase=2, kM=0.001. Thus a comparison of the solutions for ncase=1,2 indicates the effect of mass transfer from the blood to the dialyzate.
- The CFL constant is 0.15, which is well below the value of 1 usually considered for the onset of instability in the numerical solution.
- The accuracy of the numerical solution could be studied in two ways.
  - The accuracy of the integration in z could be inferred by increasing the number of grid points, e.g., n=21 to n=41 (h refinement), and by changing the spatial derivative approximation, e.g., another value of ifd (p refinement).
  - The accuracy of the integration in t could be inferred by decreasing the step, e.g., h=14.4 to h=14.4/2 (h refinement), and by changing the integration algorithm, e.g., fourth order Runge Kutta method to a higher order Runge Kutta method (p refinement).

- The total calls to pde_1 is ncall = 2000 which results from (four calls to pde_1/RK step in t)(ten RK steps in t/output)(50 outputs for the complete solution to $t = 2$ h) = 2000.

Additional features of the numerical solution are evident in Figs. 5.3 and 5.4.

In Fig. 5.3, the two solutions, $u_{1R}(t)$ and $u_2(z = 0, t)$, are close (both have the same entering values, u1L=u2zL=1). They are not exactly the same because of the entering and exiting headers for the blood flow (Fig. 5.1). As expected, the response of the blood concentration, $u_1(z,t)$ (with headers), slightly lags that for the dialyzate, $u_2(z,t)$ (no headers). Both solutions approach 1 with increasing t as expected (the unit entering concentrations move through and exit the system when there is no mass transfer (kM=0 for ncase=1).

To explain further, both solutions reflect a traveling wave that results from the ICs set in pde_1_main (with u10=u20=0).

```
%
% Initial condition
  for i=1:n
      u(i)=u10;
    u(i+n)=u20;
  end
  u(2*n+1)=u10;
  t=0;
```

That is, all of the $21 + 21 + 1 = 43$ ODEs start at zero. The entering concentrations are set to 1 in pde_1_main, u1L=1;u2zL=1; (for ncase=1). These unit values travel through the dialyzer and eventually reach the exits, at which time the solutions move

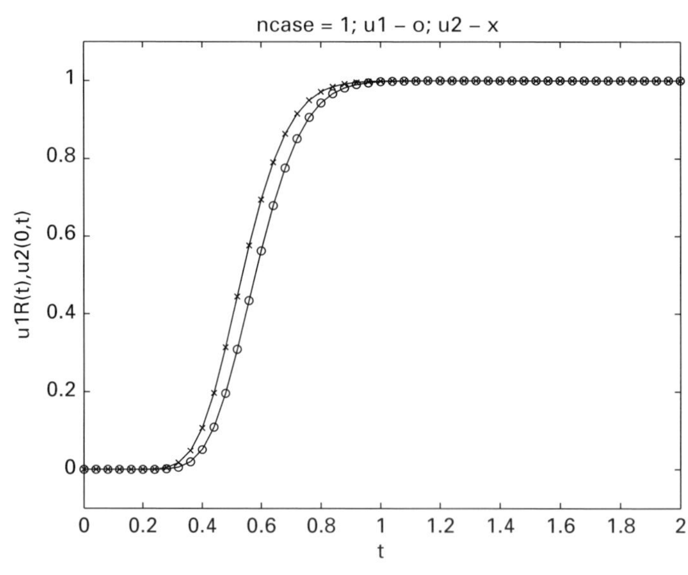

Figure 5.3 Solution from pde_1_main, pde_1 for ncase=1

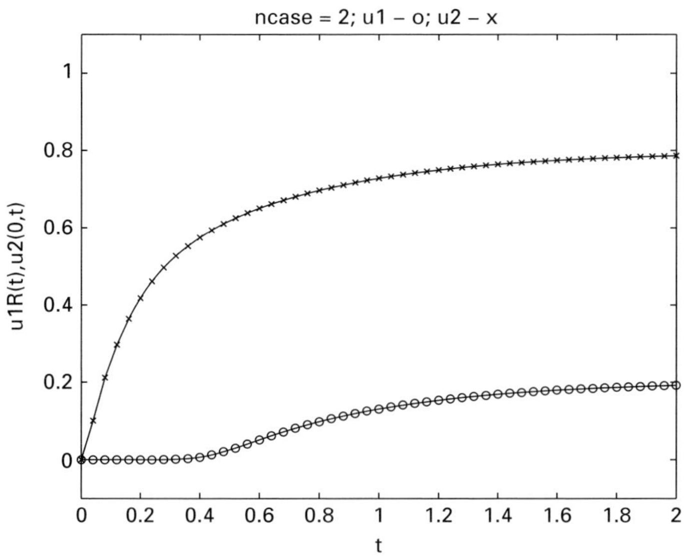

Figure 5.4 Solution from `pde_1_main`, `pde_1` for `ncase=2`

from the zero ICs to the unit BCs. The step is not instantaneous because of the numerical diffusion from the two point upwinding of the derivatives in z of eqs. (5.2) and (5.3) (`ifd=1`). The time of the arrival at the exit (right end, $z = z_L$) for u_1 can be estimated as $z_L/v_1 = 50/0.025 = 2000\text{ s} = 0.555\text{ h}$. Similarly for u_2, since $v_2 = -v_1$ the time of arrival at the left end ($z = 0$) is also approximately 0.555 h. These arrival times are reflected in Fig. 5.3; they are not exact because of the numerical diffusion from `ifd=1` and the delay in the u_1 response due to the two headers.

In Fig. 5.4, the exiting blood and dialyzate concentrations at $t = 2$ h are `2.00 0.1918 0.7863` (from Table 5.3), and these concentrations appear to be changing only slightly with t. Thus, for `kM=0.001` (`ncase=2`), the dialyzer removed about `(1-0.1918)(100) = 81%` of the blood impurities. If `kM` is increased, e.g., to `kM=0.0025`, the exiting blood impurities are reduced further.

The details of the solutions are somewhat more complicated than in Fig. 5.3. Again, all 43 ODEs start at a zero IC (with `u10=u20=0`). The u_1 response to `u1L=1;` (set in `pde_1_main`) arrives at the right end ($z = z_L$) at approximately 0.555 h, as in Fig. 5.3, but because of the mass transfer to the dialyzate ($k_M = 0.001$ for `ncase=2`), the response is reduced and eventually the exiting u_1 concentration ($u_{1R}(t)$) reaches `0.1918` at `t=2 hr` (from Table 5.3).

The u_2 response is immediate (just after $t = 0$) because the exiting dialyzate "sees" the unit entering blood concentration at $z = 0$ immediately (across the membrane) and responds accordingly. Note also that for `ncase=2`, the entering u_2 concentration ($u_2(z = z_L, t)$) is `u2zL=0;` (set in `pde_1_main`) so that the exiting u_2 concentration (at $z = 0$) is determined entirely by the blood concentration on the other side of the membrane (no impurities enter in the dialyzate at $z = z_L$). At $t = 2$ h, this exiting u_2 ($u_2(z = 0, t)$) reaches 0.7863 (from Table 5.3).

Finally, to conclude this discussion of the dialyzer model, we briefly consider the output for ifd=4 set in pde_1_main (the van Leer limiter in place of two point upwinding ifd=1 for the z derivatives in eqs. (5.2) and (5.3)). The numerical output is indicated in Table 5.4.

Table 5.4. Abbreviated numerical output for eqs. (5.2) to (5.7) from pde_1_main and pde_1, ifd=4

```
D = 5.0  A = 19.6  q1 = 0.25  q2 = 0.25  eps = 0.50

v1 = 0.025  v2 = -0.025  u1L = 1.000  u2zL = 1.00  kM = 0.000

u10 = 0.00  u20 = 0.00  zL = 50.0  n =  21

ifd =  4   ncase =  1   h = 1.440e+001  CFL = 0.15
```

t	u1R(t)	u2(0,t)
0.00	0.0000	0.0000
0.04	0.0000	0.0000
0.08	0.0000	0.0000
0.12	0.0000	0.0000
0.16	0.0000	0.0000
0.20	0.0000	0.0000
0.24	0.0000	0.0000
0.28	0.0000	0.0000
0.32	0.0000	0.0000
0.36	0.0000	0.0000
0.40	0.0000	0.0000
0.44	0.0002	0.0071
0.48	0.0131	0.1008
0.52	0.1133	0.3595
0.56	0.3462	0.6490
0.60	0.6108	0.8433
0.64	0.8061	0.9398
0.68	0.9160	0.9793
0.72	0.9673	0.9935
0.76	0.9883	0.9981
0.80	0.9961	0.9995
0.84	0.9988	0.9998
0.88	0.9996	0.9999
0.92	0.9999	1.0000
0.96	1.0000	1.0000
1.00	1.0000	1.0000
1.04	1.0000	1.0000
1.08	1.0000	1.0000
1.12	1.0000	1.0000
1.16	1.0000	1.0000
1.20	1.0000	1.0000

```
1.24     1.0000     1.0000
1.28     1.0000     1.0000
  .                   .
  .                   .
  .                   .
(output for t = 1.32 to
     1.92 deleted)
  .                   .
  .                   .
  .                   .
1.96     1.0000     1.0000
2.00     1.0000     1.0000

ncall = 2000

D = 5.0  A = 19.6  q1 = 0.25  q2 = 0.25  eps = 0.50

v1 = 0.025  v2 = -0.025  u1L = 1.000  u2zL = 0.00  kM = 0.001

u10 = 0.00  u20 = 0.00  zL = 50.0  n =  21

ifd =  4   ncase =  2   h = 1.440e+001  CFL = 0.15

   t      u1R(t)    u2(0,t)
0.00     0.0000     0.0000
0.04     0.0000     0.0983
0.08     0.0000     0.1974
0.12     0.0000     0.2729
0.16     0.0000     0.3354
0.20     0.0000     0.3874
0.24     0.0000     0.4306
0.28     0.0000     0.4666
0.32     0.0000     0.4970
0.36     0.0000     0.5230
0.40     0.0000     0.5454
  .                   .
  .                   .
  .                   .
(output for t = 0.44 to
     1.76 deleted)
  .                   .
  .                   .
  .                   .
1.80     0.1768     0.7718
1.84     0.1785     0.7734
1.88     0.1800     0.7749
1.92     0.1814     0.7762
1.96     0.1827     0.7775
2.00     0.1840     0.7787

ncall = 2000
```

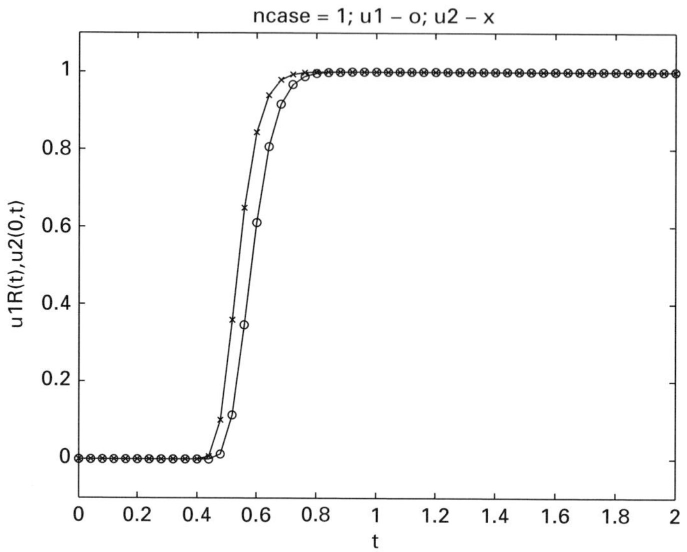

Figure 5.5 Solution from pde_1_main, pde_1 for ncase=1, ifd=4

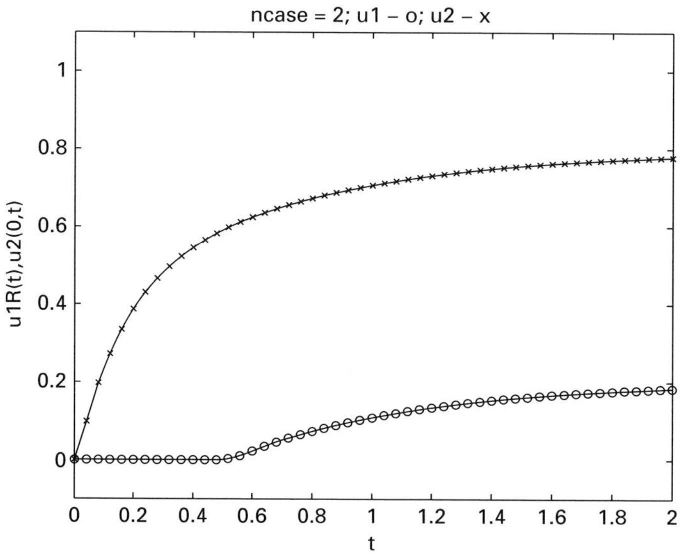

Figure 5.6 Solution from pde_1_main, pde_1 for ncase=2, ifd=4

For ifd=4, ncase=2, t=2, the values are slightly different than from Table 5.3.

```
Table 5.3

 2.00     0.1918     0.7863
```

```
Table 5.4

 2.00     0.1840     0.7787
```

These differences may result from the limited spatial resolution for `n=21` and the fact that the 2*pu* approximation (`ifd=1`, Table 5.3) and the van Leer limiter (`ifd=4`, Table 5.4) are of different orders in z; this point could be investigated with h refinement (increase `n=21`) and using other limiters (`ifd=5,6`).

Figure 5.5 indicates that van Leer gives a slightly better (sharper) resolution of the moving front solutions for `ncase=1`, that is, less numerical diffusion (compare Figs. 5.3 and 5.5) which is to be expected since the purpose of the van Leer limiter is to resolve moving fronts (as well as the limiters for `ifd=5,6`).

Figure 5.6 also indicates that van Leer gives a slightly different transient response than two point upwinding in Fig. 5.4 (including the values at 2 h as reflected in the numbers just discussed).

We will not carry the discussion further, e.g., for all six differentiators, to conserve space; generally the results conform to those in Section 1.2.4, including the oscillations for `ifd=2,3`. Particularly significant parameters in the model are the mass transfer coefficient, k_M, and mass transfer area per unit length of the dialyzer, A_M (which will be determined by membrane selection and the number of parallel membrane fibers). Other important design parameters that will affect the impurity removal from the blood stream include the diameter and length of the dialyzer, D and z_L, and the flow rates, q_1 and q_2. The model is intended to facilitate the experimentation with and selection of the design parameters.

References

[1] Bazaev, N. A., Grinvald, V. M., and Selishchev, S. V. (2010), A mathematical model for a biotechnological hemodialysis system, *Biomed. Eng.*, **44** (3), 1–7

[2] Eloot, S. (2004), *Experimental and Numerical Modeling of Dialysis*, PhD dissertation, Ghent University, Ghent, Belgium

6 Epidermal wound healing

The PDE models discussed in this chapter pertain to wound healing. We consider two models ([3]), based on one PDE and two PDEs, respectively. To start with the one-PDE model, the movement of epithelial cells across the wound is modeled by the following nonlinear form of the 1D diffusion equation with an additional nonlinear logistic (algebraic) term.

6.1 One-PDE model

$$\frac{\partial u}{\partial t} = D\frac{\partial \left((1-u/u_0)^p \frac{\partial u}{\partial r} \right)}{\partial r} + s_c u(1-u/u_0), \tag{6.1}$$

where

Variable, parameter set:	Interpretation, units
u	density of epithelial cells (cells/cm^3)
r	lateral position across the wound (cm)
t	time (s)
u_0	normal (unwounded) cell density (cells/cm^3)
D	cell diffusivity (cm^2/s)
p	parameter in the function for nonlinear diffusion (dimensionless)
s_c	coefficient of the nonlinear logistic source term (1/s)

A detailed discussion of this model in given in [3].[1] We use r as the spatial independent variable because of this choice in [3]; eq. (6.1) is in Cartesian coordinates, not radial coordinates.

[1] The original variable diffusivity $(u/u_0)^p$ is changed to $(1-u/u_0)^p$ to avoid computational problems such as the indeterminate form 0^0 (with $u=p=0$) and a zero RHS of eq. (6.1) when $u=0$ so that $(\partial u/\partial t)=0$ and therefore $u(r,t)$ does not change with t. The computational approach to the variable diffusivity is the principal focus here, and is illustrated with the alternate form of the diffusivity. This alternate form $((1-u/u_0)^p)$ can also take the indeterminate form 0^0 with $u=u_0, p=0$, but this is less likely ($u=u_0$ is less likely than $u=0$ in the model and the numerical analysis that follows).

The solution of eq. (6.1) is the cell density $u(r,t)$, which we take as a normalized variable with $u_0 = 1$. The model can easily be restated in terms of a cell density with an absolute value (and units).

Equation (6.1) is first order in t and second order in r so that it requires one IC and two BCs.

$$u(r,t=0)=0, \tag{6.2}$$

$$u(r=0,t)=u_0=1, \quad \frac{\partial u(r=r_0,t)}{\partial r}=0, \tag{6.3a,b}$$

where $r = r_0$ is the lateral half width of the wound (cm). Initial condition (6.2) states that the wound initially has no epithelial cells. Boundary condition (6.3a) specifies that the density of epithelial cells at the left end (edge) of the wound is a normal (unit) value and BC (6.3b) specifies a zero-flux condition, which can be interpreted as a symmetry condition at the midpoint of the wound, $r = r_0$ (an IC and BCs for eq. (6.1) were not given in [3], so these auxiliary conditions are inferred from the plotted solutions in this reference). We next develop a MOL solution to eqs. (6.1) to (6.3) that expresses the diffusion and regeneration of epithelial cells during the healing process.

6.1.1 Main program

A main program for the solution of eqs. (6.1) to (6.3) is given in Listing 6.1.

```
%
% Wound healing
%
% Clear previous files
  clear all
  clc
  global     nr      r0      r      u0...
              D       p      sc   ncall
%
% Model parameters
  r0=0.5; u0=1; D=2.0e-09; sc=      0; p=0;
% r0=0.5; u0=1; D=2.0e-09; sc=8.0e-06; p=0;
% r0=0.5; u0=1; D=2.0e-09; sc=8.0e-06; p=1;
% r0=0.5; u0=1; D=2.0e-09; sc=8.0e-06; p=5;
%
% Spatial grid
  nr=101;
  dr=r0/(nr-1);
  for j=1:nr
    r(j)=(j-1)*dr;
  end
%
% Independent variable for ODE integration
  tf=60*60*24*30;
  tout=[0:tf/10:tf]';
  nout=11;
  ncall=0;
```

```
%
% Initial condition
  for i=1:nr u0w(i)=0; end
%
% ODE integration
  reltol=1.0e-04; abstol=1.0e-04;
  options=odeset('RelTol',reltol,'AbsTol',abstol);
  [t,u]=ode15s(@pde_1,tout,u0w,options);
%
% Display a heading and t at output
  fprintf('\n  nr = %2d\n',nr);
  for it=1:nout
    u(it,1)=u0;
    fprintf('\n t (s) = %6.2e   t (days) = %6.2f',...
            t(it),t(it)/(60*60*24));
  end
  fprintf('\n\n ncall = %5d\n',ncall);
%
% Plot the solution as u(r,t) vs r with t as a parameter
  plot(r,u(2:nout,:),'-');
  axis([0 0.5 0 1])
  xlabel('r (cm)'); ylabel('u(r,t)');
  title('u(r,t);t = 3, 6,..., 30 days')
```

Listing 6.1 Main program pde_1_main for the MOL solution of eqs. (6.1) to (6.3)

We can note the following points about pde_1_main.

- Previous files are cleared and a global area is defined.

```
%
% Wound healing
%
% Clear previous files
  clear all
  clc
  global     nr     r0     r    u0...
              D      p     sc  ncall
```

  Also, documentation comments are not included for the model equations since they change when the single-PDE model of this section is extended to a two-PDE model in a subsequent section.
- Four sets of model parameters are programmed, and are deactivated through the use of a comment (with beginning %). Here the first set (line) of comments is active.

```
%
% Model parameters
  r0=0.5; u0=1; D=2.0e-09; sc=      0; p=0;
% r0=0.5; u0=1; D=2.0e-09; sc=8.0e-06; p=0;
% r0=0.5; u0=1; D=2.0e-09; sc=8.0e-06; p=1;
% r0=0.5; u0=1; D=2.0e-09; sc=8.0e-06; p=5;
```

An alternative for the selection of the parameters would be to use an `if` or `switch case` construct (but using the comment is just as easy).

For the first line of parameters, eq. (6.1) reduces to the 1D diffusion equation (1.18). Then eqs. (6.1) to (6.3) have a well-known analytical (infinite series) solution, but we will not use it here for the evaluation of the numerical solution since the PDE problem of eqs. (6.1) to (6.3) is a straightforward MOL application (the reader may wish to add an extension with the analytical solution).

The value of the diffusivity `D` is small (2×10^{-9} cm/s) but is not unusual for a biological system, and accounts for a time scale of one month (discussed subsequently).

- A spatial grid in r of `101` points is defined with grid spacing `dr` over the interval $0 \le r \le r_0$.

```
%
% Spatial grid
  nr=101;
  dr=r0/(nr-1);
  for j=1:nr
    r(j)=(j-1)*dr;
  end
```

- The interval in t is $0 \le t \le (60)(60)(24)(30)$, which is one month in seconds (s). The time scale in t is in s because the diffusivity D in eq. (6.1) has the units cm^2/s.

```
%
% Independent variable for ODE integration
  tf=60*60*24*30;
  tout=[0:tf/10:tf]';
  nout=11;
  ncall=0;
```

The output interval is 1/10 of the total interval (`tf/10`) for a total of `11` output points (including $t = 0$). The counter for the number of calls to the ODE routine is initialized to zero.

- The IC of eq. (6.2) is set.

```
%
% Initial condition
  for i=1:nr u0w(i)=0; end
```

- The integration of the `101` ODEs is by `ode15s`.

```
%
% ODE integration
  reltol=1.0e-04; abstol=1.0e-04;

  options=odeset('RelTol',reltol,'AbsTol',abstol);
  [t,u]=ode15s(@pde_1,tout,u0w,options);
```

The sparse version of `ode15s` is not used since the full-matrix version executes quickly.

- A heading is displayed with the number of grid points `nr`. Then the running values of t are displayed to indicate the progress in the solution (the solution `u` could also be displayed, but this would give 101 numbers for each value of t; this probably too many numbers to easily assimilate but could be visualized in a single plot, programmed next).

```
%
% Display a heading and t at output
  fprintf('\n  nr = %2d\n',nr);
  for it=1:nout
    u(it,1)=u0;
    fprintf('\n t (s) = %6.2e   t (days) = %6.2f',...
            t(it),t(it)/(60*60*24));
  end
  fprintf('\n\n ncall = %5d\n',ncall);
```

The running values of t are displayed in both seconds and days. Note also that the boundary value specified by BC (6.3a) is stored in `u(it,1)`, since this value is not computed by an ODE and therefore is not returned from the ODE routine `pde_1` via `ode15s`. The final value of the counter for the calls to `pde_1` is also displayed to give an indication of the total effort required to compute the complete numerical solution.

- The solution is plotted as $u(r,t)$ against r with t as a parameter.

```
%
% Plot the solution as u(r,t) vs r with t as a parameter
  plot(r,u(2:nout,:),'-');
  axis([0 0.5 0 1])
  xlabel('r (cm)'); ylabel('u(r,t)');
  title('u(r,t);t = 3, 6,..., 30 days')
```

The starting value of t is 3 days, since the solution at $t = 0$ undergoes a discontinuity at $r = 0$, that is, $u(r = 0, t = 0) = 0$ to $u(r = 0, t > 0) = u_0$, that is not well suited for plotting. However, the smoothness of the plotted solution for $t > 0$ in Fig. 6.1 (discussed subsequently) illustrates an important feature of parabolic PDEs such as eq. (6.1), that is, they tend to smooth discontinuities (which is not the case for hyperbolic PDEs, as demonstrated in Section 1.2.4); this property is suggested by the name of eq. (6.1), the diffusion equation, since it tends to diffuse (or smooth) discontinuities.

6.1.2 ODE routine

The ODE routine `pde_1` called by `ode15s` in `pde_1_main` is listed next.

```
  function ut=pde_1(t,u)
%
% Global area
  global    nr     r0     r     u0...
            D      p     sc  ncall
%
% BC at r = 0
  u(1)=u0; nl=1;
```

```
%
% ur
  ur=dss004(0,r0,nr,u);
%
% BC ar r = r0
  ur(nr)=0; nu=2;
%
% urr
  urr=dss044(0,r0,nr,u,ur,nl,nu);
%
% ut
  for i=2:nr
    ut(i)=D*((1-u(i)/u0)^p*urr(i)+p*(1-u(i)/u0)^(p-1)*(-1/u0)*ur(i)^2)+...
           sc*u(i)*(1-u(i)/u0);
  end
  ut(1)=0;
%
% Transpose and counter
  ut=ut';
  ncall=ncall+1;
```

Listing 6.2 ODE routine pde_1 for eqs. (6.1) to (6.4)

We can note the following details of pde_1.

- The function and a global area are defined.

```
  function ut=pde_1(t,u)
%
% Global area
  global     nr      r0       r      u0...
              D       p      sc   ncall
```

- Boundary condition (6.3a) is programmed as a Dirichlet BC (with nl=1). Note that this BC resets u at $r = 0$, which comes into pde_1 as a (RHS) argument.

```
%
% BC at r = 0
  u(1)=u0; nl=1;
```

- The derivative $(\partial u/\partial r)$ is computed by a call to dss004.

```
%
% ur
  ur=dss004(0,r0,nr,u);
```

- Boundary condition (6.3b) is programmed as a Neumann BC (with nu=2), which resets the derivative $(\partial u/\partial r)$ from dss004 at the right boundary ($r = r_0$).

```
%
% BC ar r = r0
  ur(nr)=0; nu=2;
```

- The second derivative $(\partial^2 u/\partial r^2)$ is computed by a call to dss044.

```
%
% urr
  urr=dss044(0,r0,nr,u,ur,nl,nu);
```

- The PDE, eq. (6.1), is programmed. First, the term in r in eq. (6.1) is expanded as the derivative of a product.

$$\frac{\partial\left((1-u/u_0)^p\dfrac{\partial u}{\partial r}\right)}{\partial r} = (1-u/u_0)^p\frac{\partial^2 u}{\partial r^2} + \frac{\mathrm{d}((1-u/u_0)^p)}{\mathrm{d}u}\frac{\partial u}{\partial r}\frac{\partial u}{\partial r}$$
$$= (1-u/u_0)^p\frac{\partial^2 u}{\partial r^2} + \left(p(1-u/u_0)^{p-1}(-1/u_0)\right)\left(\frac{\partial u}{\partial r}\right)^2. \tag{6.4}$$

The programming of eq. (6.1), with the substitution of eq. (6.4), follows directly.

```
%
% ut
  for i=2:nr
    ut(i)=D*((1-u(i)/u0)^p*urr(i)+p*(1-u(i)/u0)^(p-1)*(-1/u0)
            *ur(i)^2)+... sc*u(i)*(1-u(i)/u0);
  end
  ut(1)=0;
```

The left end derivative in t, $(\partial u(r=0,t)/\partial t)$, is set to zero so that the boundary value remains at $u_0 = 1$, as specified by eq. (6.3a).

- The transpose required by `ode15s` and incrementing of the counter for the calls to `pde_1` concludes `pde_1`.

```
%
% Transpose and counter
  ut=ut';
  ncall=ncall+1;
```

This completes the programming of eqs. (6.1) to (6.4).

6.1.3 Model output

We now consider the output for successive lines of the programming of the parameters in `pde_1`, starting with the linear case $p = s = 0$.

Linear diffusion equation

The numerical output is given in Table 6.1 (again, for the first line of the parameters in `pde_1_main`), and the graphical output is in Fig. 6.1. Only the running value of t appears in the numerical output of Table 6.1, to conserve space.

The solution is computed with modest effort (`ncall=196`).

The plotted solution in Fig. 6.1 is for the diffusion equation (eq. (6.1) with $p = s = 0$) with a constant Dirichlet BC at $r = 0$ and a homogeneous Neumann BC at $r = r_0$. It is offered as a point of reference for subsequent solutions that have a much different form, due to changes in p and s.

Table 6.1. Output from `pde_1_main` and `pde_1` for `r0=0.5; u0=1; D=2.0e-09; sc=0; p=0;`

```
nr = 101
```

```
t (s) = 0.00e+000   t (days) =   0.00
t (s) = 2.59e+005   t (days) =   3.00
t (s) = 5.18e+005   t (days) =   6.00
t (s) = 7.78e+005   t (days) =   9.00
t (s) = 1.04e+006   t (days) =  12.00
t (s) = 1.30e+006   t (days) =  15.00
t (s) = 1.56e+006   t (days) =  18.00
t (s) = 1.81e+006   t (days) =  21.00
t (s) = 2.07e+006   t (days) =  24.00
t (s) = 2.33e+006   t (days) =  27.00
t (s) = 2.59e+006   t (days) =  30.00

ncall =   196
```

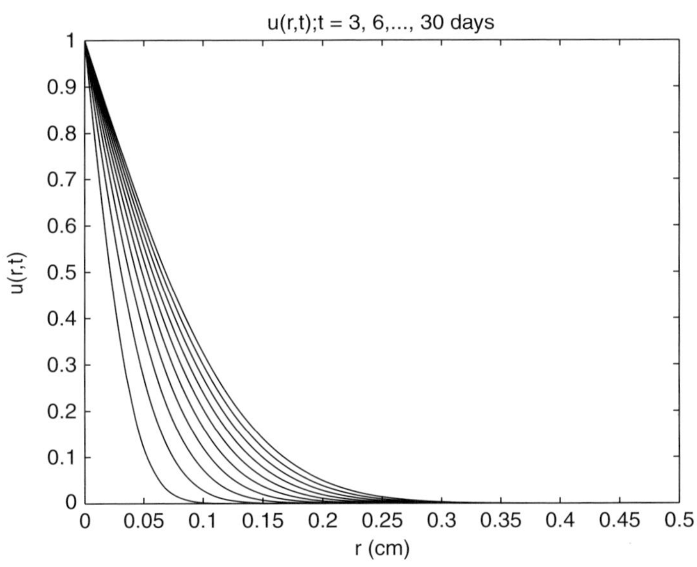

Figure 6.1 Solution to eqs. (6.1) to (6.4) for $p = s_c = 0$

This solution has the limiting value $u(r, t \to \infty) = 1$ since the left boundary defines a constant value $u_0 = 1$ and the right boundary has a no-flux condition (mass cannot leave the system). However, the final value of $t = 30$ days is not long enough to approach this limiting solution, and the time scale in `pde_1_main` would have to be increased substantially to approach the limiting solution. We do not do that here, since a final value $t = 30$ days is more appropriate for the solutions that follow.

Table 6.2. Output from `pde_1_main` and `pde_1` for `r0=0.5; u0=1; D=2.0e-09; sc=8.0 e-06; p=0;`

```
nr = 101

t (s) = 0.00e+000   t (days) =   0.00
t (s) = 2.59e+005   t (days) =   3.00
t (s) = 5.18e+005   t (days) =   6.00
t (s) = 7.78e+005   t (days) =   9.00
t (s) = 1.04e+006   t (days) =  12.00
t (s) = 1.30e+006   t (days) =  15.00
t (s) = 1.56e+006   t (days) =  18.00
t (s) = 1.81e+006   t (days) =  21.00
t (s) = 2.07e+006   t (days) =  24.00
t (s) = 2.33e+006   t (days) =  27.00
t (s) = 2.59e+006   t (days) =  30.00

ncall =    319
```

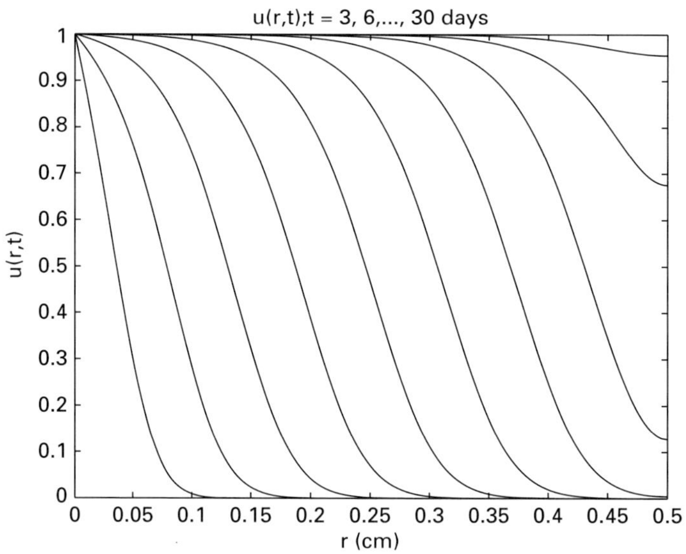

Figure 6.2 Solution to eqs. (6.1) to (6.4) for $p = 0, s_c = 8 \times 10^{-6}$

Fisher–Kolmogorov equation

For the second line of the parameter values in `pde_1_main`,

```
r0=0.5; u0=1; D=2.0e-09; sc=8.0e-06; p=0;
```

the nonlinear logistic source term of eq. (6.1), $s_c u(1 - u/u_0)$, is introduced (owing to the nonzero value of s_c). The resulting PDE is the Fisher–Kolmogorov equation ([2].

Table 6.3. Output from `pde_1_main` and `pde_1` for `r0=0.5; u0=1; D=2.0e-09; sc=8.0e-06; p=1;`

```
nr = 101

t (s) = 0.00e+000   t (days) =   0.00
t (s) = 2.59e+005   t (days) =   3.00
t (s) = 5.18e+005   t (days) =   6.00
t (s) = 7.78e+005   t (days) =   9.00
t (s) = 1.04e+006   t (days) =  12.00
t (s) = 1.30e+006   t (days) =  15.00
t (s) = 1.56e+006   t (days) =  18.00
t (s) = 1.81e+006   t (days) =  21.00
t (s) = 2.07e+006   t (days) =  24.00
t (s) = 2.33e+006   t (days) =  27.00
t (s) = 2.59e+006   t (days) =  30.00

ncall =    437
```

Chapter 8). All of the other coding in `pde_1_main` and `pde_1` remains unchanged. The numerical output is in Table 6.2 and the graphical output is in Fig. 6.2.

The solution is computed with modest effort (`ncall=319`).

The plotted solution in Fig. 6.2 is quite different from the solution in Fig. 6.1 because of the inclusion of the logistic source term. Specifically, the solution is now more like a traveling wave with $p = 0, s_c = 8 \times 10^{-6}$. In other words, the logistic source term has a major effect on the form of the solution (even though it does not include a spatial derivative such as $(\partial u/\partial r)$ for convection, which might be expected considering the form of the traveling wave solution in Fig. (6.2)). Clearly, s_c in eq. (6.1) is a sensitive parameter.

Nonlinear diffusion

For the third line of parameter values in `pde_1_main`,

```
r0=0.5; u0=1; D=2.0e-09; sc=8.0e-06; p=1;
```

p in eq. (6.1) is now nonzero and thus makes the diffusion term in eq. (6.1) nonlinear. This change does not produce a substantial variation in the solution of Fig. 6.2. The numerical and graphical output are in Table 6.3 and Fig. 6.3, respectively.

The solution is computed with modest effort (`ncall=437`). The plotted solution in Fig. 6.3 is similar to the solution in Fig. 6.2 so that p appears to not be a sensitive parameter.

To further examine the effect of p, we consider the fourth line of parameter values in `pde_1_main`.

```
r0=0.5; u0=1; D=2.0e-09; sc=8.0e-06; p=5;
```

This change ($p = 1$ to $p = 5$) does not produce a substantial variation in the solutions of Figs. 6.2 and 6.3. The numerical and graphical output are in Table 6.4 and Fig. 6.4, respectively.

Table 6.4. Output from `pde_1_main` and `pde_1` for `r0=0.5; u0=1; D=2.0e-09; sc=8.0e-06; p=5;`

```
nr = 101

t (s) = 0.00e+000   t (days) =   0.00
t (s) = 2.59e+005   t (days) =   3.00
t (s) = 5.18e+005   t (days) =   6.00
t (s) = 7.78e+005   t (days) =   9.00
t (s) = 1.04e+006   t (days) =  12.00
t (s) = 1.30e+006   t (days) =  15.00
t (s) = 1.56e+006   t (days) =  18.00
t (s) = 1.81e+006   t (days) =  21.00
t (s) = 2.07e+006   t (days) =  24.00
t (s) = 2.33e+006   t (days) =  27.00
t (s) = 2.59e+006   t (days) =  30.00

ncall =    558
```

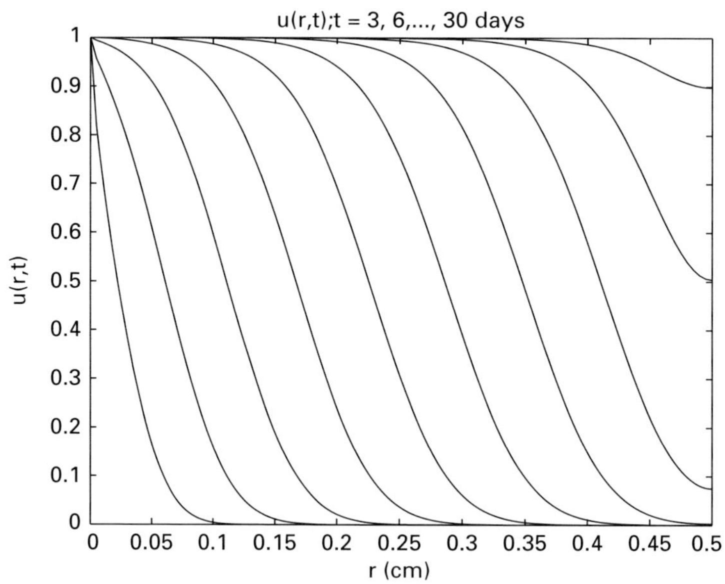

Figure 6.3 Solution to eqs. (6.1) to (6.4) for $p = 1, s_c = 8 \times 10^{-6}$

The solution is computed with modest effort (`ncall=558`). Figure 6.4 has small differences from Figs. 6.2 and 6.3 so that again p appears to not be a sensitive parameter.

To conclude this discussion, we consider an estimation of the apparent velocity of the moving front in Fig. 6.2 for the Fisher–Kolmogorov equation (linear diffusion with $p = 0$ in eq. (6.1)), which gives an indication of the speed of wound healing.

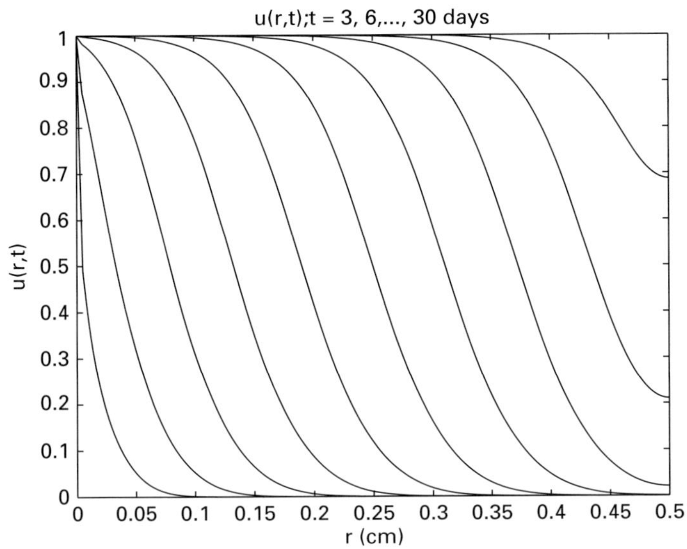

Figure 6.4 Solution to eqs. (6.1) to (6.4) for $p = 5, s_c = 8 \times 10^{-6}$

Velocity of wound healing

To investigate the velocity of wound healing, we add some additional lines of code to pde_1_main in Listing 6.1 (just before the plotting at the end).

```
%
% Estimated velocity for p = 0
  for it=4:5
    fprintf('\n\n t = %6.2f',t(it));
    for i=1:nr
      fprintf('\n r = %5.3f   u(r,t) = %5.3f',r(i),u(it,i));
    end
  end
  vs=1.0e+04*(0.175-0.120)/(1036800-777600);
  fprintf('\n\n velocity = %7.5f microns/s\n',vs);
  vday=(0.175-0.120)/(1036800-777600)*3600*24;
  fprintf('\n velocity = %6.4f cm/day\n',vday);
  rmon=(0.175-0.120)/(1036800-777600)*3600*24*30;
  fprintf('\n distance/month = %6.3f cm/mo\n',rmon);
  fprintf('\n wound half width = %6.3f cm\n',r0);
  fprintf('\n ncall = %5d\n',ncall);
```

Listing 6.3 Additional coding added to pde_1_main to compute the velocity of the moving front in Fig. 6.2 (p = 0)

We can note the following details about this code.

- Figure 6.2 indicates that the solution to eqs. (6.1) to (6.4) is a moving front that retains an essentially constant form or shape over much of the solution for $0 \le t \le 30$. We can estimate the effective velocity of the moving front by observing how far it moves in a selected interval of time. To do this, we need a more detailed display of the solution. This is done at the fourth and fifth outputs corresponding to $t = 9$ and $t = 12$ days, respectively, in a `for` loop `for it=4:5` (refer to Table 6.2 or Table 6.5 (next) for the corresponding t).

```
%
% Estimated velocity for p = 0
  for it=4:5
    fprintf('\n\n t = %6.2f',t(it));
    for i=1:nr
      fprintf('\n r = %5.3f   u(r,t) = %5.3f',r(i),u(it,i));
    end
  end
```

- From Table 6.5, for `t = 777600.00` s, $u(r,t) = 0.6 \approx 0.594$ is at `r = 0.120`.

```
t = 777600.00
r = 0.120   u(r,t) = 0.594
```

  (a portion of the output in Table 6.5 was deleted for clarity).
- Similarly, from Table 6.5 for `t = 1036800.00` s, $u(r,t) = 0.6 \approx 0.601$ is at `r = 0.175`

```
t = 1036800.00
r = 0.175   u(r,t) = 0.601
```

- Thus the velocity of the front at $u(r,t) \approx 0.6$ is $(0.175 - 0.120/1036800 - 777600)$ cm/s. This calculation is programmed as

```
vs=1.0e+04*(0.175-0.120)/(1036800-777600);
fprintf('\n\n velocity = %7.5f microns/s\n',vs);
```

  where the factor `1.0e+04` is used to convert from cm to μm. Thus, the velocity `vs` is in μm/s.
- Similarly, the velocity in cm/day is computed as

```
vday=(0.175-0.120)/(1036800-777600)*3600*24;
fprintf('\n velocity = %6.4f cm/day\n',vday);
```

- The total distance in cm traveled by the front in a month is given by

```
rmon=(0.175-0.120)/(1036800-777600)*3600*24*30;
fprintf('\n distance/month = %6.3f cm/mo\n',rmon);
```

  which gives an indication of the healing after one month.
- For reference, the wound half width r_0 is displayed along with the number of calls to `pde_1` (as included in previous examples).

```
fprintf('\n wound half width = %6.3f cm\n',r0);
fprintf('\n ncall = %5d\n',ncall);
```

We can now consider the output from the additional code in Listing 6.3 as given in Table 6.5

We can note the following points about the output in Table 6.5.

Table 6.5. Abbreviated output from additional code in Listing 6.3 in `pde_1_main`

```
nr = 101

t (s) = 0.00e+000   t (days) =   0.00
t (s) = 2.59e+005   t (days) =   3.00
t (s) = 5.18e+005   t (days) =   6.00
t (s) = 7.78e+005   t (days) =   9.00
t (s) = 1.04e+006   t (days) =  12.00
t (s) = 1.30e+006   t (days) =  15.00
t (s) = 1.56e+006   t (days) =  18.00
t (s) = 1.81e+006   t (days) =  21.00
t (s) = 2.07e+006   t (days) =  24.00
t (s) = 2.33e+006   t (days) =  27.00
t (s) = 2.59e+006   t (days) =  30.00

t = 777600.00
r = 0.000   u(r,t) = 1.000
r = 0.005   u(r,t) = 0.996
r = 0.010   u(r,t) = 0.992
     .                 .
     .                 .
     .                 .
r = 0.115   u(r,t) = 0.635
r = 0.120   u(r,t) = 0.594
r = 0.125   u(r,t) = 0.550
     .                 .
     .                 .
     .                 .
r = 0.490   u(r,t) = 0.000
r = 0.495   u(r,t) = 0.000
r = 0.500   u(r,t) = 0.000

t = 1036800.00
r = 0.000   u(r,t) = 1.000
r = 0.005   u(r,t) = 0.999
r = 0.010   u(r,t) = 0.998
     .                 .
     .                 .
     .                 .
r = 0.170   u(r,t) = 0.640
r = 0.175   u(r,t) = 0.601
r = 0.180   u(r,t) = 0.560
     .                 .
     .                 .
     .                 .
r = 0.490   u(r,t) = 0.000
r = 0.495   u(r,t) = 0.000
r = 0.500   u(r,t) = 0.000

velocity = 0.00212 microns/s
```

```
velocity = 0.0183 cm/day

distance/month =  0.550 cm/mo

wound half width =  0.500 cm

ncall =   319
```

- The summary of t at the 11 outputs for $0 \le t \le 30$ days is the same as in Fig. 6.1 to 6.4.
- Abbreviated tabular output for `it=4,5` (9 and 12 days) is included, particularly for $u(r,t) \approx 0.6$, as discussed previously.
- The two computed velocities are

```
velocity = 0.00212 microns/s
velocity = 0.0183 cm/day
```

  In particular, the second velocity gives an indication of the time in days required for effectively complete wound healing. This point is illustrated for a total healing time of one month.

```
distance/month =  0.550 cm/mo
wound half width =  0.500 cm
```

  which indicates that the moving front solution covers the wound half width in approximately one month.

  As a point of comparison, an experimental velocity of 8.6×10^{-3} mm/h is reported in [3], p34. From the preceding result (for $p = 0$ in eq. (6.1)), 0.0183 cm/day = $(0.0183)(1/24)(10) = 7.63 \times 10^{-3}$ mm/h. This value is in better agreement with the experimental value than 6×10^{-2} mm/h from [3] for $p = 0$ (linear diffusion). Also, for $p = 4$, the velocity from [3] is 9×10^{-3} mm/h so that there is a significant variation with p (using the original diffusion function $D(u/u_0)^p$), while with the present formulation based on the diffusion function $D(1 - u/u_0)^p$, the variation with p is substantially smaller.

Of course, these results are defined by the specific values of the model parameters, particularly the diffusivity `D=2.0e-09` cm^2/s in the second line of parameter values in `pde_1_main`.

This completes the discussion of the one-PDE model of eqs. (6.1) to (6.4). We now consider a two-PDE model.

6.2 Two-PDE model

The two-PDE model ([1, 3], p35) is an extension of the preceding one-PDE model (eqs. (6.1) to (6.4)) in which the production of epidermal cells through the action of an activator

Table 6.6. Variables, parameters, and terms in the PDEs

Variable, parameter, term	Interpretation
u_1	cell density
u_2	activator or inhibitor concentration
t	time
$\nabla^2 = (\partial^2/\partial r^2) + 1/r(\partial/\partial r)$	laplacian operator (in one dimension)
r	radial direction across the wound
$D_{u_1}\nabla^2 u_1$ $D_{u_2}\nabla^2 u_2$	net rate of diffusion into or out of a differential volume due to Fickian diffusion for components u_1 and u_2, respectively
$s_c(u_2)u_1(2-u_1)$	volumetric rate of cell mitosis (division)
$-u_1$	volumetric rate of cell depletion
$\lambda g(u_1)$	volumetric rate of chemical (activator or inhibitor) production by the cells
$-\lambda u_2$	volumetric rate of chemical (activator or inhibitor) consumption

and inhibitor is taken into account. The concentration of the activator or inhibitor is the dependent variable for the second PDE. The model PDEs are

$$\frac{\partial u_1}{\partial t} = D_{u_1}\nabla^2 u_1 + s_c(u_2)u_1(2-u_1) - u_1,$$

$$\frac{\partial u_2}{\partial t} = D_{u_2}\nabla^2 u_2 + \lambda g(u_1) - \lambda u_2.$$

The variables, parameters, and terms of these PDEs are listed in Table 6.6. These equations are dimensionless and therefore no dimensions are indicated for the variables, parameters or terms (they are also dimensionless).

If the wound is considered circular, the Laplacian can be expressed in cylindrical coordinates (r,θ,z) in 3D or polar coordinates (r,θ) in 2D. If we consider polar coordinates with no angular dependency, the PDEs become

$$\frac{\partial u_1}{\partial t} = D_{u_1}\left(\frac{\partial^2 u_1}{\partial r^2} + \frac{1}{r}\frac{\partial u_1}{\partial r}\right) + s_c(u_2)u_1(2-u_1) - u_1, \tag{6.5a}$$

$$\frac{\partial u_2}{\partial t} = D_{u_2}\left(\frac{\partial^2 u_2}{\partial r^2} + \frac{1}{r}\frac{\partial u_2}{\partial r}\right) + \lambda g(u_1) - \lambda u_2. \tag{6.5b}$$

The terms described in Table 6.6 indicate that eqs. (6.5) are time-dependent balances on the epidermal cells and the concentration of the activator or inhibitor (two cases). The functions $g(u_1)$ and $s_c(u_2)$ in eqs. (6.5) are different for the activator and inhibitor.

- Activator:

$$g(u_1) = \frac{u_1(1+\alpha^2)}{u_1^2+\alpha^2}, \tag{6.5c}$$

$$s_c(u_2) = \frac{2c_m(h-\beta)u_2}{c_m^2 + u_2^2} + \beta, \tag{6.5d}$$

$$\beta = \frac{1 + c_m^2 - 2hc_m}{(1-c_m)^2}. \tag{6.5e}$$

- Inhibitor:

$$g(u_1) = u_1, \tag{6.5f}$$

$$s_c(u_2) = \frac{(h-1)u_2 + h}{2(h-1)u_2 + 1}. \tag{6.5g}$$

α, c_m and h are constants set in the main program (discussed next). Equations (6.5) are first order in t and second order in r; therefore, each PDE requires one IC and two BCs. These auxiliary conditions will be taken as

$$u_1(r,t=0) = 0; u_2(r,t=0) = 0, \tag{6.6a,b}$$

$$u_1(r=1,t) = 1; u_2(r=1,t) = 1, \tag{6.7a,b}$$

$$\frac{\partial u_1(r=0,t)}{\partial r} = 0; \frac{\partial u_2(r=0,t)}{\partial r} = 0. \tag{6.7c,d}$$

Boundary conditions (6.7a) and (6.7b) indicate that the system responds to a unit step in $u_1(r=1,t), u_2(r=1,t)$, starting from the zero IC of eqs. (6.6). Boundary conditions (6.7c,d) can be considered as symmetry conditions at the center of the wound (the BCs for eqs. (6.5) at $r=0$ were not given in [1, 3] so eqs. (6.7c,d), are inferred from the plotted solutions in these references).

6.2.1 Main program

A main program, pde_2_main, for eqs. (6.5) to (6.7) follows in Listing 6.4.

```
%
% Wound healing
%
% Clear previous files
  clear all
  clc
%
% Global area
  global      h      cm  alpha   beta...
             u10    Du1     la       ...
             u20    Du2     li       ...
              nr      r  ncase  ncall
%
% Case
%
%   ncase = 1: Activator
%
%   ncase = 2: Inhibitor
  ncase=1;
```

```
%
% Model parameters
  la=30; li=5; h=10; cm=40; alpha=0.1;
  beta=(1+cm^2-2*h*cm)/(1-cm)^2;
  if(ncase==1) Du1=5.0e-04; Du2=0.45; end
  if(ncase==2) Du1=1.0e-04; Du2=0.85; end
  fprintf('\n ncase = %2d\n',ncase);
  fprintf('\n  la = %5.1f      li = %5.1f       h = %5.1f\n',la,li,h);
  fprintf('\n  cm = %5.1f  alpha = %5.3f    beta = %5.3f\n',cm,...
          alpha,beta);
  fprintf('\n Du1 = %8.3e    Du2 = %8.3e\n',Du1,Du2);
%
% Spatial grid
  nr=101; dr=1/(nr-1);
  for j=1:nr
    r(j)=(j-1)*dr;
  end
  u10=1; u20=1;
%
% Independent variable for ODE integration
  if(ncase==1) tf=25; end
  if(ncase==2) tf=50; end
  tout=[0:tf/20:tf]'; nout=21;
  ncall=0;
%
% Initial condition
  for i=1:nr u0(i)=0; u0(i+nr)=0; end
%
% ODE integration
  reltol=1.0e-04; abstol=1.0e-04;
  options=odeset('RelTol',reltol,'AbsTol',abstol);
  [t,u]=ode15s(@pde_2,tout,u0,options);
%
% Display a heading and t at output
  fprintf('\n  nr = %2d\n',nr);
  for it=1:nout
    for i=1:nr
      u1(it,i)=u(it,i);
      u2(it,i)=u(it,nr+i);
    end
    u1(it,nr)=u10; u2(it,nr)=u20;
    fprintf('\n t = %6.2e',t(it));
%
%   Detailed solution
%   for i=1:nr
%     fprintf('\n i = %3d  %5.3f  %5.3f  %5.3f  ',...
%             i,r(i),u1(it,i),u2(it,i));
%   end
  end
  fprintf('\n\n ncall = %5d\n',ncall);
%
```

```
% Plot the solution as u1(r,t), u2(r,t) vs r with t as a parameter
  figure(1)
  plot(r,u1(2:nout,:),'-');
  xlabel('r'); ylabel('u1(r,t)');
  title('u1(r,t)vs r')
  figure(2)
  plot(r,u2(2:nout,:),'-');
  xlabel('r'); ylabel('u2(r,t)');
  title('u2(r,t) vs r')
```

Listing 6.4 Main program pde_2_main for eqs. (6.5) to (6.7)

We can note the following details about this code.

- Previous files are cleared and a global area is defined.

```
%
% Wound healing
%
% Clear previous files
  clear all
  clc
%
% Global area
  global      h     cm  alpha   beta...
            u10    Du1     la        ...
            u20    Du2     li        ...
             nr      r  ncase  ncall
```

- The case is selected.

```
%
% Case
%
%    ncase = 1: Activator
%
%    ncase = 2: Inhibitor
  ncase=1;
```

- The parameters in eqs. (6.5) to (6.7) are defined numerically and displayed.

```
%
% Model parameters
  la=30; li=5; h=10; cm=40; alpha=0.1;
  beta=(1+cm^2-2*h*cm)/(1-cm)^2;
  if(ncase==1) Du1=5.0e-04; Du2=0.45; end
  if(ncase==2) Du1=1.0e-04; Du2=0.85; end
  fprintf('\n ncase = %2d\n',ncase);
  fprintf('\n  la = %5.1f      li = %5.1f       h = %5.1f\n',la,li,h);
  fprintf('\n  cm = %5.1f  alpha = %5.3f    beta = %5.3f\n',cm,...
          alpha,beta);
  fprintf('\n Du1 = %8.3e    Du2 = %8.3e\n',Du1,Du2);
```

An explanation of these numerical values follows. pde_2_main executes two cases: ncase=1 for activation and ncase=2 for inhibition. Equations (6.5) to (6.7) are stated in terms of dimensionless variables and parameters, e.g., $r, t, u_1(r,t), u_2(r,t)$ are dimensionless.

- la: λ in eq. (6.5b) for ncase=1
- li: λ in eq. (6.5b) for ncase=2
- h: h in eqs. (6.5d,e,g)
- cm: c_m in eqs. (6.5d,e)
- alpha: α in eq. (6.5c)
- beta: β in eq. (6.5d)
- Du1: D_{u_1} in eq. (6.5a) for ncase=1,2
- Du2: D_{u_2} in eq. (6.5b) for ncase=1,2

- A spatial grid in r is defined for 101 points (counting the two end points $r = 0, 1$).

```
%
% Spatial grid
  nr=101; dr=1/(nr-1);

  for j=1:nr
    r(j)=(j-1)*dr;
  end
  u10=1; u20=1;
```

The right boundary values (at $r = 1$) in eqs. (6.7a,b) are also defined numerically.

- A time scale in t is defined as $0 \le t \le 25$ with 21 output points for ncase=1 (counting both end points t=0,tf). Similarly, a time scale in t is defined as $0 \le t \le 50$ with 21 output points for ncase=2. A longer time scale is required for ncase=2 to resolve the solution in two plots (discussed subsequently). The longer scale in t was required because of the differences in the parameters for the two cases, particularly li, which is smaller than la so that the ncase=2 response is slower.

```
%
% Independent variable for ODE integration
  if(ncase==1) tf=25; end
  if(ncase==2) tf=50; end
  tout=[0:tf/20:tf]'; nout=21;
  ncall=0;
```

The counter for the number of calls to the ODE routine, pde_2, is also initialized.

- Initial conditions (6.6) are placed in a single vector u0 of length $2(101) = 202$. This programming therefore defines the number of ODEs as 202 for the ODE integrator ode15s (as the length of u0).

```
%
% Initial condition
  for i=1:nr u0(i)=0; u0(i+nr)=0; end
```

- The integration of the $2(nr) = 2(101) = 202$ ODEs is over the interval in t prescribed in tout, with the solution returned for the 21 values of t in tout. Note that ode15s calls the ODE routine, pde_2.

```
%
% ODE integration
  reltol=1.0e-04; abstol=1.0e-04;
  options=odeset('RelTol',reltol,'AbsTol',abstol);
  [t,u]=ode15s(@pde_2,tout,u0,options);
```

The numerical ODE solution is returned in u, an array with dimensions u(21,202). t is returned in array t of length t(21).

- The solution in u is placed in two arrays, u1,u2. The boundary values u1(it,nr), u2(it,nr) (from BCs (6.7a,b)) are set since these values are not returned by ode15s (they are not computed as the solutions to two ODEs at $r = 1$ from the programming in the ODE routine pde_2).

```
%
% Display a heading and t at output
  fprintf('\n  nr = %2d\n',nr);
  for it=1:nout
    for i=1:nr
      u1(it,i)=u(it,i);
      u2(it,i)=u(it,nr+i);
    end
    u1(it,nr)=u10; u2(it,nr)=u20;
    fprintf('\n t = %6.2e',t(it));
%
%   Detailed solution
%   for i=1:nr
%     fprintf('\n i = %3d  %5.3f  %5.3f  %5.3f  ',...
%             i,r(i),u1(it,i),u2(it,i));
%   end
  end
  fprintf('\n\n ncall = %5d\n',ncall);
```

Numerical output is restricted to just the 21 values of t (to give an indication of the progress of the solution). If a more detailed solution is required (at all values of r), the concluding for loop can be activated (uncommented). The total number of calls to the ODE routine pde_2 is also displayed as a measure of the computational effort required to compute the solution.

- The solution is also plotted as u_1, u_2 in two figures.

```
%
% Plot the solution as u1(r,t), u2(r,t) vs r with t as a parameter
  figure(1)
  plot(r,u1(2:nout,:),'-');
  xlabel('r'); ylabel('u1(r,t)');
  title('u1(r,t)vs r')
  figure(2)
  plot(r,u2(2:nout,:),'-');
```

```
  xlabel('r'); ylabel('u2(r,t)');
  title('u2(r,t) vs r')
```

6.2.2 ODE routine

The ODE routine, pde_2, is listed next.

```
  function ut=pde_2(t,u)
%
% Global area
  global      h     cm  alpha   beta...
            u10    Du1      la        ...
            u20    Du2      li        ...
             nr      r  ncase  ncall
%
% One vector to two vectors
  for i=1:nr
    u1(i)=u(i);
    u2(i)=u(i+nr);
  end
%
% BCs at r = 1
  u1(nr)=u10; u2(nr)=u20; nu=1;
%
% ur
  u1r=dss004(0,1,nr,u1);
  u2r=dss004(0,1,nr,u2);
%
% BCs ar r = 0
  u1r(1)=0; u2r(1)=0; nl=2;
%
% urr
  u1rr=dss044(0,1,nr,u1,u1r,nl,nu);
  u2rr=dss044(0,1,nr,u2,u2r,nl,nu);
%
% ut
  for i=1:nr-1
    if(ncase==1) lam=la; sc=sa(u2(i)); g=ga(u1(i)); end
    if(ncase==2) lam=li; sc=si(u2(i)); g=gi(u1(i)); end
    if(i==1)
      u1t(i)=Du1*2*u1rr(i)+sc*u1(i)*(2-u1(i))-u1(i);
      u2t(i)=Du2*2*u2rr(i)+lam*g-lam*u2(i);
    else
    u1t(i)=Du1*(u1rr(i)+(1/r(i))*u1r(i))+sc*u1(i)*(2-u1(i))-u1(i);
    u2t(i)=Du2*(u2rr(i)+(1/r(i))*u2r(i))+lam*g-lam*u2(i);
    end
  end
  u1t(nr)=0; u2t(nr)=0;
%
% Two vectors to one vector
  for i=1:nr
```

```
    ut(i)    =u1t(i);
    ut(i+nr)=u2t(i);
  end
%
% Transpose and counter
  ut=ut';
  ncall=ncall+1;
```

Listing 6.5 ODE routine pde_2 for eqs. (6.5) to (6.7)

We can note the following details about pde_2.

- The function and a global area are defined.

```
  function ut=pde_2(t,u)
%
% Global area
  global      h      cm  alpha    beta...
            u10     Du1     la        ...
            u20     Du2     li        ...
             nr       r  ncase  ncall
```

- The single vector u of length 202 that is an input (RHS) argument of pde_2 is placed in two vectors u1,u2 to facilitate the programming of eqs. (6.5) to (6.7).

```
%
% One vector to two vectors
  for i=1:nr
    u1(i)=u(i);
    u2(i)=u(i+nr);
  end
```

- Boundary conditions (5.7a,b) are programmed as Dirichlet (nu=1) at $r = 1$ (point nr).

```
%
% BCs at r = 1
  u1(nr)=u10; u2(nr)=u20; nu=1;
```

- The first derivatives $(\partial u_1/\partial r), (\partial u_2/\partial r)$ are computed by dss004 (u1r,u2r).

```
%
% ur
  u1r=dss004(0,1,nr,u1);
  u2r=dss004(0,1,nr,u2);
```

  Note that in calling dss044, $0 \leq r \leq 1$.
- The first derivatives are reset as Neumann (nl=2) at $r = 0$ according to BCs (6.7c,d).

```
%
% BCs ar r = 0
  u1r(1)=0; u2r(1)=0; nl=2;
```

- The second derivatives $(\partial^2 u_1/\partial r^2), (\partial^2 u_2/\partial r^2)$ are computed by dss044 (u1rr,u2rr).

```
%
% urr
  u1rr=dss044(0,1,nr,u1,u1r,nl,nu);
  u2rr=dss044(0,1,nr,u2,u2r,nl,nu);
```

- The first derivatives $(\partial u_1/\partial t), (\partial u_2/\partial t)$ are computed according to eqs. (6.5a,b).

```
%
% ut
  for i=1:nr-1
    if(ncase==1) lam=la; sc=sa(u2(i)); g=ga(u1(i)); end
    if(ncase==2) lam=li; sc=si(u2(i)); g=gi(u1(i)); end
    if(i==1)
      u1t(i)=Du1*2*u1rr(i)+sc*u1(i)*(2-u1(i))-u1(i);
      u2t(i)=Du2*2*u2rr(i)+lam*g-lam*u2(i);
    else
    u1t(i)=Du1*(u1rr(i)+(1/r(i))*u1r(i))+sc*u1(i)*(2-u1(i))-u1(i);
    u2t(i)=Du2*(u2rr(i)+(1/r(i))*u2r(i))+lam*g-lam*u2(i);
    end
  end
  u1t(nr)=0; u2t(nr)=0;
```

The programming of the derivatives in t is done in several steps.

- At each point in r (each `i`), λ, s_c, g in eqs. (6.5a,b) are computed for `ncase=1` (activation) or `ncase=2` (inhibition).

```
%
% ut
  for i=1:nr-1
    if(ncase==1) lam=la; sc=sa(u2(i)); g=ga(u1(i)); end
    if(ncase==2) lam=li; sc=si(u2(i)); g=gi(u1(i)); end
```

  `ga,sa` are functions for g, s_c for `ncase=1` from eqs. (6.5c,d) discussed subsequently. `gi,si` are functions for g, s_c for `ncase=2` from eqs. (6.5f,g).
- At $r = 0$ (`i=1`), the first derivative radial groups in r of eqs. (6.5a,b) are indeterminate. They are modified according to l'Hospital's rule.

$$\lim_{r \to 0} \frac{1}{r}\frac{\partial u_1}{\partial r} = \frac{\partial^2 u_1}{\partial r^2},$$

$$\lim_{r \to 0} \frac{1}{r}\frac{\partial u_2}{\partial r} = \frac{\partial^2 u_2}{\partial r^2}.$$

Thus, the radial groups in eqs. (6.5a,b) become

$$\frac{\partial^2 u_1}{\partial r^2} + \frac{1}{r}\frac{\partial u_1}{\partial r} = 2\frac{\partial^2 u_1}{\partial r^2}, \tag{6.7e}$$

$$\frac{\partial^2 u_2}{\partial r^2} + \frac{1}{r}\frac{\partial u_2}{\partial r} = 2\frac{\partial^2 u_2}{\partial r^2}. \tag{6.7f}$$

Equations (6.7e,f) are programmed (at $r = 0$ or `i=1`) as

```
if(i==1)
  u1t(i)=Du1*2*u1rr(i)+sc*u1(i)*(2-u1(i))-u1(i);
  u2t(i)=Du2*2*u2rr(i)+lam*g-lam*u2(i);
```

– Equations (6.5a,b) for $r \neq 0$ are programmed as

```
else
u1t(i)=Du1*(u1rr(i)+(1/r(i))*u1r(i))+sc*u1(i)*(2-u1(i))-u1(i);
u2t(i)=Du2*(u2rr(i)+(1/r(i))*u2r(i))+lam*g-lam*u2(i);
end
end
u1t(nr)=0; u2t(nr)=0;
```

The derivatives $(\partial u_1(r=1,t)/\partial t), (\partial u_1(r=1,t)/\partial t)$ are set to zero in accordance with BCs (6.7c,d).

- All 202 derivatives in t are now programmed (the LHS of eqs. (6.5a,b)), so they can be placed in a single vector `ut` to be returned to `ode15s` as a LHS argument of `pde_2`.

```
%
% Two vectors to one vector
  for i=1:nr
    ut(i)    =u1t(i);
    ut(i+nr)=u2t(i);
  end
```

- A transpose of `ut` required by `ode15s` and an increment in the counter `ncall` concludes `pde_2`.

```
%
% Transpose and counter
  ut=ut';
  ncall=ncall+1;
```

The four functions for g, s_c called in `pde_2` are the remaining programming (Listings 6.5a to 6.5d).

```
function ga=gf(u1)
global alpha
ga=u1*(1+alpha^2)/(u1^2+alpha^2);
```

Listing 6.5a Function ga from eq. (6.5c)

The programming in ga follows directly from eq. (6.5c). Note that a file with the name `ga.m` is required to use (call) this function (the name of the function in the first line, `gf`, is not used).

```
function sa=sf(u2)
global     h     cm    beta
sa=2*cm*(h-beta)*u2/(cm^2+u2^2)+beta;
```

Listing 6.5b Function `sa` from eq. (6.5d)

Again, a file named `sa.m` is required to use (call) this function. `beta` is a constant computed once in `pde_2_main` according to eq. (6.5e) before `sa` is called from `pde_2`.

```
function gi=gf(u1)
gi=u1;
```

Listing 6.5c Function gi from eq. (6.5f)

```
function si=sf(u2)
global h
si=((h-1)*u2+h)/(2*(h-1)*u2+1);
```

Listing 6.5d Function si from eq. (6.5g)

This completes the programming of eqs. (6.5) to (6.7). The output from the main program pde_2_main is considered next.

6.2.3 Two-PDE model output

The output from pde_2_main is in two sections for ncase=1,2.

ncase = 1

The numerical and graphical output is in Table 6.7 and Figs 6.5 and 6.6.

We note that to compute a complete solution, $0 \leq t \leq 25$, 14483 calls to pde_2 were required. This is not a prohibitively large number and the solution was computed in a few minutes on a modest desktop computer.

The plotted solutions are given in Fig. 6.5 ($u_1(r,t)$) and Fig. 6.6 ($u_2(r,t)$).

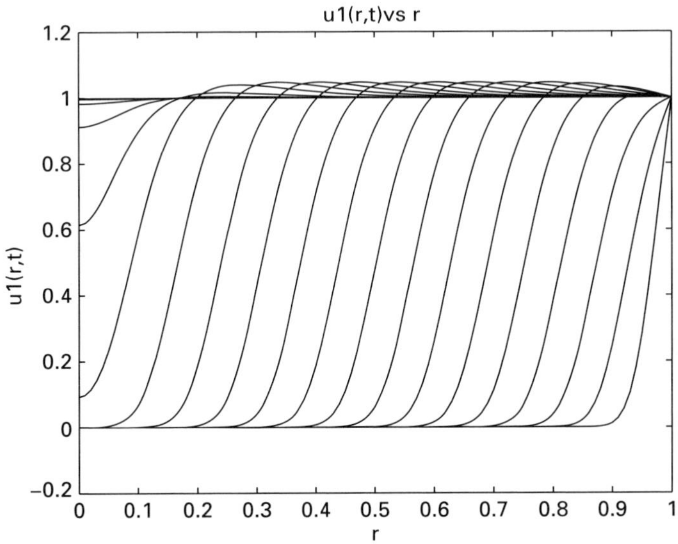

Figure 6.5 $u_1(r,t)$ from eqs. (6.5) to (6.7) for ncase=1

Table 6.7. Numerical output from `pde_2_main` of Listing 6.4 for `ncase=1`

```
  la =   30.0      li =    5.0        h =   10.0

  cm =   40.0  alpha = 0.100   beta = 0.527

 Du1 = 5.000e-004    Du2 = 4.500e-001

  nr = 101

 t = 0.00e+000
 t = 1.25e+000
 t = 2.50e+000
 t = 3.75e+000
 t = 5.00e+000
 t = 6.25e+000
 t = 7.50e+000
 t = 8.75e+000
 t = 1.00e+001
 t = 1.13e+001
 t = 1.25e+001
 t = 1.38e+001
 t = 1.50e+001
 t = 1.63e+001
 t = 1.75e+001
 t = 1.88e+001
 t = 2.00e+001
 t = 2.13e+001
 t = 2.25e+001
 t = 2.38e+001
 t = 2.50e+001

 ncall = 14483
```

The moving front characteristic of $u_1(r,t)$ as the wound closes is clear. Also, these solutions appear to essentially reproduce the solutions in [1], although a direct comparison is not possible since numerical output from [1] is not given, and the plotted output does not include the parametric values of t.

ncase = 2

The numerical and graphical output is in Table 6.8 and Figs 6.7 and 6.8.

We note that to compute a complete solution, $0 \le t \le 50$, `1287` calls to `pde_2` were required, less than $1/10$ the number for `ncase=1`. This large reduction in the calls can be attributed simply to parameter changes between `ncase=1` and `ncase=2` since all of the code is the same for both cases. In other words, the change in the value of `ncall`

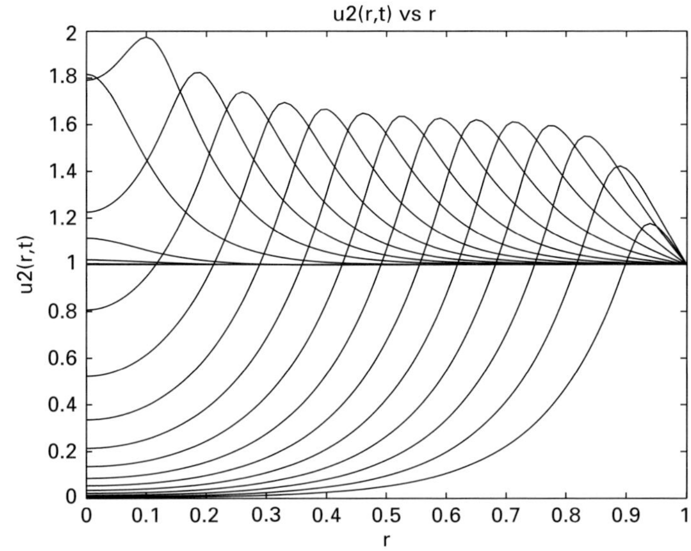

Figure 6.6 $u_2(r,t)$ from eqs. (6.5) to (6.7) for `ncase=1`

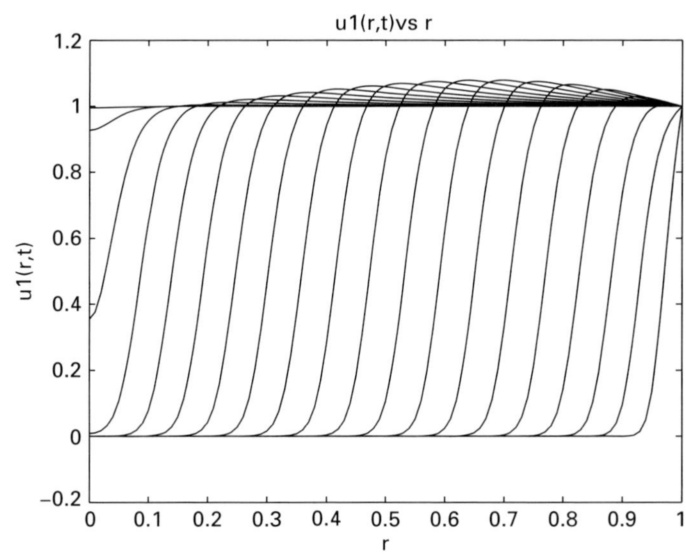

Figure 6.7 $u_1(r,t)$ from eqs. (6.5) to (6.7) for `ncase=2`

clearly indicates the sensitivity of the numerical calculations to the particular parameter values.

The plotted solutions are given in Figs. 6.7 ($u_1(r,t)$) and Figs. 6.8 ($u_2(r,t)$).

Again, the moving front characteristic of $u_1(r,t)$ as the wound closes is clear. The velocity is lower for `ncase=2`, thereby necessitating a longer time scale (to $t = 50$ for `ncase=2` rather than $t = 25$ for `ncase=1`). As before for `ncase=1`, these solutions appear

Table 6.8. Numerical output from `pde_2_main` of Listing 6.4 for `ncase=2`

```
  la =   30.0      li =    5.0        h =   10.0

  cm =   40.0  alpha = 0.100    beta = 0.527

 Du1 = 1.000e-004    Du2 = 8.500e-001

  nr = 101

 t = 0.00e+000
 t = 2.50e+000
 t = 5.00e+000
 t = 7.50e+000
 t = 1.00e+001
 t = 1.25e+001
 t = 1.50e+001
 t = 1.75e+001
 t = 2.00e+001
 t = 2.25e+001
 t = 2.50e+001
 t = 2.75e+001
 t = 3.00e+001
 t = 3.25e+001
 t = 3.50e+001
 t = 3.75e+001
 t = 4.00e+001
 t = 4.25e+001
 t = 4.50e+001
 t = 4.75e+001
 t = 5.00e+001

 ncall =  1287
```

to essentially reproduce the solutions in [1], although a direct comparison is not possible since numerical output from [1] is not given, and the plotted output does not include the parametric values of t.

This completes the discussion of the two-PDE model. The main features of this model are two simultaneous (coupled), nonlinear PDEs, which would most likely be beyond analytical methods, but which are straightforward with a numerical approach. We conclude this chapter with a few additional observations.

6.3 Conclusions concerning space and time discretizations

The preceding discussion indicates that the MOL programming of the PDE models required two basic decisions: (1) the selection of a discretization in space, and (2) the

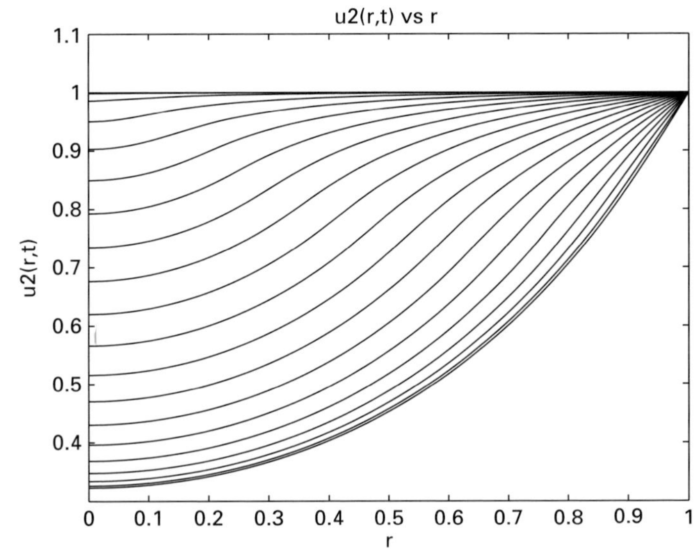

Figure 6.8 $u_2(r,t)$ from eqs. (6.5) to (6.7) for ncase=2

selection of an ODE integrator; the latter is also a form of discretization (the ODE integrator takes discrete steps in t). The process of selecting these two discretizations is generally by experimentation, with no guarantee of success in advance. In the present case, the spatial discretization was by dss004 and dss044 ($O(h^4)$ where h is the spatial grid spacing), which are our usual choice, at least to start. Then some experimentation with the order of the spatial discretization is easily carried out just by calling two alternative routines, e.g., dss006 and dss046, which are $O(h^6)$. This form of p refinement is recommended, although unexpectedly, using higher order FD approximations may cause the calculation to fail (since these higher order FD approximations are based on higher order polynomials that can oscillate more than lower order polynomials and therefore cause the calculations to fail).

Another test would be to change the spatial grid spacing by varying the number of grid points (nr = 101 in the present case). Since for ncase=1, the number of calls to pde_2 was relatively large (14483), we decided to reduce nr to reduce the computational effort. Therefore nr was reduced from 101 to 51. This had two unexpected effects:

- The plotted profiles in r had a nonsmooth appearance, indicating the grid was too coarse.
- The ODE integration by ode15s failed for ncase=2. Specifically, the integration stopped with an error message before the final value of t was reached, to warn that indicated the specified error tolerances (abserr, relerr set in pde_2_main before the call to ode15s) could not be achieved.

Clearly, neither of these outcomes is acceptable; they are presented as an example of what might go wrong with h (and p) refinement.

The t discretization can also be done in two ways. The order of the ODE integrator can be changed, such as changing from the modified Euler method $(O(h^2))$ to the Runge Kutta integrator $(O(h^4))$, as discussed in Chapter 1. p refinement is actually done automatically and internally within `ode15s` as the integration proceeds from order 1 to order 5 (which is the reason for the `15` designation in the name `ode15s`). h refinement is also carried out automatically and internally by `ode15s` in attempting to meet the specified error tolerances.

`ode15s` is a high quality integrator, and is therefore the basis for much of our MOL analysis, especially when the sparse option is included. However, it can fail, as when `nr` was changed from `101` to `51` for `ncase=2`, typically for no apparent reason, and therefore with no apparent remedy. Since `ode15s` is a large routine with hundreds of lines of code, trying to determine what went wrong is nearly impossible (except by the authors who wrote it). When this happens, we often next go to a simpler integrator, even a fixed-step Euler integrator. This has the advantage of our knowing in detail what it is doing, possibly with printing intermediate output to try to identify the underlying problem. But there is no guarantee that this will find the source of the computational problem, and additional experimentation and investigation might be required, such as taking just one small step away from the initial condition.

In summary, the development of a new MOL code usually requires some experimentation. This was true for the PDE models and codes discussed in this book. Then once some numerical output is produced, a critical review, usually with an error analysis such as h and p refinement, is essential. On the other hand, the success rate for developing MOL solutions to complex PDE problems (which are usually beyond analytical methods) is quite high.

References

[1] Murray, J. D. (2003), *Mathematical Biology, II: Spatial Models and Biomedical Applications*, 3rd Edn, 444–454

[2] Schiesser, W. E. and Griffiths, G. W, (2009), *A Compendium of Partial Differential Equation Models*, Cambridge, UK: Cambridge University Press

[3] Sherratt, J. A. and Murray, J. D. (1990), Models of epidermal wound healing, *Proc. R. Soc. Lond. B*, **241** (1300), 29–36

7 Drug distribution from a polymer matrix

In this concluding example application, we consider features of the model that broaden the coverage of concepts and topics in the previous examples. In particular, the following model is based on simultaneous 2D PDEs (the previous examples were 1D). The model is represented in Fig. 7.1 as a cylindrical system, which typically could be a polymer matrix (PM) [1, 2]. A drug is initially embedded in the PM, and the computational problem then is to determine how fast the drug will leave the PM and enter the surroundings, typically tissue that is treated by the drug. The movement of the drug within the PM is modeled by diffusion, and the transfer rate to the surroundings is expressed in term of a mass transfer coefficient. The equations that express these concepts are discussed next.

7.1 Linear model

The diffusion equation in cylindrical coordinates (r,z,θ) is taken from [3], eq. (A.1.14), p 389

$$\frac{\partial u}{\partial t} = D\left[\frac{\partial^2 u}{\partial r^2} + \frac{1}{r}\frac{\partial u}{\partial r} + \frac{1}{r^2}\frac{\partial^2 u}{\partial \theta^2} + \frac{\partial^2 u}{\partial z^2}\right]. \tag{7.1}$$

The analysis of the system in Fig. 7.1 is based on symmetry in θ so that the angular terms in eq. (7.1) are dropped; this symmetry comes about from a uniform external concentration, as explained next.

Two components will be considered: u_1, u_2 designate H_2O and a drug concentration, respectively. Therefore, eq. (7.1) applied to two components gives

$$\frac{\partial u_1}{\partial t} = D_{u_1}\left[\frac{\partial^2 u_1}{\partial r^2} + \frac{1}{r}\frac{\partial u_1}{\partial r} + \frac{\partial^2 u_1}{\partial z^2}\right], \tag{7.2a}$$

$$\frac{\partial u_2}{\partial t} = D_{u_2}\left[\frac{\partial^2 u_2}{\partial r^2} + \frac{1}{r}\frac{\partial u_2}{\partial r} + \frac{\partial^2 u_2}{\partial z^2}\right]. \tag{7.2b}$$

Equations (7.2) are first order in t and second order in r and z, and they therefore each require one initial condition (IC) in t and two boundary conditions (BCs) in r and z. The ICs are

$$u_1(r,z,t=0) = u_{10};\ u_2(r,z,t=0) = u_{20}, \tag{7.3a,b}$$

where u_{10}, u_{20} are specified constants.

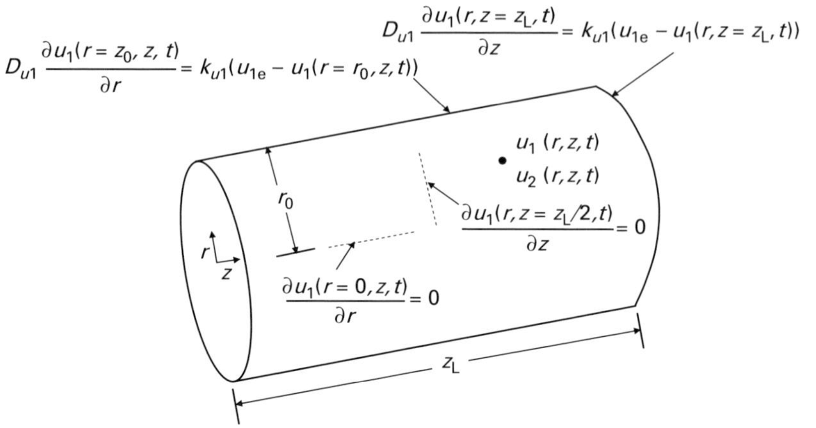

Figure 7.1 Diagram of a drug delivery system

Two homogeneous (zero) Neumann BCs (see Section 1.3.2) for eqs. (7.2) at $r=0$ specify symmetry in r.

$$\frac{\partial u_1(r=0,z,t)}{\partial r}=\frac{\partial u_2(r=0,z,t)}{\partial r}=0. \tag{7.4a,b}$$

Two third type BCs (see Section 1.3.3) at the exterior surface $r=r_0$ are based on mass transfer coefficients k_{u_1},k_{u_2} for u_1,u_2, respectively.

$$D_{u_1}\frac{\partial u_1(r=r_0,z,t)}{\partial r}=k_{u_1}(u_{1\mathrm{e}}-u_1(r=r_0,z,t)), \tag{7.5a}$$

$$D_{u_2}\frac{\partial u_2(r=r_0,z,t)}{\partial r}=k_{u_2}(u_{2\mathrm{e}}-u_2(r=r_0,z,t)). \tag{7.5b}$$

The external concentrations $u_{1\mathrm{e}},u_{2\mathrm{e}}$ are specified constants, which give the symmetry in θ (these concentrations are uniform with respect to θ). Equations (7.5) equate the mass fluxes at the surface $r=r_0$, $D_{u_1}(\partial u_1(r=r_0,z,t)/\partial r)$, and $D_{u_1}(\partial u_1(r=r_0,z,t)/\partial r)$ (according to Fick's first law), to the fluxes due to concentration differences at $r=r_0$, $k_{u_1}(u_{1\mathrm{e}}-u_1(r=r_0,z,t))$, and $k_{u_2}(u_{2\mathrm{e}}-u_2(r=r_0,z,t))$. Two special cases can be mentioned:

- $D_{u_1}=D_{u_2}=0$ These are no-flux or zero-flux BCs and correspond to no H_2O and no drug leaving the PM.
- $D_{u_1}\to\infty; D_{u_2}\to\infty$ These BCs correspond to no resistance to mass transfer at the surface $r=r_0$, in which case $u_1(r=r_0,z,t)=u_{1\mathrm{e}}; u_2(r=r_0,z,t)=u_{2\mathrm{e}}$.

Other combinations are possible; for example, $D_{u_1}\to\infty$ (or $u_1(r=r_0,z,t)=u_{1\mathrm{e}}$) while D_{u_2} finite (so that $u_2(r=r_0,z,t)\neq u_{2\mathrm{e}}$).

Two BCs in z at $z=z_L/2$ reflect symmetry in z, that is, the solution for $0\le z\le z_L/2$ is the mirror image of the solution for $z_L/2\le z\le z_L$ so that only half of the system in

Fig. 7.1 has to be considered with respect to z; here we use the right half, corresponding to $z_L/2 \le z \le z_L$.

$$D_{u_1}\frac{\partial u_1(r,z=z_L/2,t)}{\partial z} = D_{u_2}\frac{\partial u_2(r,z=z_L/2,t)}{\partial z} = 0. \quad (7.6a,b)$$

The symmetry in z again comes about from the constant values of u_{1e}, u_{2e}.

The BCs at $z = z_L$ specify the fluxes in terms of the same mass transfer coefficients as in eqs. (7.5) (they could have different values).

$$D_{u_1}\frac{\partial u_1(r,z=z_L,t)}{\partial z} = k_{u_1}(u_{1e} - u_1(r,z=z_L,t)) \quad (7.7a)$$

$$D_{u_2}\frac{\partial u_2(r,z=z_L,t)}{\partial z} = k_{u_2}(u_{1e} - u_2(r,z=z_L,t)) \quad (7.7b)$$

Equations (7.2) to (7.7) constitute the first form of the model for the system of Fig. 7.1. We can note three features of this model.

- Equations (7.2) to (7.7) are linear, that is, u_1, u_2, and all of their derivatives are to the first power or first degree. This linearity might suggest that an analytical solution should be available. While this may be true in principle, in practice, the derivation of the solution would be quite involved and therefore we will pursue a numerical solution to eqs. (7.2) to (7.7).
- The parameters are taken as constants, that is, $D_{u_1}, D_{u_2}, k_{u_1}, k_{u_2}, u_{1e}, u_{2e}$ are constant. Again, this would suggest that an analytical solution is feasible but we will pursue a numerical approach to produce a solution with reasonable effort. Also, for this case of constant parameters, the model cannot be described as a constant coefficient because eqs. (7.2) have variable coefficients in r, owing to the use of cylindrical coordinates; the $1/r$ variable coefficients would further complicate the derivation of an analytical solution, but as we should observe, they do not present any difficulty when using a numerical approach.
- Equations (7.2) are uncoupled, that is, we could solve these two PDEs separately (since u_1 appears in only eq. (7.2a) and its associated IC and BCs, while u_2 appears only in eq. (7.2b) and its associated IC and BCs). In a subsequent version of the model, we will consider the case for which the PDEs are coupled.

To conclude this section, Table 7.1 summarizes the model variables and parameters

Note that for concentrations, we use normalized values, $0 \le u_1, u_2, u_{10}, u_{20}, u_{1e}, u_{2e} \le 1$. This choice of the range of these variables and parameters facilitates their interpretation (e.g., their departure from one). This scaling of the concentrations is feasible because of the linearity of eqs. (7.2) to (7.7), which provides the useful property that the absolute values of the variables is inconsequential so that we can select a convenient scale (such as 0 to 1). In the case of the nonlinear model to be considered subsequently, the use of absolute values of the variables is required.

To conclude this discussion of the model, eqs. (7.2) to (7.7), we should understand that certain assumptions are implied when stating the equations. For example, the porosity

Table 7.1. Summary of the variables and parameters of eqs. (7.2) to (7.7)

Variable, parameter	Interpretation and representative units
u_1, u_2	concentrations of water, drug (normalized)
r	radial position in the PM (cm)
z	axial position in the PM (cm)
t	time (s)
r_0	PM radius (cm)
z_L	PM length (cm)
u_{10}, u_{20}	initial values of u_1, u_2 (normalized)
u_{1e}, u_{2e}	exterior values of u_1, u_2 (normalized)
D_{u_1}, D_{u_2}	diffusivities (cm^2/s)
k_{u_1}, k_{u_2}	mass transfer coefficients (cm/s)

of the PM is considered constant (this is reflected in the constant diffusivities), and the dimensions of the PM are considered constant (i.e., z_L and r_0 do not change). These assumptions are not required, and a PM with variable porosity (changing with time) and dimensions (also changing with time) could be included in the numerical approach, which might make the model more realistic (better conform to the actual behavior of the PM). We have not included these effects, in order to keep the model basic and of modest complexity. In other words, the emphasis is on an introduction to the MOL solution, and not on attempting to include all of the complexity that might be part of a more detailed and realistic analysis of the drug delivery system. We thereby intend to explain the MOL methodology through this example application (which can then be applied to more complex models).

We next consider the MOL solution of eqs. (7.2) to (7.7).

7.1.1 Main program

A main program for the MOL solution of eqs. (7.2) to (7.7) is given in Listing 7.1.

```
%
% Dynamic analysis of drug delivery
%
% Clear previous files
  clear all
  clc
%
% Global area
%
% Global area
  global     nr     nz     dr     dz     drs    dzs...
              r     r0      z     zL     Du1    Du2...
             u1     u2    u1e    u2e     ku1    ku2...
          ncall
```

```
%
% Model parameters
  u10=0.5; u20=1;
  u1e=1; u2e=0;
  r0=1; zL=2;
  Du1=1.0e-06; Du2=1.0e-06;
  ku1=1.0e-01; ku2=1.0e-01;
%
% Grid in axial direction
  nz=11;
  dz=zL/(2*(nz-1));
  for i=1:nz
    z(i)=zL/2+(i-1)*dz;
  end
  dzs=dz^2;
%
% Grid in radial direction
  nr=11;
  dr=r0/(nr-1);
  for j=1:nr
    r(j)=(j-1)*dr;
  end
  drs=dr^2;
%
% Independent variable for ODE integration
  tf=2*3600*24;
  tout=[0.0:2*900*24:tf]';
  nout=5;
  ncall=0;
%
% Initial condition
  for i=1:nz
  for j=1:nr
    u1(i,j)=u10;
    u2(i,j)=u20;
    u0((i-1)*nr+j)=u1(i,j);
    u0((i-1)*nr+j+nz*nr)=u2(i,j);
  end
  end
%
% ODE integration
  reltol=1.0e-04; abstol=1.0e-04;
  options=odeset('RelTol',reltol,'AbsTol',abstol);
  mf=1;
  if(mf==1)[t,u]=ode15s(@pde_1,tout,u0,options);end
  if(mf==2)[t,u]=ode15s(@pde_2,tout,u0,options);end
  if(mf==3)[t,u]=ode15s(@pde_3,tout,u0,options);end
  if(mf==4)[t,u]=ode15s(@pde_4,tout,u0,options);end
%
% 1D to 2D matrices
  for it=1:nout
```

```
  for i=1:nz
  for j=1:nr
    u1(it,i,j)=u(it,(i-1)*nr+j);
    u2(it,i,j)=u(it,(i-1)*nr+j+nz*nr);
  end
  end
  end
%
% Display a heading and radial profiles
%
% z=zL/2
  fprintf('\n  nr = %2d    nz = %2d\n',nr,nz);
  for it=1:nout
    fprintf('\n t = %4.1f    z = %3.1f\n',t(it)/3600,z(1));
  for j=1:nr
    fprintf(...
        ' r = %4.2f   u1(r,z,t) = %6.3f   u2(r,z,t) = %6.3f\n',...
        r(j),u1(it,1,j),u2(it,1,j));
  end
    fprintf('\n ku2*(u2(r=r0,z=zL/2,t)-u2e) = %8.3e\n\n',...
            3600*ku2*(u2(it,1,nr)-u2e));
  end
  fprintf('\n ncall = %5d\n',ncall);
%
% Parametric plots, radial profiles, z=zL/2
%
% 2D plots
  figure(1);
  subplot(2,2,1)
  for j=1:nr u1plot(j)=u1(2,1,j); u2plot(j)=u2(2,1,j); end
  plot(r,u1plot,'-o',r,u2plot,'-x'); axis([0 r0 0 1]);
  title('u1,u2(r,z=zL/2,t=12hr),o-u1,x-u2');
  xlabel('r'); ylabel('u1,u2(r,z=zL/2,t=12hr)')
  subplot(2,2,2)
  for j=1:nr u1plot(j)=u1(3,1,j); u2plot(j)=u2(3,1,j); end
  plot(r,u1plot,'-o',r,u2plot,'-x'); axis([0 r0 0 1]);
  title('u1,u2(r,z=zL/2,t=24hr),o-u1,x-u2');
  xlabel('r'); ylabel('u1,u2(r,z=zL/2,t=24hr)')
  subplot(2,2,3)
  for j=1:nr u1plot(j)=u1(4,1,j); u2plot(j)=u2(4,1,j); end
  plot(r,u1plot,'-o',r,u2plot,'-x'); axis([0 r0 0 1]);
  title('u1,u2(r,z=zL/2,t=36hr),o-u1,x-u2');
  xlabel('r'); ylabel('u1,u2(r,z=zL/2,t=36hr)')
  subplot(2,2,4)
  for j=1:nr u1plot(j)=u1(5,1,j); u2plot(j)=u2(5,1,j); end
  plot(r,u1plot,'-o',r,u2plot,'-x'); axis([0 r0 0 1]);
  title('u1,u2(r,z=zL/2,t=48hr),o-u1,x-u2');
  xlabel('r'); ylabel('u1,u2(r,z=zL/2,t=48hr)')
%
% 3D plots
  for it=1:nout
```

```
  for j=1:nr u1surf(it,j)=u1(it,1,j); end
  for j=1:nr u2surf(it,j)=u2(it,1,j); end
end
figure(2)
surf(r,t/(3600*24),u1surf);
xlabel('r (cm)'); ylabel('t (day)'); zlabel('u1(r,z=zL/2,t)');
figure(3)
surf(r,t/(3600*24),u2surf);
view(-20,60)
xlabel('r (cm)'); ylabel('t (day)'); zlabel('u2(r,z=zL/2,t)');
```

Listing 7.1 Main program `pde_1_main` for the MOL solution of eqs. (7.2) to (7.7)

We can note the following details about `pde_1_main`.

- Previous files are cleared and selected variables and parameters are declared global so they can be shared with other routines.

```
%
% Dynamic analysis of drug delivery
%
% Clear previous files
  clear all
  clc
%
% Global area
%
% Global area
  global     nr      nz      dr      dz      drs     dzs...
              r      r0       z      zL      Du1     Du2...
             u1      u2     u1e     u2e      ku1     ku2...
          ncall
```

  Documentation comments for eqs. (7.2) to (7.7) have not been included to conserve space (they are in the code that can be downloaded).
- The model parameters are defined numerically.

```
%
% Model parameters
  u10=0.5; u20=1;
  u1e=1; u2e=0;
  r0=1; zL=2;
  Du1=1.0e-06; Du2=1.0e-06;
  ku1=1.0e-01; ku2=1.0e-01;
```

  Note in particular:

  – The initial values of the water and drug concentrations,

    ```
    u10=0.5; u20=1;
    ```

    Thus, the water concentration is 0.5 of the surrounding value (listed next), and the drug concentration has its highest value initially (1).

– The surrounding concentrations are

```
u1e=1; u2e=0;
```

Thus, water has its maximum value (1) in the surroundings and there is no drug due to utilization (e.g., in the surrounding tissue). Of course, these values can be changed, and even programmed as a function of t. As an extension of the model, mass conservation balances (additional PDEs) applied to the surroundings could be used to compute changes in u_{1e}, u_{2e} as a function of time and position.

– The drug delivery PM of Fig 7.1 is 1 cm in radius and 2 cm in length.

```
r0=1; zL=2;
```

– The diffusivities in eqs. (7.2), (7.5), (7.6) and (7.7) are 1×10^{-6} cm^2/s, which is rather typical for liquids. Smaller values reflecting retarded diffusion due to the PM structure or large drug molecules could be considered, which would reduce the rate of drug delivery.

```
Du1=1.0e-06; Du2=1.0e-06;
```

Also, the diffusivities could change with time, owing to changes in the porosity of the PM or the effect of changes in one component, for example, water, on the other component, that is, the drug. An important advantage of the numerical approach to the solution of the model equations is that effects like these can easily be included; this would be difficult to achieve analytically. A subsequent variation in the model demonstrates how the diffusivities can be programmed as an explicit function of t.

– The mass transfer coefficients in eqs. (7.7) (in cm/s) were selected to give significant resistance to mass transfer at $r = r_0$.

```
ku1=1.0e-01; ku2=1.0e-01;
```

In practice, these would be relatively difficult to estimate and would be dependent on the features of the surroundings. They therefore would probably require estimation from experimental data. An alternative would be to set them to ∞ so that the surface concentrations equal the surrounding concentrations (no resistance to mass transfer at $r = r_0, z = z_L$).

- An 11 point grid in z and r is defined.

```
%
% Grid in axial direction
  nz=11;
  dz=zL/(2*(nz-1));
  for i=1:nz
    z(i)=zL/2+(i-1)*dz;
  end
  dzs=dz^2;
%
% Grid in radial direction
  nr=11;
  dr=r0/(nr-1);
  for j=1:nr
```

```
    r(j)=(j-1)*dr;
  end
  drs=dr^2;
```

Thus, there are $11 \times 11 \times 2 = 242$ ODEs (the factor of two results from two PDEs, eqs. (7.2)) in the MOL approximation of eqs. (7.2) to (7.7); this is a modest ODE problem. Also, the rapid increase in the number of ODEs as the number of grid points is increased is clear; this $nr \times nz$ scaling is usually termed the curse of dimensionality, and of course, it is even more of a curse in 3D. Note also that several of the parameters, i.e. `nz, nr, dz, dr, dzs, drs`, are passed as global variables to the ODE routine `pde_1`, considered next.

- The interval in t is defined as $0 \le t \le 2$ days. Since the model parameters are in s (seconds), (the diffusivities and mass transfer coefficients), the model is executed in s with five outputs (including $t = 0$) at intervals of `2*900*24` s.

```
%
% Independent variable for ODE integration
  tf=2*3600*24;
  tout=[0.0:2*900*24:tf]';
  nout=5;
  ncall=0;
```

- A single IC vector, `u0`, is formed as required by the ODE integrator `ode15s`. Note in particular the subscripting to form this vector from the two ICs of eqs. (7.2) (according to ICs (7.3)). Also, the nested `for` loops in `i,j` define a total of $11 \times 11 \times 2 = 242$ ICs. The resulting dimension of `u0` (a 242-vector) is the way the number of ODEs is conveyed to `ode15s`.

```
%
% Initial condition
  for i=1:nz
  for j=1:nr
    u1(i,j)=u10;
    u2(i,j)=u20;
    u0((i-1)*nr+j)=u1(i,j);
    u0((i-1)*nr+j+nz*nr)=u2(i,j);
  end
  end
```

The subscripting illustrated for eqs. (7.2) can be readily extended to systems of n PDEs (with $n = 2$ in the present case).

- `ode15s` is called for four different cases, `mf=1,2,3,4` with four different ODE routines, `pde_1` to `pde_4`. Presently, `mf=1`; the other three cases are discussed subsequently.

```
%
% ODE integration
  reltol=1.0e-04; abstol=1.0e-04;
  options=odeset('RelTol',reltol,'AbsTol',abstol);
  mf=1;
  if(mf==1)[t,u]=ode15s(@pde_1,tout,u0,options);end
  if(mf==2)[t,u]=ode15s(@pde_2,tout,u0,options);end
```

```
  if(mf==3)[t,u]=ode15s(@pde_3,tout,u0,options);end
  if(mf==4)[t,u]=ode15s(@pde_4,tout,u0,options);end
```

- ode15s returns a solution vector u(5,242), where the first dimension, 5, corresponds to the five values of t specified previously for the output of the numerical solution and the second dimension, 242, corresponds to the 242 ODEs ordered as previously discussed when the IC vector u0 was defined.

```
%
% 1D to 2D matrices
  for it=1:nout
  for i=1:nz
  for j=1:nr
    u1(it,i,j)=u(it,(i-1)*nr+j);
    u2(it,i,j)=u(it,(i-1)*nr+j+nz*nr);
  end
  end
  end
```

Note that the three nested for loops produce two arrays, u1(5,11,11), u2(5,11,11), where the first dimension 5 refers to t, the second, 11, refers to z, and the third, 11, refers to r. The use of these two arrays facilitates the numerical and graphical display of the solution is discussed next.

- Since ode15s returns $5 \times 242 = 1210$ numbers, some selection is required in order to display the solution in a comprehensible format. Here we display the numerical solution at the midpoint $z = z_L/2$ as a function of r (from the for loop in j) for $t = 0, 0.5, 1, 1.5, 2$ h (from the for loop in it); note the use of r(j),u1(it,1,j),u2(it,1,j) in the third fprintf statement where the second subscript 1 corresponds to $z = z_L/2$ and the third subscript j corresponds to $0 \leq r \leq r_0$.

```
%
% Display a heading and radial profiles
%
% z=zL/2
  fprintf('\n  nr = %2d   nz = %2d\n',nr,nz);
  for it=1:nout
    fprintf('\n t = %4.1f   z = %3.1f\n',t(it)/3600,z(1));
  for j=1:nr
    fprintf(...
        ' r = %4.2f   u1(r,z,t) = %6.3f   u2(r,z,t) = %6.3f\n',...
        r(j),u1(it,1,j),u2(it,1,j));
  end
    fprintf('\n ku2*(u2(r=r0,z=zL/2,t)-u2e) = %8.3e\n\n',...
            3600*ku2*(u2(it,1,nr)-u2e));
  end
  fprintf('\n ncall = %5d\n',ncall);
```

The scale $0 \leq t \leq 48$ h is defined with the conversion 1/3600 (s converted to h). The surface flux for the drug, ku2*(u2(r=r0,z=zL/2,t)-u2e) is also displayed at each t. Finally, the number of calls to pde_1 is displayed as an indication of the total effort required to compute the solution (`ncall` is incremented by 1 each time `pde_1` is executed by `ode15s`).

- A composite of four plots corresponding to $t = 12, 24, 36, 48$ h is plotted.

```
%
% Parametric plots, radial profiles, z=zL/2
%
% 2D plots
  figure(1);
  subplot(2,2,1)
  for j=1:nr u1plot(j)=u1(2,1,j); u2plot(j)=u2(2,1,j); end
  plot(r,u1plot,'-o',r,u2plot,'-x'); axis([0 r0 0 1]);
  title('u1,u2(r,z=zL/2,t=12hr),o-u1,x-u2');
  xlabel('r'); ylabel('u1,u2(r,z=zL/2,t=12hr)')
  subplot(2,2,2)
  for j=1:nr u1plot(j)=u1(3,1,j); u2plot(j)=u2(3,1,j); end
  plot(r,u1plot,'-o',r,u2plot,'-x'); axis([0 r0 0 1]);
  title('u1,u2(r,z=zL/2,t=24hr),o-u1,x-u2');
  xlabel('r'); ylabel('u1,u2(r,z=zL/2,t=24hr)')
  subplot(2,2,3)
  for j=1:nr u1plot(j)=u1(4,1,j); u2plot(j)=u2(4,1,j); end
  plot(r,u1plot,'-o',r,u2plot,'-x'); axis([0 r0 0 1]);
  title('u1,u2(r,z=zL/2,t=36hr),o-u1,x-u2');
  xlabel('r'); ylabel('u1,u2(r,z=zL/2,t=36hr)')
  subplot(2,2,4)
  for j=1:nr u1plot(j)=u1(5,1,j); u2plot(j)=u2(5,1,j); end
  plot(r,u1plot,'-o',r,u2plot,'-x'); axis([0 r0 0 1]);
  title('u1,u2(r,z=zL/2,t=48hr),o-u1,x-u2');
  xlabel('r'); ylabel('u1,u2(r,z=zL/2,t=48hr)')
```

$u_1(r, z = z_L/2, t), u_2(r, z = z_L/2, t)$ are plotted as a function of r with t as a parameter. The `ylabel` identifies the four plots for $t = 12, 24, 36, 48$ h.

- Two 3D plots for $u_1(r, z = z_L/2, t), u_1(r, z = z_L/2, t)$ are then plotted with `surf`. The nested `for` loops first put the solution at $z = z_L/2$ in 2D arrays, `u1surf(it,j)`, `u2surf(it,j)` for use by `surf`.

```
%
% 3D plots
  for it=1:nout
    for j=1:nr u1surf(it,j)=u1(it,1,j); end
    for j=1:nr u2surf(it,j)=u2(it,1,j); end
  end
  figure(2)
  surf(r,t/(3600*24),u1surf);
  xlabel('r (cm)'); ylabel('t (day)'); zlabel('u1(r,z=zL/2,t)');
  figure(3)
  surf(r,t/(3600*24),u2surf);
  view(-20,60)
  xlabel('r (cm)'); ylabel('t (day)'); zlabel('u2(r,z=zL/2,t)');
```

The `view` gives a better perspective of the u_2 plot than the defaults for `surf`. The conversion `t/(3600*24)` sets the scale in t as $0 \leq t \leq 2$ days.

The numerical and graphical output from `pde_1_main` are considered after the following discussion of the ODE routine, `pde_1`.

7.1.2 ODE routine with FD explicit programming

The ODE routine `pde_1` called by `ode15s` in Listing 7.1 is listed next.

```
 function ut=pde_1(t,u)
%
% Global area
  global     nr      nz      dr      dz     drs     dzs...
              r      r0       z      zL     Du1     Du2...
             u1      u2     u1e     u2e      ku1    ku2...
          ncall
%
% 1D to 2D matrices
  for i=1:nz
  for j=1:nr
    ij=(i-1)*nr+j;
    u1(i,j)=u(ij);
    u2(i,j)=u(ij+nr*nz);
  end
  end
%
% Step through the grid points in r and z
  for i=1:nz
  for j=1:nr
%
%   (1/r)*u1r, (1/r)*u2r
    if(j==1)
      u1r(i,j)=2*(u1(i,j+1)-u1(i,j))/drs;
      u2r(i,j)=2*(u2(i,j+1)-u2(i,j))/drs;
    elseif(j==nr)
      u1r(i,j)=(1/r(j))*(ku1/Du1)*(u1e-u1(i,j));
      u2r(i,j)=(1/r(j))*(ku2/Du2)*(u2e-u2(i,j));
    else
      u1r(i,j)=(1/r(j))*(u1(i,j+1)-u1(i,j-1))/(2*dr);
      u2r(i,j)=(1/r(j))*(u2(i,j+1)-u2(i,j-1))/(2*dr);
    end
%
%   u1rr, u2rr
    if(j==1)
      u1rr(i,j)=2*(u1(i,j+1)-u1(i,j))/drs;
      u2rr(i,j)=2*(u2(i,j+1)-u2(i,j))/drs;
    elseif(j==nr)
      u1f=u1(i,j-1)+2*dr*ku1/Du1*(u1e-u1(i,j));
      u1rr(i,j)=(u1f-2*u1(i,j)+u1(i,j-1))/drs;
      u2f=u2(i,j-1)+2*dr*ku2/Du2*(u2e-u2(i,j));
      u2rr(i,j)=(u2f-2*u2(i,j)+u2(i,j-1))/drs;
    else
      u1rr(i,j)=(u1(i,j+1)-2*u1(i,j)+u1(i,j-1))/drs;
```

```
        u2rr(i,j)=(u2(i,j+1)-2*u2(i,j)+u2(i,j-1))/drs;
      end
%
%     u1zz, u2zz
      if(i==1)
        u1zz(i,j)=2*(u1(i+1,j)-u1(i,j))/dzs;
        u2zz(i,j)=2*(u2(i+1,j)-u2(i,j))/dzs;
      elseif(i==nz)
        u1f=u1(i-1,j)+2*dz*ku1/Du1*(u1e-u1(i,j));
        u1zz(i,j)=(u1f-2*u1(i,j)+u1(i-1,j))/dzs;
        u2f=u2(i-1,j)+2*dz*ku2/Du2*(u2e-u2(i,j));
        u2zz(i,j)=(u2f-2*u2(i,j)+u2(i-1,j))/dzs;
      else
        u1zz(i,j)=(u1(i+1,j)-2*u1(i,j)+u1(i-1,j))/dzs;
        u2zz(i,j)=(u2(i+1,j)-2*u2(i,j)+u2(i-1,j))/dzs;
      end
%
%     PDEs
        u1t(i,j)=Du1*(u1rr(i,j)+u1r(i,j)+u1zz(i,j));
        u2t(i,j)=Du2*(u2rr(i,j)+u2r(i,j)+u2zz(i,j));
    end
    end
%
% 2D to 1D matrices
    for i=1:nz
    for j=1:nr
      ij=(i-1)*nr+j;
      ut(ij)=u1t(i,j);
      ut(ij+nr*nz)=u2t(i,j);
    end
    end
%
% Transpose and count
    ut=ut';
    ncall=ncall+1;
```

Listing 7.2 ODE routine pde_1 with FDs from explicit programming

Next pde_1 of Listing 7.2 is discussed in some detail, including the associated mathematics and associated finite difference (FD) approximations.

- The function is defined and selected variables and parameters are declared global so they can be shared with the main program pde_1_main of Listing 7.1.

```
  function ut=pde_1(t,u)
%
% Global area
  global   nr    nz    dr    dz    drs    dzs...
            r    r0     z    zL    Du1    Du2...
           u1    u2   u1e   u2e    ku1    ku2...
        ncall
```

- The single dependent variable vector u, which is a RHS input argument of pde_1, is placed in two dependent variable vectors, u1,u2, to facilitate the programming of eqs. (7.2) to (7.7).

```
%
% 1D to 2D matrices
  for i=1:nz
  for j=1:nr
    ij=(i-1)*nr+j;
    u1(i,j)=u(ij);
    u2(i,j)=u(ij+nr*nz);
  end
  end
```

Note in particular the subscript arithmetic based on i and j for z and r, respectively.

- Two nested for loops are used to cover the domain in z and r.

```
%
% Step through the grid points in r and z
  for i=1:nz
  for j=1:nr
```

The final requirement is to compute the two arrays with the derivatives in t, u1t,u2t, defined by eqs. (7.2). These arrays are then combined at the end of pde_1 to form a single vector ut, which is a LHS output argument of pde_1 that is passed to ode15s for the ODE integration through t.

- The two first order derivative terms in eqs. (7.2), $(1/r)(\partial u_1/\partial r)$ and $(1/r)(\partial u_2/\partial r)$, are computed by FDs.

```
%
%   (1/r)*u1r, (1/r)*u2r
    if(j==1)
      u1r(i,j)=2*(u1(i,j+1)-u1(i,j))/drs;
      u2r(i,j)=2*(u2(i,j+1)-u2(i,j))/drs;
    elseif(j==nr)
      u1r(i,j)=(1/r(j))*(ku1/Du1)*(u1e-u1(i,j));
      u2r(i,j)=(1/r(j))*(ku2/Du2)*(u2e-u2(i,j));
    else
      u1r(i,j)=(1/r(j))*(u1(i,j+1)-u1(i,j-1))/(2*dr);
      u2r(i,j)=(1/r(j))*(u2(i,j+1)-u2(i,j-1))/(2*dr);
    end
```

A brief explanation of the three sections in the if follows.

  - j=1 corresponds to $r=0$ so that BCs (7.4) apply. The radial term $(1/r)(\partial u_1/\partial r)$ is indeterminate (0/0) and therefore l'Hospital's rule is applied.

$$\lim_{r\to 0}\frac{1}{r}\frac{\partial u_1}{\partial r}=\frac{\partial^2 u_1}{\partial r^2}. \tag{7.8a}$$

Then a FD approximation for the second derivative in eq. (7.8a) is used (at `j=1`).

$$\frac{\partial^2 u_1}{\partial r^2} \approx \frac{u_1(2) - 2u_1(1) + u_1(0)}{\Delta r^2}, \tag{7.8b}$$

where $u_1(0)$ is a fictitious value corresponding to $r = -\Delta r$ (since $0 \leq r \leq r_0$). However, from the FD approximation of BC (7.4a),

$$\frac{\partial u_1}{\partial r} \approx \frac{u_1(2) - u_1(0)}{2\Delta r} = 0, \tag{7.8c}$$

or

$$u_1(0) \approx u_1(2). \tag{7.8d}$$

Substitution of eq. (7.8d) in eq. (7.8b) gives

$$\frac{\partial^2 u_1}{\partial r^2} \approx 2\frac{u_1(2) - u_1(1)}{\Delta r^2}, \tag{7.8e}$$

which is programmed as

```
if(j==1)
  u1r(i,j)=2*(u1(i,j+1)-u1(i,j))/drs;
```

The same result follows for u_2 with 1 replaced by 2.

```
u2r(i,j)=2*(u2(i,j+1)-u2(i,j))/drs;
```

Note in this programming that `i` does not change. This follows from the concept of a partial derivative in r so that z is constant (and therefore `i` does not change).

- `j=nr` corresponds to $r = r_0$, where BCs (7.5) apply. The programming of these BCs is straightforward.

```
elseif(j==nr)
   u1r(i,j)=(1/r(j))*(ku1/Du1)*(u1e-u1(i,j));
   u2r(i,j)=(1/r(j))*(ku2/Du2)*(u2e-u2(i,j));
```

- $j \neq 1, nr$ corresponds to the interior points in r for which the terms $(1/r)(\partial u_1/\partial r)$ and $(1/r)(\partial u_2/\partial r)$ in eqs. (7.2) are programmed directly.

```
else
  u1r(i,j)=(1/r(j))*(u1(i,j+1)-u1(i,j-1))/(2*dr);
  u2r(i,j)=(1/r(j))*(u2(i,j+1)-u2(i,j-1))/(2*dr);
```

The first derivatives in r are approximated as

$$\frac{\partial u_1}{\partial r} \approx \frac{u_1(j+1) - u_1(j-1)}{2\Delta r}; \quad \frac{\partial u_2}{\partial r} \approx \frac{u_2(j+1) - u_2(j-1)}{2\Delta r}. \tag{7.8f,g}$$

- The second derivatives in r in eqs. (7.2), $(\partial^2 u_1/\partial r^2)$ and $(\partial^2 u_2/\partial r^2)$, are programmed as

```
%
%   u1rr, u2rr
```

```
if(j==1)
  u1rr(i,j)=2*(u1(i,j+1)-u1(i,j))/drs;
  u2rr(i,j)=2*(u2(i,j+1)-u2(i,j))/drs;
elseif(j==nr)
  u1f=u1(i,j-1)+2*dr*ku1/Du1*(u1e-u1(i,j));
  u1rr(i,j)=(u1f-2*u1(i,j)+u1(i,j-1))/drs;
  u2f=u2(i,j-1)+2*dr*ku2/Du2*(u2e-u2(i,j));
  u2rr(i,j)=(u2f-2*u2(i,j)+u2(i,j-1))/drs;
else
  u1rr(i,j)=(u1(i,j+1)-2*u1(i,j)+u1(i,j-1))/drs;
  u2rr(i,j)=(u2(i,j+1)-2*u2(i,j)+u2(i,j-1))/drs;
end
```

A brief explanation of each of the three sections in the `if` follows.

- `j=1` corresponds to $r = 0$ where BCs (7.4) apply. The second derivative in u_1 is approximated as

$$\frac{\partial^2 u_1}{\partial r^2} \approx \frac{u_1(j=2) - 2u_1(j=1) + u_1(j=0)}{\Delta r^2}, \tag{7.9a}$$

where $u_1(j=0)$ is a fictitious value (at $r = -\Delta r$) and is given by eq. (7.8d). Then the second derivative in u_1 is approximated as

$$\frac{\partial^2 u_1}{\partial r^2} \approx 2\frac{u_1(j=2) - u_1(j=1)}{\Delta r^2}, \tag{7.9b}$$

which is programmed (for u_1 and u_2) as

```
if(j==1)
  u1rr(i,j)=2*(u1(i,j+1)-u1(i,j))/drs;
  u2rr(i,j)=2*(u2(i,j+1)-u2(i,j))/drs;
```

- `j=nr` corresponds to $r = r_0$ where BCs (7.5) apply. The FD of these BCs requires the use of a fictitious point. For example, BC (7.5a) is approximated as

$$D_{u1}\frac{\partial u_1}{\partial r} \approx D_{u1}\frac{u_{1f} - u_1(j=nr-1)}{2\Delta r} = k_1(u_{1e} - u_1(j=nr)), \tag{7.9c}$$

where u_{1f} is a fictitious value (at $r = r_0 + \Delta r$). Solving eq. (7.9c) for u_{1f}, we have

$$u_{1f} = u_1(j=nr-1) + 2\Delta r(k_1/D_{u1})(u_{1e} - u_1(j=nr)), \tag{7.9d}$$

which is expressed as the first line of code in `i==nr`.

```
elseif(j==nr)
  u1f=u1(i,j-1)+2*dr*ku1/Du1*(u1e-u1(i,j));
```

Then the second derivative in u_1 is approximated as

$$\frac{\partial^2 u_1}{\partial r^2} \approx \frac{u_1(j+1) - 2u_1(j) + u_1(j-1)}{\Delta r^2}, \tag{7.9e}$$

where $u_1(j+1)$ is the fictitious value given by eq. (7.9d). Therefore, eqs. (7.9d) and (7.9e) are combined and programmed as the second line of `j==nr`

```
u1rr(i,j)=(u1f-2*u1(i,j)+u1(i,j-1))/drs;
```

Note the use of the fictitious value `u1f`. The second derivative in u_2 is programmed in the same way.

```
u2f=u2(i,j-1)+2*dr*ku2/Du2*(u2e-u2(i,j));
u2rr(i,j)=(u2f-2*u2(i,j)+u2(i,j-1))/drs;
```

– For the interior points in r, the second derivative, $(\partial^2 u_1/\partial r^2)$, is approximated as a three point centered FD

$$\frac{\partial^2 u_1}{\partial r^2} \approx \frac{u(j+1) - 2u(j) + u(j-1)}{\Delta r^2} \tag{7.9f}$$

and programmed (for u_1 and u_2) as

```
else
  u1rr(i,j)=(u1(i,j+1)-2*u1(i,j)+u1(i,j-1))/drs;
  u2rr(i,j)=(u2(i,j+1)-2*u2(i,j)+u2(i,j-1))/drs;
```

- The second derivatives in z in eqs. (7.2), $(\partial^2 u_1/\partial z^2)$ and $(\partial^2 u_2/\partial z^2)$, are programmed in a similar fashion to those in r.

```
%
% u1zz, u2zz
  if(i==1)
    u1zz(i,j)=2*(u1(i+1,j)-u1(i,j))/dzs;
    u2zz(i,j)=2*(u2(i+1,j)-u2(i,j))/dzs;
  elseif(i==nz)
    u1f=u1(i-1,j)+2*dz*ku1/Du1*(u1e-u1(i,j));
    u1zz(i,j)=(u1f-2*u1(i,j)+u1(i-1,j))/dzs;
    u2f=u2(i-1,j)+2*dz*ku2/Du2*(u2e-u2(i,j));
    u2zz(i,j)=(u2f-2*u2(i,j)+u2(i-1,j))/dzs;
  else
    u1zz(i,j)=(u1(i+1,j)-2*u1(i,j)+u1(i-1,j))/dzs;
    u2zz(i,j)=(u2(i+1,j)-2*u2(i,j)+u2(i-1,j))/dzs;
  end
```

A brief explanation of each of the three sections in the `if` follows.

– `i=1` corresponds to $z = z_L/2$ where BCs (7.6) apply. The second derivative in u_1 is approximated as

$$\frac{\partial^2 u_1}{\partial z^2} \approx \frac{u_1(i=2) - 2u_1(i=1) + u_1(i=0)}{\Delta z^2}, \tag{7.10a}$$

where $u_1(i=0)$ is a fictitious value at $z = z_L/2 - \Delta z$ (since $z_L/2 \le z \le z_L$) and can be approximated as

$$u_1(i=0) \approx u_1(i=2), \tag{7.10b}$$

in analogy with eq. (7.8d). The second derivative in u_1 is therefore approximated as

$$\frac{\partial^2 u_1}{\partial z^2} \approx 2\frac{u_1(i=2)-u_1(i=1)}{\Delta z^2}, \tag{7.10c}$$

in analogy with eq. (7.9b). The programming (for u_1 and u_2) is

```
if(i==1)
  u1zz(i,j)=2*(u1(i+1,j)-u1(i,j))/dzs;
  u2zz(i,j)=2*(u2(i+1,j)-u2(i,j))/dzs;
```

Note that in this programming `j` does not change. This follows from the concept of a partial derivative in z for which r is constant (and therefore `j` does not change).

- `i=nz` corresponds to $z = z_L$, where BCs (7.7) apply. The FD of these BCs requires the use of a fictitious point. For example, BC (7.7a) is approximated as

$$D_{u1}\frac{\partial u_1}{\partial z} \approx D_{u1}\frac{u_{1f}-u_1(i=nz-1)}{2\Delta z} = k_1(u_{1e}-u_1(i=nz)), \tag{7.10d}$$

where u_{1f} is a fictitious value (at $z = z_L + \Delta z$). Solving eq. (7.10d) for u_{1f}, we have

$$u_{1f} = u_1(i=nz-1) + 2\Delta z(k_1/D_{u1})(u_{1e}-u_1(i=nz)), \tag{7.10e}$$

which is expressed as the first line of code in `i==nz`.

```
elseif(i==nz)
  u1f=u1(i-1,j)+2*dz*ku1/Du1*(u1e-u1(i,j));
```

Then the second derivative in u_1 is approximated as

$$\frac{\partial^2 u_1}{\partial z^2} \approx \frac{u_1(i+1)-2u_1(i)+u_1(i-1)}{\Delta z^2}, \tag{7.10f}$$

where $u_1(i+1)$ is the fictitious value given by eq. (7.10e). Therefore, eqs. (7.10e) and (7.10f) are combined and programmed as the second line of `j==nr`

```
u1zz(i,j)=(u1f-2*u1(i,j)+u1(i-1,j))/dzs;
```

Note the use of the fictitious value `u1f`.
The second derivative in u_2 is programmed in the same way.

```
u2f=u2(i-1,j)+2*dz*ku2/Du2*(u2e-u2(i,j));
u2zz(i,j)=(u2f-2*u2(i,j)+u2(i-1,j))/dzs;
```

- For the interior points in z, the second derivative, $(\partial^2 u_1/\partial z^2)$, is approximated as a three point centered FD.

$$\frac{\partial^2 u_1}{\partial z^2} \approx \frac{u(i+1)-2u(i)+u(i-1)}{\Delta z^2}, \tag{7.10g}$$

and programmed (for u_1 and u_2) as

```
      else
         u1zz(i,j)=(u1(i+1,j)-2*u1(i,j)+u1(i-1,j))/dzs;
         u2zz(i,j)=(u2(i+1,j)-2*u2(i,j)+u2(i-1,j))/dzs;
```

- The programming of PDEs (7.2) is straightforward.

```
%
%   PDEs
      u1t(i,j)=Du1*(u1rr(i,j)+u1r(i,j)+u1zz(i,j));
      u2t(i,j)=Du2*(u2rr(i,j)+u2r(i,j)+u2zz(i,j));
  end
  end
```

The two ends terminate the loops in i and j.

This completes the programming for the derivative in t (the LHS of eqs. (7.2)). The preceding programming of the PDEs indicates one of the important features of the MOL approach, that is, the programming is similar in appearance to the PDEs.

- The two derivative arrays, u1t and u2t, are placed in a single vector, ut, which is returned as a LHS argument of pde_1.

```
%
% 2D to 1D matrices
  for i=1:nz
  for j=1:nr
    ij=(i-1)*nr+j;
    ut(ij)=u1t(i,j);
    ut(ij+nr*nz)=u2t(i,j);
  end
  end
```

ut is of length $11 \times 11 \times 2 = 242$. We point this out to emphasize that all 242 derivatives in t must be assigned a numerical value before the end of pde_1. If even one derivative is overlooked (which is easy to do), the numerical solution of eqs. (7.2) to (7.7) will generally be incorrect. This suggests that an effective way to check the programming of the PDEs is to display the 242 values of ut (which could be done by listing ut at the end of pde_1 without a semicolon). However, as a word of caution, we would want to do this at most only a few times because of the number of values in ut.

- pde_1 concludes with a transpose of ut as required by ode15s and the incrementing of the counter ncall (returned to pde_1 as a global variable).

```
%
% Transpose and count
  ut=ut';
  ncall=ncall+1;
```

This completes the programming of eqs. (7.2) to (7.7). We now consider the numerical and graphical output from pde_1_main of Listing 7.1.

Table 7.2. Abbreviated output from `pde_1_main` and `pde_1`

```
 nr = 11   nz = 11

t =  0.0   z = 1.0
r = 0.00   u1(r,z,t) =  0.500   u2(r,z,t) =  1.000
r = 0.10   u1(r,z,t) =  0.500   u2(r,z,t) =  1.000
r = 0.20   u1(r,z,t) =  0.500   u2(r,z,t) =  1.000
r = 0.30   u1(r,z,t) =  0.500   u2(r,z,t) =  1.000
r = 0.40   u1(r,z,t) =  0.500   u2(r,z,t) =  1.000
r = 0.50   u1(r,z,t) =  0.500   u2(r,z,t) =  1.000
r = 0.60   u1(r,z,t) =  0.500   u2(r,z,t) =  1.000
r = 0.70   u1(r,z,t) =  0.500   u2(r,z,t) =  1.000
r = 0.80   u1(r,z,t) =  0.500   u2(r,z,t) =  1.000
r = 0.90   u1(r,z,t) =  0.500   u2(r,z,t) =  1.000
r = 1.00   u1(r,z,t) =  0.500   u2(r,z,t) =  1.000

ku2*(u2(r=r0,z=zL/2,t)-u2e) = 3.600e+002

          .                   .
          .                   .
          .                   .
    Output for t = 12, 24, 36 removed
          .                   .
          .                   .
          .                   .

t = 48.0   z = 1.0
r = 0.00   u1(r,z,t) =  0.761   u2(r,z,t) =  0.479
r = 0.10   u1(r,z,t) =  0.764   u2(r,z,t) =  0.472
r = 0.20   u1(r,z,t) =  0.774   u2(r,z,t) =  0.453
r = 0.30   u1(r,z,t) =  0.790   u2(r,z,t) =  0.421
r = 0.40   u1(r,z,t) =  0.811   u2(r,z,t) =  0.378
r = 0.50   u1(r,z,t) =  0.838   u2(r,z,t) =  0.325
r = 0.60   u1(r,z,t) =  0.868   u2(r,z,t) =  0.265
r = 0.70   u1(r,z,t) =  0.900   u2(r,z,t) =  0.199
r = 0.80   u1(r,z,t) =  0.934   u2(r,z,t) =  0.131
r = 0.90   u1(r,z,t) =  0.968   u2(r,z,t) =  0.064
r = 1.00   u1(r,z,t) =  1.000   u2(r,z,t) =  0.000

ku2*(u2(r=r0,z=zL/2,t)-u2e) = 2.194e-003

ncall =   395
```

7.1.3 Model output

Abbreviated tabulated numerical output from `pde_1_main` is listed in Table 7.2.

We can note the following details about this output.

- The initial values $u_1(r,z,t=0)=0.5, u_2(r,z,t=0)=1$ assigned in `pde_1_main` are confirmed in the $t=0$ output.
- The surface values of u_1, u_2 (at $r=r_0=1$) for $t=48$ h are close to the surrounding values. The concentration profile for u_1 reflects the diffusion of H_2O into the PM (as expected with $u_{1e}=1$ and $u_1(r,z=z_L/2,t=48) > u_1(r,z=z_L/2,t=0)=0.5$) and the concentration profile for u_2 reflects the diffusion of the drug out of the PM (as expected with $u_{2e}=0$ and $u_2(r,z=z_L/2,t=48) < u_2(r,z=z_L/2,t=0)=1$).
- The initial flux at the surface, `ku2*(u2(r=r0,z=zL/2,t)-u2e) = 3.600e+002` is uncharacteristically large because of the large difference $u_2(r=r_0,z=z_L/2,t=0)-u_{2e}=1-0$. For $t>0$, this difference is much smaller. For example, at $t=48$ h, $u_2(r=r0,z=z_L/2,t=48)-u_{2e}=0.000-0$; that is, the drug surface concentration is close to the surrounding concentration (but the difference is not exactly zero which accounts for the flux 2.194×10^3).
- The surface flux could be numerically integrated over the entire surface in Fig. 7.1 to obtain the total rate at which the drug leaves the PM at a particular value of t.
- The total amount of the drug in the PM at t, $Q_{u_1}(t)$, can be calculated from volume integration in r and z, e.g., by Simpson's rule.

$$Q_{u_1}(t)=(2)2\pi\int_{z_L/2}^{z_L}\int_0^{r_0}u_2(z,r,t)r\mathrm{d}r\mathrm{d}z. \tag{7.11a}$$

  Note that the lower limit of the integration in z is $z_L/2$ and therefore the integral is multiplied by two. Then the total amount of the drug that has left the PM at t, $Q_e(t)$, is

$$Q_e(t)=(2)\pi r_0^2(z_L/2)u_{20}-Q_{u_1}(t). \tag{7.11b}$$

  The double integral of eq. (7.11a) could be evaluated numerically from the numerical solution $u_2(r,z,t)$.
- The total effort to compute the numerical solution is modest, with `ncall = 395`.

The 2D plot from `pde_1_main` is in Fig. 7.2.

The four plots reflect the preceding conclusions, that is, $u_1(r,z=z_L/2,t)$ increases with t from the initial value $u_1(r,z=z_L/2,t=0)=0.5$ and $u_2(r,z=z_L/2,t)$ decreases with t from the initial value $u_2(r,z=z_L/2,t=0)=1$

The 3D plot of $u_1(r,z=z_L/2,t)$ from `pde_1_main` is in Fig. 7.3.

Figure 7.3 indicates that the H_2O content in the PM increases with t, which could possibly lead to the PM dissolution over time.

The 3D plot of $u_2(r,z=z_L/2,t)$ from `pde_1_main` is in Fig. 7.4.

Figure 7.4 indicates that the drug content in the PM decreases with t (the drug is delivered to the surroundings such as the surrounding tissue).

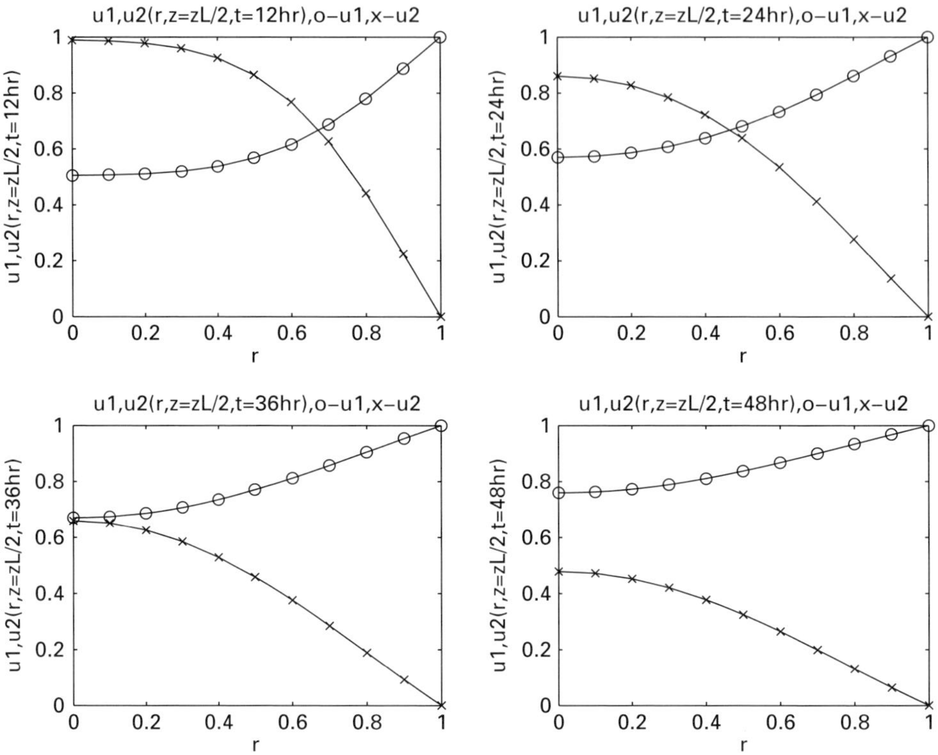

Figure 7.2 Composite plot of $u_1(r, z = z_L/2, t), u_2(r, z = z_L/2, t)$ for $t = 12, 24, 36, 48$ h

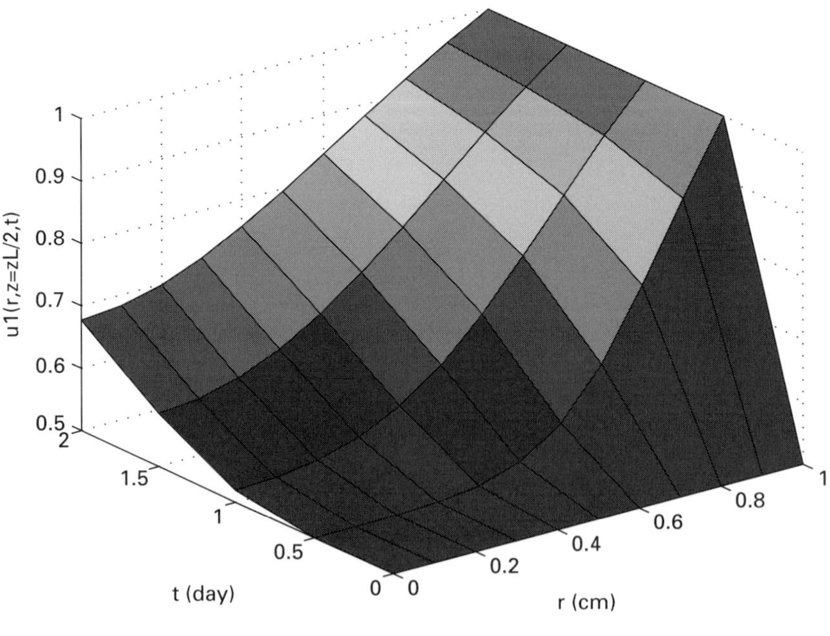

Figure 7.3 Plot of $u_1(r, z = z_L/2, t)$

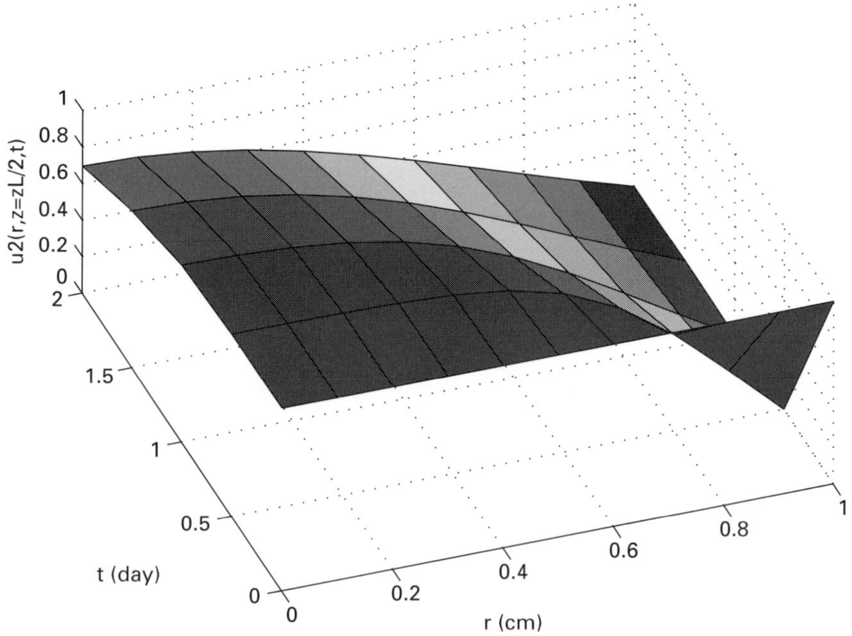

Figure 7.4 Plot of $u_2(r, z = z_L/2, t)$

7.1.4 ODE routine with FDs from library routines

Equations (7.2) to (7.7) were programmed in pde_1 of Listing 7.2 with the spatial derivatives in r and z approximated by FDs that were programmed explicitly. A second approach would be to calculate the spatial derivatives with library routines that are designed specifically for this purpose. This approach is illustrated by pde_2, listed next.

```
  function ut=pde_2(t,u)
%
% Global area
  global      nr      nz      dr      dz     drs     dzs...
               r      r0       z      zL     Du1     Du2...
              u1      u2     u1e     u2e     ku1     ku2...
           ncall
%
% 1D to 2D matrices
  for i=1:nz
  for j=1:nr
    ij=(i-1)*nr+j;
    u1(i,j)=u(ij);
    u2(i,j)=u(ij+nr*nz);
  end
  end
%
% Step through the grid points in r
  for i=1:nz
```

```
    u1_1d=u1(i,:);
    u2_1d=u2(i,:);
%
%   u1r, u2r
    u1r_1d=dss004(0,r0,nr,u1_1d);
    u1r(i,:)=u1r_1d;
    u1r(i,1)= 0.0;
    u1r(i,nr)=(ku1/Du1)*(u1e-u1(i,nr));
    u2r_1d=dss004(0,r0,nr,u2_1d);
    u2r(i,:)=u2r_1d;
    u2r(i,1)= 0;
    u2r(i,nr)=(ku2/Du2)*(u2e-u2(i,nr));
%
%   u1rr, u2rr
    u1r_1d( 1)=0;
    u1r_1d(nr)=(ku1/Du1)*(u1e-u1_1d(nr));
    nl=2; nu=2;
    u1rr_1d=dss044(0,r0,nr,u1_1d,u1r_1d,nl,nu);
    u1rr(i,:)=u1rr_1d;
    u2r_1d( 1)=0;
    u2r_1d(nr)=(ku2/Du2)*(u2e-u2_1d(nr));
    nl=2; nu=2;
    u2rr_1d=dss044(0,r0,nr,u2_1d,u2r_1d,nl,nu);
    u2rr(i,:)=u2rr_1d;
%
%   (1/r)*u1r, (1/r)*u2r
    for j=1:nr
      if(j~=1)
        u1r(i,j)=(1.0/r(j))*u1r(i,j);
        u2r(i,j)=(1.0/r(j))*u2r(i,j);
      elseif(j==1)
        u1rr(i,j)=2.0*u1rr(i,j);
        u2rr(i,j)=2.0*u2rr(i,j);
      end
%
%   Next j
    end
%
% Next i
  end
%
% Step through the grid points in z
  for j=1:nr
    u1_1d=u1(:,j);
    u2_1d=u2(:,j);
%
%   u1zz, u2zz
    u1z_1d( 1)=0.0;
    u1z_1d(nz)=(ku1/Du1)*(u1e-u1_1d(nz));
    nl=2; nu=2;
    u1zz_1d=dss044(zL/2,zL,nz,u1_1d,u1z_1d,nl,nu);
```

```
    u1zz(:,j)=u1zz_1d;
    u2z_1d( 1)=0.0;
    u2z_1d(nz)=(ku2/Du2)*(u2e-u2_1d(nz));
    nl=2; nu=2;
    u2zz_1d=dss044(zL/2,zL,nz,u2_1d,u2z_1d,nl,nu);
    u2zz(:,j)=u2zz_1d;
%
% Next j
  end
%
% PDEs
  for i=1:nz
  for j=1:nr
      u1t(i,j)=Du1*(u1rr(i,j)+u1r(i,j)+u1zz(i,j));
      u2t(i,j)=Du2*(u2rr(i,j)+u2r(i,j)+u2zz(i,j));
  end
  end
%
% 2D to 1D matrices
  for i=1:nz
  for j=1:nr
    ij=(i-1)*nr+j;
    ut(ij)=u1t(i,j);
    ut(ij+nr*nz)=u2t(i,j);
  end
  end
%
% Transpose and count
  ut=ut';
  ncall=ncall+1;
```

Listing 7.3 pde_2 with calculation of the spatial derivatives in eqs. (7.2) to (7.7) by library routines

We can note the following details about pde_2.

- The beginning of pde_2 is the same as pde_1 in Listing 7.2 and therefore is not discussed here (the routine definition, global area, and transfer to two 2D arrays, u_1, u_2).
- pde_2 is based on the use of the library routines dss004,dss044, which compute numerical derivatives of 1D arrays. Since u_1, u_2 are 2D arrays, a 2D to 1D mapping and the inverse are required in order to use the library routines and this is the essential difference between pde_1 and pde_2. We now consider the details of how dss004,dss044 are used.

```
%
% Step through the grid points in r
  for i=1:nz
    u1_1d=u1(i,:);
    u2_1d=u2(i,:);
```

The `for` steps along in z (with index `i`). At each z, the radial profiles in r are placed in 1D arrays, `u1_1d,u2_1d`. Note the use of `:` to transfer all of the values of u_1, u_2 with respect to r at a particular z.

- Now that 1D arrays are available, the differentiation routines can be used.

```
%
%   u1r, u2r
    u1r_1d=dss004(0,r0,nr,u1_1d);
    u1r(i,:)=u1r_1d;
    u1r(i,1)= 0.0;
    u1r(i,nr)=(ku1/Du1)*(u1e-u1(i,nr));
    u2r_1d=dss004(0,r0,nr,u2_1d);
    u2r(i,:)=u2r_1d;
    u2r(i,1)= 0;
    u2r(i,nr)=(ku2/Du2)*(u2e-u2(i,nr));
```

For the first derivatives in r, `dss004` is called to differentiate `u1_1d` to the derivative in r, `u1r_1d`. Note the use of `r` in the name of the derivative, `u1r_1d`, to denote a first derivative in `r`). Also, `1d` is used to indicate the derivative is a 1D array (a vector of length `nr`).

The 1D derivative is then placed in a 2D array, `u1r(i,:)=u1r_1d;`. The first derivative at $r = 0$ is reset by BC (7.4a), `u1r(i,1)=0.0;`, and the first derivative at $r = r_0$ is reset by BC (7.5a), `u1r(i,nr)=(ku1/Du1)*(u1e-u1(i,nr));`. The code is then repeated by u_2, including the use of BCs (7.4b) and (7.5b) to complete the first derivatives in r for u_1 and u_2.

- The second derivatives in r are then computed by `dss044`. Since BCs (7.4a) and (7.5a) are Neumann (the first derivative in r is specified), the flags for this type of BC used by `dss044` are set as `nl=2; nu=2;`. The first call to `dss044` computes the second derivative, `u1rr_1d`, directly from `u1_1d`, using the boundary first derivatives in `u1r_1d`. Note again the use of `r` and `rr` in the array names to denote first and second derivatives in r. Finally, the 1D second derivative is returned to a 2D array, `u1rr(i,:)=u1rr_1d;`.

```
%
%   u1rr, u2rr
    u1r_1d( 1)=0;
    u1r_1d(nr)=(ku1/Du1)*(u1e-u1_1d(nr));
    nl=2; nu=2;
    u1rr_1d=dss044(0,r0,nr,u1_1d,u1r_1d,nl,nu);
    u1rr(i,:)=u1rr_1d;
    u2r_1d( 1)=0;
    u2r_1d(nr)=(ku2/Du2)*(u2e-u2_1d(nr));
    nl=2; nu=2;
    u2rr_1d=dss044(0,r0,nr,u2_1d,u2r_1d,nl,nu);
    u2rr(i,:)=u2rr_1d;
```

The code is then repeated for u_2 to complete the second derivatives in r for u_1 and u_2.

- The radial groups in eqs. (7.2), $(1/r)(\partial u_1/\partial r)$ and $(1/r)(\partial u_2/\partial r)$, are computed from the previously computed first derivatives.

```
%
%    (1/r)*u1r, (1/r)*u2r
     for j=1:nr
       if(j~=1)
         u1r(i,j)=(1.0/r(j))*u1r(i,j);
         u2r(i,j)=(1.0/r(j))*u2r(i,j);
       elseif(j==1)
         u1rr(i,j)=2.0*u1rr(i,j);
         u2rr(i,j)=2.0*u2rr(i,j);
       end
%
%    Next j
     end
%
% Next i
  end
```

Note that for $r = 0$ (j==1), eqs. (7.8a) and (7.8e) are used for the indeterminate form. The final end statement terminates the loop through z with index i.

- All of the terms in r in eqs. (7.2) are now computed and the derivatives in z are computed next.

```
%
% Step through the grid points in z
  for j=1:nr
    u1_1d=u1(:,j);
    u2_1d=u2(:,j);
%
%   u1zz, u2zz
    u1z_1d( 1)=0.0;
    u1z_1d(nz)=(ku1/Du1)*(u1e-u1_1d(nz));
    nl=2; nu=2;
    u1zz_1d=dss044(zL/2,zL,nz,u1_1d,u1z_1d,nl,nu);
    u1zz(:,j)=u1zz_1d;
    u2z_1d( 1)=0.0;
    u2z_1d(nz)=(ku2/Du2)*(u2e-u2_1d(nz));
    nl=2; nu=2;
    u2zz_1d=dss044(zL/2,zL,nz,u2_1d,u2z_1d,nl,nu);
    u2zz(:,j)=u2zz_1d;
%
% Next j
  end
```

The for in j steps through successive values of r. At each r, the second derivative in z is computed by dss044 after application of (Neumann) BCs (7.6a) and (7.7a). The final result is the second derivative in a 2D array, u1zz(:,j) for u_1 and u2zz(:,j) for u_2.

- This completes all of the RHS terms in eqs. (7.2) so that PDEs can then be programmed (as in `pde_1`).

```
%
% PDEs
  for i=1:nz
  for j=1:nr
      u1t(i,j)=Du1*(u1rr(i,j)+u1r(i,j)+u1zz(i,j));
      u2t(i,j)=Du2*(u2rr(i,j)+u2r(i,j)+u2zz(i,j));
  end
  end
```

  Note again the use of `t` in the arrays `u1t(i,j)`, `u2t(i,j)` to denote a first derivative in t (LHS of eqs. (7.2)).
- Finally, the two 2D arrays are placed in a single 1D array (vector), `ut`, which is returned as a LHS argument of `pde_2` for use by `ode15s`, followed by the usual transpose required by `ode15s`.

The combination of `pde_1_main` of Listing 7.1 and `pde_2` of Listing 7.3 (`mf=2`) produces a solution that is essentially identical to the solution from `pde_1` (`mf=1`) in Table 7.1 and Figs. 7.2 to 7.4 and therefore the `pde_2` output is not discussed here. This agreement provides some assurance that the solutions are accurate. This also suggests that an error analysis could be performed to evaluate the numerical solution. For example, grid points could be added in r and z and the resulting solution compared with the previous solution with $nr = nz = 11$; this is termed h refinement since the grid spacing is often designated in the literature as h, i.e., the preceding Δr and Δz.

Also, the order of the FDs used to calculate the spatial derivatives in r and z could be varied and the resulting solutions compared with that of Table 7.1 and Figs. 7.2 to 7.4. For example, `dss006` and `dss046`, which have sixth order FDs could be used in place of `dss004` and `dss044`, which have fourth order FDs. The degree of agreement of the two solutions (fourth and sixth order FDs) would then give some indication of the accuracy of the solutions. This procedure of varying the order of the FD approximations is termed p refinement, since the order of the approximation is generally designated as p in the literature; for example, the FDs in `pde_1` are $O(\Delta r^2), O(\Delta z^2)$ so $p = 2$, while for `dss004` and `dss044`, $p = 4$.

This concludes the discussion of the MOL solution of eqs. (7.2) to (7.7). We now consider some extensions of these equations to illustrate how numerical methods can be used to investigate postulated physical and chemical phenomena. First we consider eqs. (7.2) with the diffusivities, D_{u1} and D_{u2}, expressed as explicit functions of t; this might represent, for example, some anticipated changes in the structure of the PM as the drug release takes place. We term this case the variable coefficient model since $D_{u1}(t)$ and $D_{u2}(t)$ are now coefficients in eqs. (7.2) varying with t (recall that eqs. (7.2) also have variable coefficients $1/r$, owing to the use of cylindrical coordinates).

7.2 Variable coefficient model

An extension to time-varying diffusivities requires a minor modification of pde_2 in Listing 7.3. The resulting ODE routine we designate as pde_3. It departs from pde_2 only where the diffusivities in eqs. (7.2) to (7.7), Du1,Du2 are replaced with variable diffusivities, Du1t,Du2t, programmed at the beginning of pde_3 as

```
%
% Variable diffusivities
  ts=24*60*60;
  Du1t=Du1*(1+t/ts);
  Du2t=Du2*(1+t/ts);
```

Note the use of t, which is an input RHS argument of pde_3.

Then, for example, eqs. (7.2) are programmed as

```
% PDEs
  for i=1:nz
  for j=1:nr
      ts=24*60*60;
      u1t(i,j)=Du1t*(u1rr(i,j)+u1r(i,j)+u1zz(i,j));
      u2t(i,j)=Du2t*(u2rr(i,j)+u2r(i,j)+u2zz(i,j));
  end
  end
```

Listing 7.4 Example of modification of pde_2 to include time-varying diffusivities, designated as pde_3

We can note the following details about pde_3.

- A time for scaling t, ts, is just the number of seconds in one day.

  ```
  ts=24*60*60;
  ```

- ts is then used to define a linear variation of the diffusivities with t, that is, Du1t=Du1*(1+t/ts),Du2t=Du2*(1+t/ts) (Du1t,Du2t replace Du1,Du2 throughout pde_3). For this case, the diffusivities have doubled when t=ts. This increase of the diffusivities might represent, for example, an increase in the porosity of the PM. This programming illustrates how virtually any variation with t could be considered and generally demonstrates how the numerical approach facilitates experimentation with time-varying diffusivities that would be difficult to achieve with an analytical approach.

As would be expected, an increase in the diffusivities leads to an increase in the rate of transfer of H_2 into the PM and an increase of the rate of transfer of the drug out of the PM. This is illustrated in Fig 7.5, which can be compared with the base case in Fig. 7.2.

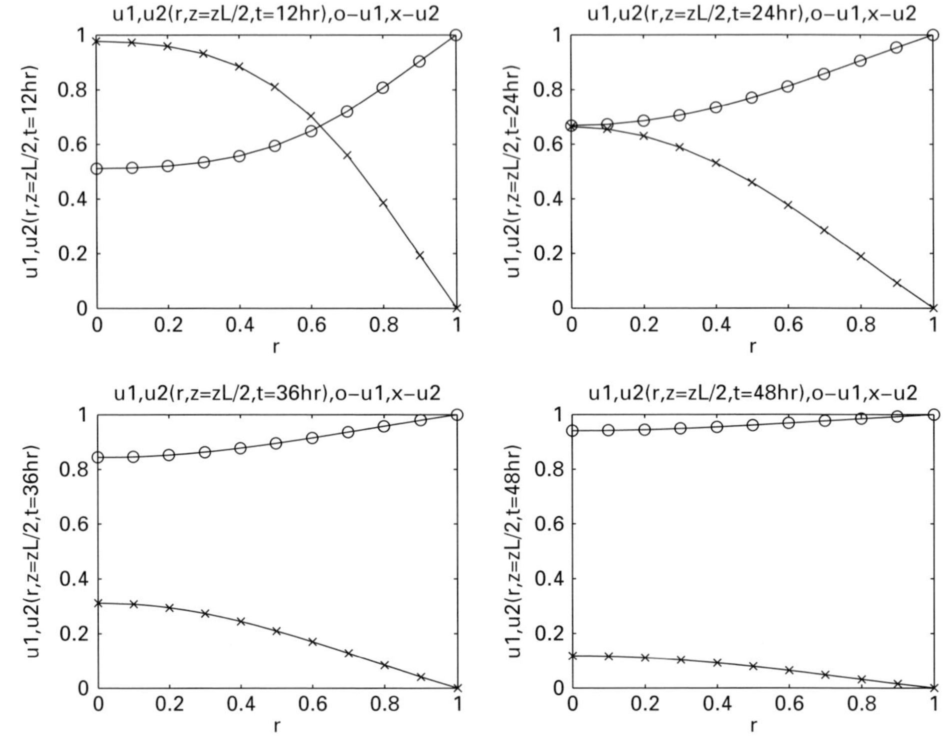

Figure 7.5 Composite plot of $u_1(r,z=z_L/2,t), u_2(r,z=z_L/2,t)$ for time-varying diffusivities

7.3 Nonlinear model

To conclude this discussion of the drug delivery system of Fig. 7.1, we now consider a nonlinear case for which the diffusivities are a function of u_1. Specifically, we consider an exponential variation of diffusivities, as reported by Aguzzi *et al.*, [1], eq. (18).

$$D_{u_1} = D_{u_{1\text{crit}}} e^{-\beta_{u_1}(1-u_1/u_{1\text{crit}})}; \; D_{u_2} = D_{u_{2\text{crit}}} e^{-\beta_{u_2}(1-u_1/u_{1\text{crit}})} \tag{7.12a,b}$$

where $u_{1\text{crit}}, u_{2\text{crit}}, \beta_{u_1}, D_{u_{1\text{crit}}}, D_{u_{2\text{crit}}}, \beta_{u_2}$ are constants typically determined by comparing the solution of the model equations with experimental data.

Since eqs. (7.12) specify exponential (nonlinear) functions of u_1, we have to consider a basic property of nonlinear models. The solution of the nonlinear model equations will be determined by the absolute values of the dependent variables, u_1, u_2. We can appreciate this point by noting that a change in the dependent variable u_1 in eqs. (12) does not give a proportional change in D_{u_1}, D_{u_2}. Rather, D_{u_1}, D_{u_2} are dependent on the absolute value of u_1.

This is in contrast with linear models, such as of eqs. (7.2) to (7.7), for which the absolute value of the dependent variables has no effect on the form of the solution. In other words, for constants c_1, c_2, the dependent variables $u_1 + c_1, u_2 + c_2$ will have the previous solution for u_1, u_2 merely shifted by c_1, c_2. Thus, for a linear model, the datum or reference for the dependent variables is inconsequential.

Therefore, we have to use absolute values of the dependent variables u_1, u_2 in eqs. (12). We will proceed in two steps.

Case 1 The constant diffusivity case of `pde_1` is used within a variable diffusivity format to test the coding in the ODE routine designated `pde_4`. In other words, `pde_4` should produce essentially the same numerical solution as `pde_1`, but it can then be applied also to the variable diffusivity case.

Case 2 `pde_4` is applied to a variable diffusivity case based on a set of constants selected for eqs. (7.12).

The details of these two cases require some explanation that follows. `pde_4` is listed next.

```
  function ut=pde_4(t,u)
%
% Global area
  global      nr      nz      dr      dz     drs     dzs...
               r      r0       z      zL     Du1     Du2...
              u1      u2     u1e     u2e     ku1     ku2...
           ncall
%
% 1D to 2D matrices
  for i=1:nz
  for j=1:nr
    ij=(i-1)*nr+j;
    u1(i,j)=u(ij);
    u2(i,j)=u(ij+nr*nz);
  end
  end
%
% Step through the grid points in r and z
  for i=1:nz
  for j=1:nr
%
%   First RHS term in r
%
%   Constant Du1, Du2
    Du1=Du1; Du2=Du2; dDu1=0; dDu2=0;
%
%   Variable Du1, Du2
%   u1crit=1; beta_u1=1; Du1crit=1.0e-06;
%             beta_u2=1; Du2crit=1.0e-06;
%   Du1=Du1crit*exp(-beta_u1*(1-u1(i,j)/u1crit));
%   Du2=Du2crit*exp(-beta_u2*(1-u1(i,j)/u1crit));
%   dDu1=Du1*(beta_u1/u1crit); dDu2=0;
    if(j==1)
      term1_1(i,j)=Du1*2*(u1(i,j+1)-u1(i,j))/drs;
      term1_2(i,j)=Du2*2*(u2(i,j+1)-u2(i,j))/drs;
    elseif(j==nr)
```

```
        u1f=u1(i,j-1)+2*dr*(ku1/Du1)*(u1e-u1(i,j));
        term1_1(i,j)=Du1*(u1f-2*u1(i,j)+u1(i,j-1))/drs;
        u2f=u2(i,j-1)+2*dr*(ku2/Du2)*(u2e-u2(i,j));
        term1_2(i,j)=Du2*(u2f-2*u2(i,j)+u2(i,j-1))/drs;
      else
        term1_1(i,j)=Du1*(u1(i,j+1)-2*u1(i,j)+u1(i,j-1))/drs;
        term1_2(i,j)=Du2*(u2(i,j+1)-2*u2(i,j)+u2(i,j-1))/drs;
      end
%
%     Second RHS term in r
      if(j==1)
        term2_1(i,j)=0;
        term2_2(i,j)=0;
      elseif(j==nr)
        u1f=u1(i,j-1)+2*dr*(ku1/Du1)*(u1e-u1(i,j));
        term2_1(i,j)=dDu1*((u1f-u1(i,j-1))/(2*dr))^2;
        u2f=u2(i,j-1)+2*dr*(ku2/Du2)*(u2e-u2(i,j));
        term2_2(i,j)=dDu2*((u2f-u2(i,j-1))/(2*dr))^2;
      else
        term2_1(i,j)=dDu1*((u1(i,j+1)-u1(i,j-1))/(2*dr))^2;
        term2_2(i,j)=dDu2*((u2(i,j+1)-u2(i,j-1))/(2*dr))^2;
      end
%
%     Third RHS term in r
      if(j==1)
        term3_1(i,j)=term1_1(i,j);
        term3_2(i,j)=term1_2(i,j);
      elseif(j==nr)
        u1f=u1(i,j-1)+2*dr*(ku1/Du1)*(u1e-u1(i,j));
        term3_1(i,j)=(Du1/r(j))*(u1f-u1(i,j-1))/(2*dr);
        u2f=u2(i,j-1)+2*dr*(ku2/Du2)*(u2e-u2(i,j));
        term3_2(i,j)=(Du2/r(j))*(u2f-u2(i,j-1))/(2*dr);
      else
        term3_1(i,j)=(Du1/r(j))*(u1(i,j+1)-u1(i,j-1))/(2*dr);
        term3_2(i,j)=(Du2/r(j))*(u2(i,j+1)-u2(i,j-1))/(2*dr);
      end
%
%     First RHS term in z
      if(i==1)
        term4_1(i,j)=Du1*2*(u1(i+1,j)-u1(i,j))/dzs;
        term4_2(i,j)=Du2*2*(u2(i+1,j)-u2(i,j))/dzs;
      elseif(i==nz)
        u1f=u1(i-1,j)+2*dz*(ku1/Du1)*(u1e-u1(i,j));
        term4_1(i,j)=Du1*(u1f-2*u1(i,j)+u1(i-1,j))/dzs;
        u2f=u2(i-1,j)+2*dz*(ku2/Du2)*(u2e-u2(i,j));
        term4_2(i,j)=Du2*(u2f-2*u2(i,j)+u2(i-1,j))/dzs;
      else
        term4_1(i,j)=Du1*(u1(i+1,j)-2*u1(i,j)+u1(i-1,j))/dzs;
        term4_2(i,j)=Du2*(u2(i+1,j)-2*u2(i,j)+u2(i-1,j))/dzs;
      end
%
```

```
%   Second RHS term in z
    if(i==1)
      term5_1(i,j)=0;
      term5_2(i,j)=0;
    elseif(i==nz)
      u1f=u1(i-1,j)+2*dz*(ku1/Du1)*(u1e-u1(i,j));
      term5_1(i,j)=dDu1*((u1f-u1(i-1,j))/(2*dz))^2;
      u2f=u2(i-1,j)+2*dz*(ku2/Du2)*(u2e-u2(i,j));
      term5_2(i,j)=dDu2*((u2f-u2(i-1,j))/(2*dz))^2;
    else
      term5_1(i,j)=dDu1*((u1(i+1,j)-u1(i-1,j))/(2*dz))^2;
      term5_2(i,j)=dDu2*((u2(i+1,j)-u2(i-1,j))/(2*dz))^2;
    end
%
% Next j
  end
%
% Next i
  end
%
%   PDEs
  for i=1:nz
  for j=1:nr
      u1t(i,j)=term1_1(i,j)+term2_1(i,j)+term3_1(i,j)...
              +term4_1(i,j)+term5_1(i,j);
      u2t(i,j)=term1_2(i,j)+term2_2(i,j)+term3_2(i,j)...
              +term4_2(i,j)+term5_2(i,j);
  end
  end
%
% 2D to 1D matrices
  for i=1:nz
  for j=1:nr
    ij=(i-1)*nr+j;
    ut(ij)=u1t(i,j);
    ut(ij+nr*nz)=u2t(i,j);
  end
  end
%
% Transpose and count
  ut=ut';
  ncall=ncall+1;
```

Listing 7.5 pde_4 for the nonlinear model

We can note the following details about pde_4.

- The beginning is the same as pde_1 in Listing (7.2) (routine definition, global area, transfer from 1D to 2D arrays, nested for loops to step through the $r-z$ domain), and therefore will not be discussed here to conserve space.

- The diffusivities in eqs. (7.1), D_{u_1} and D_{u_2}, are computed for one of the two cases, constant or variable diffusivities. Note that we use comments to activate one case and deactivate the other, to preserve all of the preceding code (in main program pde_1_main and the global areas).

```
%
%   First RHS term in r
%
%   Constant Du1, Du2
    Du1=Du1; Du2=Du2; dDu1=0; dDu2=0;
%
%   Variable Du1, Du2
%   u1crit=1; beta_u1=1; Du1crit=1.0e-06;
%             beta_u2=1; Du2crit=1.0e-06;
%   Du1=Du1crit*exp(-beta_u1*(1-u1(i,j)/u1crit));
%   Du2=Du2crit*exp(-beta_u2*(1-u1(i,j)/u1crit));
%   dDu1=Du1*(beta_u1/u1crit); dDu2=0;
```

For the case of constant diffusivities, the output from pde_4 should essentially duplicate the output from pde_1.

The associated mathematics for pde_4 requires some explanation before continuing with the discussion of the coding. The diffusion equation for the variable diffusivity case ([3], eq. (A.1.13), p 388) is

$$\frac{\partial u}{\partial t}=\frac{\partial\left(rD_{rr}\dfrac{\partial u}{\partial r}\right)}{r\partial r}+\frac{\partial\left(D_{\theta\theta}\dfrac{\partial u}{r\partial\theta}\right)}{r\partial\theta}+\frac{\partial\left(D_{zz}\dfrac{\partial u}{\partial z}\right)}{\partial z}. \tag{7.13a}$$

Note that the diffusivities $D_{rr}, D_{\theta\theta}, D_{zz}$ are inside derivatives and it is this generalization that is discussed next, including the computer code.

We again assume angular symmetry so that the term in θ in eq. (7.13a) is dropped. The group in r can be expanded (with application to u_1).

$$\begin{aligned}
\frac{1}{r}\frac{\partial\left(rD_{u1}\dfrac{\partial u_1}{\partial r}\right)}{\partial r}&=\frac{1}{r}\left[r\frac{\partial\left(D_{u1}\dfrac{\partial u_1}{\partial r}\right)}{\partial r}+\left(D_{u1}\frac{\partial u_1}{\partial r}\right)\frac{\partial r}{\partial r}\right]\\
&=\frac{\partial\left(D_{u1}\dfrac{\partial u_1}{\partial r}\right)}{\partial r}+\frac{1}{r}\left(D_{u1}\frac{\partial u_1}{\partial r}\right)\\
&=D_{u1}\frac{\partial^2 u_1}{\partial r^2}+\frac{\partial u_1}{\partial r}\frac{\partial D_{u1}}{\partial r}+\frac{D_{u1}}{r}\left(\frac{\partial u_1}{\partial r}\right)\\
&=D_{u1}\frac{\partial^2 u_1}{\partial r^2}+\frac{\partial u_1}{\partial r}\frac{dD_{u1}}{du_1}\frac{\partial u_1}{\partial r}+\frac{D_{u1}}{r}\left(\frac{\partial u_1}{\partial r}\right)\\
&=D_{u1}\frac{\partial^2 u_1}{\partial r^2}+\frac{dD_{u1}}{du_1}\left(\frac{\partial u_1}{\partial r}\right)^2+\frac{D_{u1}}{r}\left(\frac{\partial u_1}{\partial r}\right).
\end{aligned} \tag{7.13b}$$

The programming of the various RHS terms in eq. (7.13b) is now considered.

- The first RHS terms of eqs. (7.13b) are programmed as `term1_1, term1_2` for u_1, u_2, respectively:

$$\text{term1\_1} = D_{u1}\frac{\partial^2 u_1}{\partial r^2},$$

$$\text{term1\_2} = D_{u2}\frac{\partial^2 u_2}{\partial r^2}.$$

```
if(j==1)
  term1_1(i,j)=Du1*2*(u1(i,j+1)-u1(i,j))/drs;
  term1_2(i,j)=Du2*2*(u2(i,j+1)-u2(i,j))/drs;
elseif(j==nr)
  u1f=u1(i,j-1)+2*dr*(ku1/Du1)*(u1e-u1(i,j));
  term1_1(i,j)=Du1*(u1f-2*u1(i,j)+u1(i,j-1))/drs;
  u2f=u2(i,j-1)+2*dr*(ku2/Du2)*(u2e-u2(i,j));
  term1_2(i,j)=Du2*(u2f-2*u2(i,j)+u2(i,j-1))/drs;
else
  term1_1(i,j)=Du1*(u1(i,j+1)-2*u1(i,j)+u1(i,j-1))/drs;
  term1_2(i,j)=Du2*(u2(i,j+1)-2*u2(i,j)+u2(i,j-1))/drs;
end
```

The three parts of this code follow in essentially the same way as discussed previously.

  - `j==1`: eq. (7.9b) and the code that follows,
  - `j==nr`: eq. (7.9d) and the code that follows,
  - Interior points: eq. (7.9f) and the code that follows.

- The second RHS terms of eqs. (7.13b) are programmed as `term2_1, term2_2` for u_1, u_2, respectively:

$$\text{term2\_1} = \frac{dD_{u1}}{du_1}\left(\frac{\partial u_1}{\partial r}\right)^2,$$

$$\text{term2\_2} = \frac{dD_{u2}}{du_2}\left(\frac{\partial u_2}{\partial r}\right)^2.$$

```
%
%   Second RHS term in r
    if(j==1)
      term2_1(i,j)=0;
      term2_2(i,j)=0;
    elseif(j==nr)
      u1f=u1(i,j-1)+2*dr*(ku1/Du1)*(u1e-u1(i,j));
      term2_1(i,j)=dDu1*((u1f-u1(i,j-1))/(2*dr))^2;
      u2f=u2(i,j-1)+2*dr*(ku2/Du2)*(u2e-u2(i,j));
      term2_2(i,j)=dDu2*((u2f-u2(i,j-1))/(2*dr))^2;
    else
      term2_1(i,j)=dDu1*((u1(i,j+1)-u1(i,j-1))/(2*dr))^2;
      term2_2(i,j)=dDu2*((u2(i,j+1)-u2(i,j-1))/(2*dr))^2;
    end
```

The three parts of this code are briefly explained next.

- j==1: $(\partial u_1/\partial r)$ (and $(\partial u_2/\partial r)$) are zero from BCs (7.4) (at $r = 0$).
- j==nr: the fictitious value u1f is given by eq. (7.9d).

```
u1f=u1(i,j-1)+2*dr*(ku1/Du1)*(u1e-u1(i,j));
```

Then the programming of the second term (at $r = r_0$) is straightforward.

```
term2_1(i,j)=dDu1*((u1f-u1(i,j-1))/(2*dr))^2;
```

The programming for u_2 follows in the same way.

```
u2f=u2(i,j-1)+2*dr*(ku2/Du2)*(u2e-u2(i,j));
term2_2(i,j)=dDu2*((u2f-u2(i,j-1))/(2*dr))^2;
```

- Interior points: the programming of the first derivatives u_1, u_2 from eq. (7.8f) (applied to u_1 and u_2) is used in the second term.

```
else
  term2_1(i,j)=dDu1*((u1(i,j+1)-u1(i,j-1))/(2*dr))^2;
  term2_2(i,j)=dDu2*((u2(i,j+1)-u2(i,j-1))/(2*dr))^2;
end
```

Note that in this programming, the derivatives of the diffusivities in eqs. (7.12) are used, that is, $(\mathrm{d}D_{u_1}/\mathrm{d}u_1)$ = dDu1,$(\mathrm{d}D_{u_2}/\mathrm{d}u_2)$ = dDu2. These derivatives were programmed previously as

```
%
%   First RHS term in r
%
%   Constant Du1, Du2
    Du1=Du1; Du2=Du2; dDu1=0; dDu2=0;
%
%   Variable Du1, Du2
%   u1crit=1; beta_u1=1; Du1crit=1.0e-06;
%             beta_u2=1; Du2crit=1.0e-06;
%   Du1=Du1crit*exp(-beta_u1*(1-u1(i,j)/u1crit));
%   Du2=Du2crit*exp(-beta_u2*(1-u1(i,j)/u1crit));
%   dDu1=Du1*(beta_u1/u1crit); dDu2=0;
```

For the constant diffusivity case, these derivatives are zero.

- The third RHS terms of eqs. (7.13b) are programmed as term3_1, term3_2 for u_1, u_2, respectively:

$$\text{term3\_1} = \frac{D_{u1}}{r}\left(\frac{\partial u_1}{\partial r}\right),$$

$$\text{term3\_2} = \frac{D_{u2}}{r}\left(\frac{\partial u_2}{\partial r}\right).$$

```
%
%   Third RHS term in r
    if(j==1)
      term3_1(i,j)=term1_1(i,j);
      term3_2(i,j)=term1_2(i,j);
    elseif(j==nr)
      u1f=u1(i,j-1)+2*dr*(ku1/Du1)*(u1e-u1(i,j));
```

```
    term3_1(i,j)=(Du1/r(j))*(u1f-u1(i,j-1))/(2*dr);
    u2f=u2(i,j-1)+2*dr*(ku2/Du2)*(u2e-u2(i,j));
    term3_2(i,j)=(Du2/r(j))*(u2f-u2(i,j-1))/(2*dr);
  else
    term3_1(i,j)=(Du1/r(j))*(u1(i,j+1)-u1(i,j-1))/(2*dr);
    term3_2(i,j)=(Du2/r(j))*(u2(i,j+1)-u2(i,j-1))/(2*dr);
  end
```

The three parts of this code are briefly explained next.

- `j==1`: $(\partial u_1/\partial r)$ and $(\partial u_2/\partial r)$ are zero from BCs (7.4) (at $r = 0$); the previous `term1_1`, `term1_2` values (from evaluation of the indeterminate values) are used to save some computation.
- `j==nr`: the fictitious value `u1f` is given by eq. (7.9d).

```
u1f=u1(i,j-1)+2*dr*(ku1/Du1)*(u1e-u1(i,j));
```

  Then the programming of the third term (at $r = r_0$) is straightforward.

```
term3_1(i,j)=(Du1/r(j))*(u1f-u1(i,j-1))/(2*dr);
```

  The programming for u_2 follows in the same way.

```
u2f=u2(i,j-1)+2*dr*(ku2/Du2)*(u2e-u2(i,j));
term3_2(i,j)=(Du2/r(j))*(u2f-u2(i,j-1))/(2*dr);
```

- Interior points: the programming of the first derivatives of u_1, u_2 from eqs. (7.8f,g) is used in the second term.

```
else
  term3_1(i,j)=(Du1/r(j))*(u1(i,j+1)-u1(i,j-1))/(2*dr);
  term3_2(i,j)=(Du2/r(j))*(u2(i,j+1)-u2(i,j-1))/(2*dr);
end
```

This completes the programming of the three terms in r of eq. (7.13b). We now consider the derivative in z of eq. (7.13a) (applied to u_1).

$$\frac{\partial\left(D_{u_1}\dfrac{\partial u_1}{\partial z}\right)}{\partial z} = D_{u_1}\frac{\partial^2 u_1}{\partial z^2} + \frac{\mathrm{d}D_{u_1}}{\mathrm{d}u_1}\left(\frac{\partial u_1}{\partial z}\right)^2. \tag{7.13c}$$

Here we assume that the diffusivity is the same with respect to r and z, $D_{rr} = D_{zz} = D_{u_1}$, that is, an isotropic system.

The coding of eq. (7.13c) follows in the same way as for r.

- The first RHS terms of eqs. (7.13c) are programmed as `term4_1,term4_2` to distinguish from the programming in r:

$$\text{term4\_1} = D_{u1}\frac{\partial^2 u_1}{\partial z^2},$$

$$\text{term4\_2} = D_{u2}\frac{\partial^2 u_2}{\partial z^2}.$$

```
%
%    First RHS term in z
     if(i==1)
       term4_1(i,j)=Du1*2*(u1(i+1,j)-u1(i,j))/dzs;
       term4_2(i,j)=Du2*2*(u2(i+1,j)-u2(i,j))/dzs;
     elseif(i==nz)
       u1f=u1(i-1,j)+2*dz*(ku1/Du1)*(u1e-u1(i,j));
       term4_1(i,j)=Du1*(u1f-2*u1(i,j)+u1(i-1,j))/dzs;
       u2f=u2(i-1,j)+2*dz*(ku2/Du2)*(u2e-u2(i,j));
       term4_2(i,j)=Du2*(u2f-2*u2(i,j)+u2(i-1,j))/dzs;
     else
       term4_1(i,j)=Du1*(u1(i+1,j)-2*u1(i,j)+u1(i-1,j))/dzs;
       term4_2(i,j)=Du2*(u2(i+1,j)-2*u2(i,j)+u2(i-1,j))/dzs;
     end
```

The three parts of this code follow in essentially the same way as discussed previously for r.

- i==1 corresponds to $z = z_L/2$, where BCs (7.6a,b) apply, so the second derivative in eq. (7.13c) is approximated as

$$\frac{\partial^2 u_1}{\partial z^2} \approx= \frac{u_1(i=2) - 2u_1(i=1) + u_1(i=0)}{\Delta z^2}.$$

$u_1(i=0)$ is a fictitious value (to the left of $z = z_L/2$); it is given by the approximation of BC (7.10b)

$$\frac{\partial u_1(z=0,t)}{\partial z} \approx \frac{u_1(i=2) - u_1(i=0)}{2\Delta z} = 0,$$

or

$$u_1(i=0) = u_1(i=2).$$

Thus,

$$\frac{\partial^2 u_1}{\partial z^2} \approx= 2\frac{u_1(i=2) - u_1(i=1)}{\Delta z^2},$$

which is programmed (for u_1 and u_2) as in eq. (7.10c)

```
%
%    First RHS term in z
     if(i==1)
       term4_1(i,j)=Du1*2*(u1(i+1,j)-u1(i,j))/dzs;
       term4_2(i,j)=Du2*2*(u2(i+1,j)-u2(i,j))/dzs;
```

- i==nz corresponds to $z = z_L$, where BCs (7.7) apply. The FD of these BCs requires the use of a fictitious point. For example, BC (7.7a) is approximated as

$$D_{u1}\frac{\partial u_1}{\partial z} \approx D_{u1}\frac{u_{1f} - u_1(i=nz-1)}{2\Delta z} = k_1(u_{1e} - u_1(i=nz)),$$

where u_{1f} is a fictitious value (to the right of $z = z_L$). Solving for u_{1f}, we have

$$u_{1f} = u_1(i=nz-1) + 2\Delta z(k_1/D_{u1})(u_{1e} - u_1(i=nz)),$$

which is expressed as the first line of code in `i==nz`.

```
u1f=u1(i-1,j)+2*dz*(ku1/Du1)*(u1e-u1(i,j));
```

Then

$$\text{term4\_1} = D_{u1}\frac{\partial^2 u_1}{\partial z^2} \approx \frac{u(i=nz+1) - 2u(i=nz) + u(i=nz-1)}{\Delta z^2}$$

is approximated as the line

```
term4_1(i,j)=Du1*(u1f-2*u1(i,j)+u1(i-1,j))/dzs;
```

Note the use of the fictitious value `u1f` in the approximation of the second derivative $(\partial^2 u_1/\partial z^2)$.

The programming for u_2 follows in the same way.

```
u2f=u2(i-1,j)+2*dz*(ku2/Du2)*(u2e-u2(i,j));
term4_2(i,j)=Du2*(u2f-2*u2(i,j)+u2(i-1,j))/dzs;
```

- For the interior points in z, the second derivative, $(\partial^2 u_1/\partial z^2)$, is approximated as a three point centered FD

$$\frac{\partial^2 u_1}{\partial z^2} \approx \frac{u(i+1) - 2u(i) + u(i-1)}{\Delta z^2},$$

programmed (for u_1 and u_2) as

```
else
  term4_1(i,j)=Du1*(u1(i+1,j)-2*u1(i,j)+u1(i-1,j))/dzs;
  term4_2(i,j)=Du2*(u2(i+1,j)-2*u2(i,j)+u2(i-1,j))/dzs;
end
```

- The second RHS terms of eqs. (7.13c) are programmed as `term5_1,term5_2` to distinguish from the programming in r.

$$\text{term5\_1} = \frac{\mathrm{d}D_{u1}}{\mathrm{d}u_1}\left(\frac{\partial u_1}{\partial z}\right)^2,$$

$$\text{term5\_2} = \frac{\mathrm{d}D_{u2}}{\mathrm{d}u_2}\left(\frac{\partial u_2}{\partial z}\right)^2.$$

```
%
%   Second RHS term in z
    if(i==1)
      term5_1(i,j)=0;
      term5_2(i,j)=0;
    elseif(i==nz)
      u1f=u1(i-1,j)+2*dz*(ku1/Du1)*(u1e-u1(i,j));
      term5_1(i,j)=dDu1*((u1f-u1(i-1,j))/(2*dz))^2;
      u2f=u2(i-1,j)+2*dz*(ku2/Du2)*(u2e-u2(i,j));
      term5_2(i,j)=dDu2*((u2f-u2(i-1,j))/(2*dz))^2;
    else
      term5_1(i,j)=dDu1*((u1(i+1,j)-u1(i-1,j))/(2*dz))^2;
```

```
        term5_2(i,j)=dDu2*((u2(i+1,j)-u2(i-1,j))/(2*dz))^2;
      end
%
% Next j
    end
%
% Next i
    end
```

A brief explanation of each of the three sections in the `if` follows.

- `i==1` corresponds to $z = z_L/2$, where BCs (7.6a,b) apply, so the terms are zero.

```
if(i==1)
  term5_1(i,j)=0;
  term5_2(i,j)=0;
```

- `i==nz` corresponds to $z = z_L$ where BCs (7.7) apply. The FD of these BCs requires the use of a fictitious point. For example, BC (7.7a) is approximated as

$$D_{u1}\frac{\partial u_1}{\partial z} \approx D_{u1}\frac{u_{1f} - u_1(i = nz - 1)}{2\Delta z} = k_1(u_{1e} - u_1(i = nz)),$$

where u_{1f} is a fictitious value (to the right of $z = z_L$). Solving for u_{1f}, we have

$$u_{1f} = u_1(i = nz - 1) + 2\Delta z(k_1/D_{u1})(u_{1e} - u_1(i = nz)),$$

which is expressed as the first line of code in `i==nz`.

```
elseif(i==nz)
  u1f=u1(i-1,j)+2*dz*(ku1/Du1)*(u1e-u1(i,j));
```

Then

$$\text{term5\_1} = \frac{\mathrm{d}D_{u1}}{\mathrm{d}u_1}\left(\frac{\partial u_1}{\partial z}\right)^2$$

is programmed as

```
  term5_1(i,j)=dDu1*((u1f-u1(i-1,j))/(2*dz))^2;
```

Note the use of `dDu1` for $(\mathrm{d}D_{u1}/\mathrm{d}u_1)$ and the fictitious value `u1f` in the approximation of the first derivative $(\partial u_1/\partial z)$.

The programming for u_2 is

```
  u2f=u2(i-1,j)+2*dz*(ku2/Du2)*(u2e-u2(i,j));
  term5_2(i,j)=dDu2*((u2f-u2(i-1,j))/(2*dz))^2;
```

- For the interior points in z, the first $(\partial u_1/\partial z)$ derivative is approximated as a two point centered FD,

$$\frac{\partial u_1}{\partial z} \approx \frac{u_1(i+1) - u_1(i-1)}{2\Delta z}.$$

Then

$$\text{term5\_1} = \frac{\mathrm{d}D_{u1}}{\mathrm{d}u_1}\left(\frac{\partial u_1}{\partial z}\right)^2.$$

The programming for u_1 and u_2 is

```
else
  term5_1(i,j)=dDu1*((u1(i+1,j)-u1(i-1,j))/(2*dz))^2;
  term5_2(i,j)=dDu2*((u2(i+1,j)-u2(i-1,j))/(2*dz))^2;
end
```

– The end statements complete the for loops in j and i for r and z, respectively.

```
%
% Next j
  end
%
% Next i
  end
```

– We note in the programming of the term4 and term5 terms that the second subscript j does not change. This again reflects a basic feature of the partial derivatives in z, that is, r is constant. In other words, the programming of the five terms proceeds in two steps: the derivatives in r with j changing and i constant, followed by the derivatives in z with i changing and j constant. Both cases are handled within the pair of nested for loops in i and j.

- The programming of all of the RHS terms in the PDEs for u_1 and u_2 over $0 \le r \le r_0$, $z_L/2 \le z \le z_L$ is now complete. The LHS derivatives in t, $(\partial u_1/\partial t)$ and $(\partial u_2/\partial t)$ are just the sum of the five terms.

```
%
%   PDEs
  for i=1:nz
  for j=1:nr
      u1t(i,j)=term1_1(i,j)+term2_1(i,j)+term3_1(i,j)...
              +term4_1(i,j)+term5_1(i,j);
      u2t(i,j)=term1_2(i,j)+term2_2(i,j)+term3_2(i,j)...
              +term4_2(i,j)+term5_2(i,j);
  end
  end
```

- The two 2D matrices u1t(i,j) and u2t(i,j) are placed in a single 1D vector, ut.

```
%
% 2D to 1D matrices
  for i=1:nz
  for j=1:nr
    ij=(i-1)*nr+j;
    ut(ij)=u1t(i,j);
    ut(ij+nr*nz)=u2t(i,j);
  end
  end
```

- pde_4 of Listing 7.5 ends with the transpose of ut required by ODE15s and incrementing of the number of calls to pde_4.

```
%
% Transpose and count
  ut=ut';
  ncall=ncall+1;
```

We now consider the output from pde_1_main of Listing 7.1 and pde_4 of Listing 7.5, first for the case of constant diffusivities programmed in pde_4.

```
%
%   Constant Du1, Du2
    Du1=Du1; Du2=Du2; dDu1=0; dDu2=0;
```

Abbreviated output in the form of Table 7.2 follows (with mf=4 in pde_1_main so that ode15s calls pde_4).

The output from pde_4 (Table 7.3) is identical to the output from pde_1 (Table 7.1). Thus, the graphical output from pde_4 will not be included here, since it is identical to Figs. 7.2 to 7.4.

We can now consider the output from pde_4 for the case of variable diffusivities. To develop the details of this case, we will first decide on the use of u_1 and u_2 over the previous intervals to facilitate a comparison with the constant diffusivity case,

$$0 \le u_1, u_2 \le 1.$$

Then, considering eq. (7.12a) with $u_{1\text{crit}} = 1, \beta_{u_1} = 1$,

- $u_1 = 0$

$$D_{u_1} = D_{u_{1\text{crit}}} \mathrm{e}^{-\beta_{u_1}(1-u_1/u_{1\text{crit}})} = D_{u_{1\text{crit}}} \mathrm{e}^{-1(1-0/1)} = D_{u_{1\text{crit}}}/\mathrm{e}. \tag{7.14a}$$

- $u_1 = 1$

$$D_{u_1} = D_{u_{1\text{crit}}} \mathrm{e}^{-\beta_{u_1}(1-u_1/u_{1\text{crit}})} = D_{u_{1\text{crit}}} \mathrm{e}^{-1(1-1/1)} = D_{u_{1\text{crit}}}. \tag{7.14b}$$

Thus, for $0 \le u_1 \le 1$, the variation in D_{u_1} with u_1 is $D_{u_{1\text{crit}}}/\mathrm{e} \le D_{u_1} \le D_{u_{1\text{crit}}}$. A similar conclusion follows for D_{u_2} (from eq. (7.12b)). Thus, for $\beta_{u_1} > 0$ and $\beta_{u_2} > 0$, the diffusivities D_{u_1}, D_{u_2} increase with increasing u_1. Physically, this might be interpreted that with increasing u_1 the H_2O and drug have a larger path for diffusion. Recall again that u_1 is the concentration of H_2O per unit volume of the total content in Fig. 7.1, that is, H_2O + drug + PM; typical units might be g/cm^3 or gmol/cm^3, where cm^3 is a volume of the total content (H_2O + drug + PM). Thus, an increase in u_1 corresponds to an increase in the amount of H_2O relative to the PM.

We can consider other cases. For example, if $\beta_{u_1} = \beta_{u_2} = 0$, there is no variation in D_{u_1} and D_{u_2} (the preceding constant diffusivity case). For $\beta_{u_1} = 5$, $D_{u_{1\text{crit}}}/\mathrm{e}^5 \le D_{u_1} \le D_{u_{1\text{crit}}}$, which is a substantially larger variation than for $\beta_{u_1} = 1$. Also, for $\beta_{u_1} < 0$ and $\beta_{u_2} < 0$, the diffusivities decrease with increasing u_1. We can then use pde_4 to study the nonlinear

Table 7.3. Abbreviated output from `pde_1_main` and `pde_4`

```
  nr = 11    nz = 11

 t =   0.0    z = 0.1
 r = 0.00    u1(r,z,t) =  0.500   u2(r,z,t) =  1.000
 r = 0.10    u1(r,z,t) =  0.500   u2(r,z,t) =  1.000
 r = 0.20    u1(r,z,t) =  0.500   u2(r,z,t) =  1.000
 r = 0.30    u1(r,z,t) =  0.500   u2(r,z,t) =  1.000
 r = 0.40    u1(r,z,t) =  0.500   u2(r,z,t) =  1.000
 r = 0.50    u1(r,z,t) =  0.500   u2(r,z,t) =  1.000
 r = 0.60    u1(r,z,t) =  0.500   u2(r,z,t) =  1.000
 r = 0.70    u1(r,z,t) =  0.500   u2(r,z,t) =  1.000
 r = 0.80    u1(r,z,t) =  0.500   u2(r,z,t) =  1.000
 r = 0.90    u1(r,z,t) =  0.500   u2(r,z,t) =  1.000
 r = 1.00    u1(r,z,t) =  0.500   u2(r,z,t) =  1.000

 ku2*(u2(r=r0,z=zL/2,t)-u2e) = 3.600e+002

          .                   .
          .                   .
          .                   .
     Output for t = 12, 24, 36 removed
          .                   .
          .                   .
          .                   .

 t = 48.0    z = 0.1
 r = 0.00    u1(r,z,t) =  0.761   u2(r,z,t) =  0.479
 r = 0.10    u1(r,z,t) =  0.764   u2(r,z,t) =  0.472
 r = 0.20    u1(r,z,t) =  0.774   u2(r,z,t) =  0.453
 r = 0.30    u1(r,z,t) =  0.790   u2(r,z,t) =  0.421
 r = 0.40    u1(r,z,t) =  0.811   u2(r,z,t) =  0.378
 r = 0.50    u1(r,z,t) =  0.838   u2(r,z,t) =  0.325
 r = 0.60    u1(r,z,t) =  0.868   u2(r,z,t) =  0.265
 r = 0.70    u1(r,z,t) =  0.900   u2(r,z,t) =  0.199
 r = 0.80    u1(r,z,t) =  0.934   u2(r,z,t) =  0.131
 r = 0.90    u1(r,z,t) =  0.968   u2(r,z,t) =  0.064
 r = 1.00    u1(r,z,t) =  1.000   u2(r,z,t) =  0.000

 ku2*(u2(r=r0,z=zL/2,t)-u2e) = 2.194e-003

 ncall =   395
```

effects due to changes in D_{u_1} and D_{u_2} from variations in u_1. Ultimately, which form of variation is selected (from eqs. (7.12) or other proposed functions) will be determined by experimental observations and perhaps theory pertaining to diffusion in a PM. For eqs. (7.12), experimental data will also determine the values of $u_{1\text{crit}}$, $D_{u_{1\text{crit}}}$, β_{u_1}, $D_{u_{2\text{crit}}}$, and β_{u_2}.

For the particular choice of the exponential function in eqs. (7.12a,b), we also have the following derivatives.

$$\frac{dD_{u_1}}{du_1} = D_{u_{1\text{crit}}} e^{-\beta_{u_1}(1-u_1/u_{1\text{crit}})} (\beta_{u_1}/u_{1\text{crit}}), \tag{7.15a}$$

$$\frac{dD_{u_2}}{du_2} = 0. \tag{7.15b}$$

Equation (7.15b) follows from eq. (7.12b), that is, D_{u_2} is a function of only u_1, and not u_2, (which provides nonlinear coupling between the PDEs when eq. (7.13a) is applied to u_1 and u_2). Physically, D_{u_2} not being a function of u_2 might be explained by a generally low concentration of the drug so that its rate of diffusion (through D_{u_2}) is not influenced by its concentration.

Equations (7.12) and (7.15) are programmed in pde_4 of Listing 7.5 with the second set of statements for variable diffusivities activated (uncommented).

```
%
%    First RHS term in r
%
%    Constant Du1, Du2
%    Du1=Du1; Du2=Du2; dDu1=0; dDu2=0;
%
%    Variable Du1, Du2
     u1crit=1; beta_u1=1; Du1crit=1.0e-06;
               beta_u2=1; Du2crit=1.0e-06;
     Du1=Du1crit*exp(-beta_u1*(1-u1(i,j)/u1crit));
     Du2=Du2crit*exp(-beta_u2*(1-u1(i,j)/u1crit));
     dDu1=Du1*(beta_u1/u1crit); dDu2=0;
```

All of the other coding in pde_1_main and pde_4 is unchanged.

Abbreviated output in the form of Table 7.4 follows (again, with mf=4 in pde_1_main so that ode15s calls pde_4 and the code in pde_4 for variable diffusivities is activated).

We can observe the following details about this output.

- The output in Table 7.4 is significantly different from that in Table 7.1 (or Table 7.2) for constant diffusivities. A comparison at $t = 48$ follows.

We can note the following details about the output in Table 7.5.

- Less H_2O has diffused into the PM for the variable diffusivity case because of the lower diffusivity D_{u_1}, e.g., compare

```
r = 0.00   u1(r,z,t) =  0.761   u2(r,z,t) =  0.479
r = 0.00   u1(r,z,t) =  0.677   u2(r,z,t) =  0.697
```

  and 0.677 < 0.761.
- Less drug has left the PM for the variable diffusivity case because of the lower diffusivity D_{u_2}, e.g., 0.697 > 0.479.

Table 7.4. Abbreviated output from `pde_1_main` and `pde_4`, variable diffusivities

```
 nr = 11    nz = 11

t =   0.0   z = 1.0
r = 0.00   u1(r,z,t) =  0.500   u2(r,z,t) =  1.000
r = 0.10   u1(r,z,t) =  0.500   u2(r,z,t) =  1.000
r = 0.20   u1(r,z,t) =  0.500   u2(r,z,t) =  1.000
r = 0.30   u1(r,z,t) =  0.500   u2(r,z,t) =  1.000
r = 0.40   u1(r,z,t) =  0.500   u2(r,z,t) =  1.000
r = 0.50   u1(r,z,t) =  0.500   u2(r,z,t) =  1.000
r = 0.60   u1(r,z,t) =  0.500   u2(r,z,t) =  1.000
r = 0.70   u1(r,z,t) =  0.500   u2(r,z,t) =  1.000
r = 0.80   u1(r,z,t) =  0.500   u2(r,z,t) =  1.000
r = 0.90   u1(r,z,t) =  0.500   u2(r,z,t) =  1.000
r = 1.00   u1(r,z,t) =  0.500   u2(r,z,t) =  1.000

ku2*(u2(r=r0,z=zL/2,t)-u2e) = 3.600e+002

          .                   .
          .                   .
          .                   .
    Output for t = 12, 24, 36 removed
          .                   .
          .                   .
          .                   .

t = 48.0   z = 1.0
r = 0.00   u1(r,z,t) =  0.677   u2(r,z,t) =  0.697
r = 0.10   u1(r,z,t) =  0.683   u2(r,z,t) =  0.687
r = 0.20   u1(r,z,t) =  0.698   u2(r,z,t) =  0.657
r = 0.30   u1(r,z,t) =  0.724   u2(r,z,t) =  0.609
r = 0.40   u1(r,z,t) =  0.757   u2(r,z,t) =  0.545
r = 0.50   u1(r,z,t) =  0.796   u2(r,z,t) =  0.466
r = 0.60   u1(r,z,t) =  0.838   u2(r,z,t) =  0.377
r = 0.70   u1(r,z,t) =  0.882   u2(r,z,t) =  0.282
r = 0.80   u1(r,z,t) =  0.924   u2(r,z,t) =  0.185
r = 0.90   u1(r,z,t) =  0.964   u2(r,z,t) =  0.089
r = 1.00   u1(r,z,t) =  1.000   u2(r,z,t) =  0.000

ku2*(u2(r=r0,z=zL/2,t)-u2e) = 3.067e-003

ncall =  1804
```

- The flux of the drug is higher at the surface $r = r_0$ for the variable diffusivity case because the gradient is larger. This is not obvious from Table 7.5, but can be observed by comparing the solution in Fig. 7.6 for the variable diffusivity case with Fig. 7.2 for the constant diffusivity case (the lower right corner plots are for $t = 48$).

Table 7.5. A comparison of the numerical solutions for $t = 48$ for constant and variable diffusivities

```
From Table 7.1 for constant diffusivities

t = 48.0   z = 0.1
r = 0.00   u1(r,z,t) =  0.761   u2(r,z,t) =  0.479
r = 0.10   u1(r,z,t) =  0.764   u2(r,z,t) =  0.472
r = 0.20   u1(r,z,t) =  0.774   u2(r,z,t) =  0.453
r = 0.30   u1(r,z,t) =  0.790   u2(r,z,t) =  0.421
r = 0.40   u1(r,z,t) =  0.811   u2(r,z,t) =  0.378
r = 0.50   u1(r,z,t) =  0.838   u2(r,z,t) =  0.325
r = 0.60   u1(r,z,t) =  0.868   u2(r,z,t) =  0.265
r = 0.70   u1(r,z,t) =  0.900   u2(r,z,t) =  0.199
r = 0.80   u1(r,z,t) =  0.934   u2(r,z,t) =  0.131
r = 0.90   u1(r,z,t) =  0.968   u2(r,z,t) =  0.064
r = 1.00   u1(r,z,t) =  1.000   u2(r,z,t) =  0.000

ku2*(u2(r=r0,z=zL/2,t)-u2e) = 2.194e-003

ncall =   395

From Table 7.4 for variable diffusivities

t = 48.0   z = 0.1
r = 0.00   u1(r,z,t) =  0.677   u2(r,z,t) =  0.697
r = 0.10   u1(r,z,t) =  0.683   u2(r,z,t) =  0.687
r = 0.20   u1(r,z,t) =  0.698   u2(r,z,t) =  0.657
r = 0.30   u1(r,z,t) =  0.724   u2(r,z,t) =  0.609
r = 0.40   u1(r,z,t) =  0.757   u2(r,z,t) =  0.545
r = 0.50   u1(r,z,t) =  0.796   u2(r,z,t) =  0.466
r = 0.60   u1(r,z,t) =  0.838   u2(r,z,t) =  0.377
r = 0.70   u1(r,z,t) =  0.882   u2(r,z,t) =  0.282
r = 0.80   u1(r,z,t) =  0.924   u2(r,z,t) =  0.185
r = 0.90   u1(r,z,t) =  0.964   u2(r,z,t) =  0.089
r = 1.00   u1(r,z,t) =  1.000   u2(r,z,t) =  0.000

ku2*(u2(r=r0,z=zL/2,t)-u2e) = 3.067e-003

ncall =  1804
```

- The computational effort is greater for the variable diffusivity case (`ncall = 1804` vs `ncall = 395`) so the variable diffusivities had a significant effect on the computation of the solution by `ode15s`. However, the computational effort is still modest.

Figures 7.2 and 7.6 suggest an advantage of using normalized variables, that is, u_1 and u_2 have the same range $0 \leq u_1, u_2 \leq 1$ which facilitates a comparison of these two dependent variables. However, absolute variables can be used just as well. This would probably require a reevaluation of the model parameters, such as the diffusivities

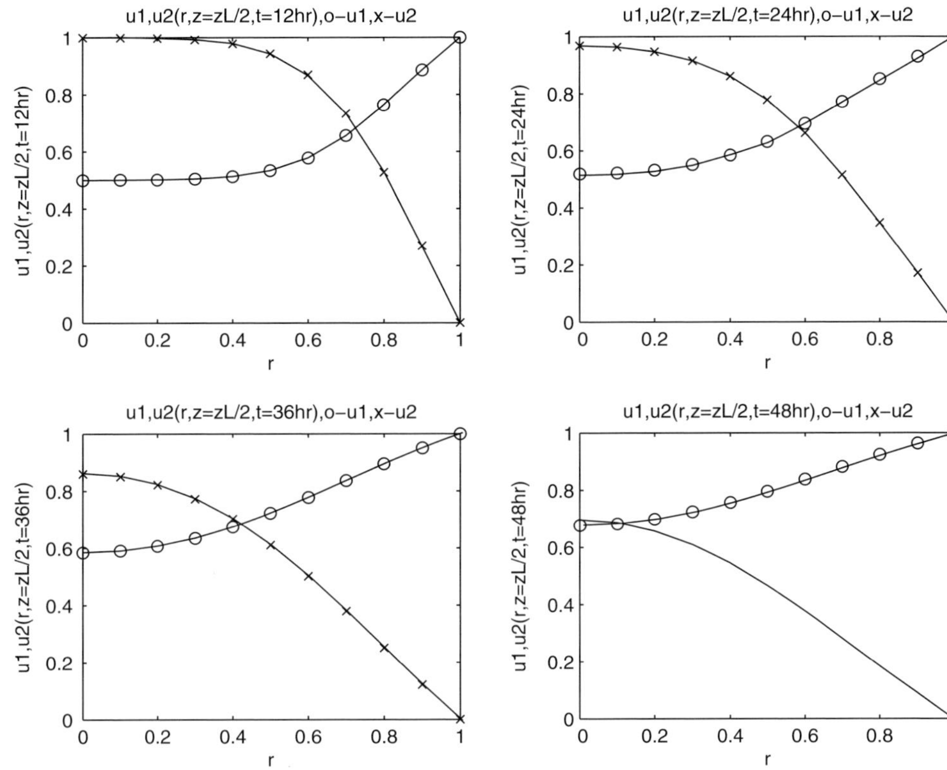

Figure 7.6 Composite plot of $u_1(r, z = z_L/2, t), u_2(r, z = z_L/2, t)$ for variable diffusivities

D_{u_1}, D_{u_2}, and therefore the parameters in eqs. (7.12). An essential requirement is to use consistent units throughout all of the model equations but otherwise the choice of units is open and can be selected to conform with the requirements of the model analysis, such as a comparison with experimental data.

Also, derivative groups such as

$$\frac{\partial\left(rD_{rr}\dfrac{\partial u}{\partial r}\right)}{r\partial r}$$

in eq. (7.13a) can be computed directly rather than after an analytical expansion, such as eq. (7.13b). This can be done in stages (and is therefore termed stagewise differentiation). For example, for the preceding r group,

- The derivative $(\partial u/\partial r)$ can be computed numerically, either by explicit programming of the FDs as in `pde_1`, or by using library routines as in `pde_2`.
- The product $rD_{rr}(\partial u/\partial r)$ can then be computed, including the use of a variable diffusivity ($D_{rr}(r, z, t, u)$).

- The derivative of this product can next be computed, either explicitly or through a library routine,

$$\frac{\partial\left(rD_{rr}\frac{\partial u}{\partial r}\right)}{\partial r}.$$

The library routine would be applied to the entire product.
- Finally, the resulting derivative would be multiplied by $1/r$ to complete the numerical evaluation of the radial group.

$$\frac{1}{r}\frac{\partial\left(rD_{rr}\frac{\partial u}{\partial r}\right)}{\partial r}.$$

This application of stagewise differentiation may seem like a more direct approach to the term in r of eq. (13.7a) than the previous approach of first analytically expanding the term (as in eq. (13.7b)), followed by application of a numerical FD approximation to each of the resulting terms (e.g., the three terms in eq. (13.7b)). However, experience has demonstrated that stagewise differentiation may be less robust than using the analytical expansion. Also, in the present case, we wanted to demonstrate that using the analytical expansion gave exactly the same solution for the constant diffusivity case as the programming based on initial use of the constant diffusivity (as demonstrated in Tables 7.1 and 7.2).

To conclude this discussion of the model, we mention one other procedure that can be quite useful in developing a mathematical model. The primary results from the model are $u_1(r,z,t)$ and $u_2(r,z,t)$ in numerical form. However, these solutions will be determined by the various terms in the PDEs and BCs, and these terms are readily available. For example, the RHS terms of the PDEs for the variable diffusivity case, `term1_1, term1_2` to `term5_1, term5_2` are all computed and can be displayed numerically and graphically. Also, the LHS derivatives in t computed in the ODE routines `pde_1` to `pde_4` are available and can be displayed. Then the magnitudes of the LHS and RHS terms can be compared to determine their relative contributions (even their signs can be interesting). A detailed examination of the various terms in the PDEs can give a complete description of why the solutions have their observed features, and modifications might be suggested in the ongoing development of the model. In other words, numerical information that elucidates the performance of the model is readily available.

Additionally, components of the various terms can be examined. For example, the exponential function in eqs. (7.12) can be studied separately (without computing a solution to the PDEs), and the magnitude of the computed diffusivities D_{u_1}, D_{u_2} compared with experimental data or estimates that may be available. Even something as basic as the sign of the component functions is an important consideration. For example, the exponential function of eq. (7.12) is nonnegative, which is an essential requirement since a negative diffusivity is physically unrealistic and mathematically causes the diffusion equation to be unstable. In other words, a detailed examination of the components and terms of a PDE such as $D_{u_1}, (\mathrm{d}D_{u_1}/\mathrm{d}u_1)$, and $D_{u_2}, (\mathrm{d}D_{u_2}/\mathrm{d}u_2)$ in `term1_1, term1_2` to `term5_1, term5_2` is worthwhile, particularly as a new model is being formulated, to understand why the observed solutions have particular features, or even to explain why the computer code does not execute as expected.

In summary, we have not attempted to present a state-of-the-art model for drug distribution from a PM. Rather, we have attempted to demonstrate the MOL solution of a PDE model with the features listed at the beginning of the chapter, e.g., two simultaneous 2D PDEs in cylindrical coordinates for linear, time variable coefficient, and nonlinear cases. Also, we have presented some alternatives for programming the model in `pde_1` to `pde_4` based on FDs. Finally, we have suggested some procedures for evaluating the accuracy of the numerical solutions, e.g., h and p refinement. We hope that the MOL procedures discussed in this and earlier chapters will be useful to the reader for the numerical study of a PDE model of interest. We will be pleased to respond to enquiries and questions to the extent possible by e-mail, including the procedure for downloading the routines (gratis) discussed in the book (directed to wes1@lehigh.edu).

References

[1] Aguzzi, C., Cerezo, P., Salcedo, I., Sanchez, R., and Viseras, C. (2010), Mathematical models describing drug release from biopolymeric delivery systems, *Mater. Technol.*, **25** (3/4) 205–211

[2] Formaggia, L., Minisini, S. and Zunino, P. (2010), Modeling polymeric controlled drug release and transport phenomena in the arterial tissue, *Math. Mod. Meth. Appl. S.*, **20** (10), 1759–1786

[3] Schiesser, W. E. and Griffiths, G. W. (2009), *A Compendium of Partial Differential Equation Models*, Cambridge, UK: Cambridge University Press

Appendix 1 Origin of convection-diffusion-reaction PDEs

Most ODE/PDE models originate from the application of conservation principles, typically the conservation of mass, momentum, and energy. In this appendix, we consider the derivation of: (1) a PDE, eq. (2.1) (and also eq. (1.18)), (2) the finite difference (FD) approximation used for the MOL solution of eq. (2.1), and (3) the FD approximation of boundary condition (BC) (2.2) for eq. (2.1).

A1.1 Derivation of a PDE from a conservation principle

We first consider the derivation of eq. (2.1) using conservation of mass.

$$\frac{\partial c}{\partial t} = D\frac{\partial^2 c}{\partial z^2}. \tag{1.18, 2.1, A1.1}$$

In the following discussion, the original equation numbers are repeated, along with a set of numbers with the designation "A1" for Appendix 1.

We start with a mass balance on an incremental cube with sides of length $\Delta x, \Delta y, \Delta z$ where x, y, z are the three directions in Cartesian coordinates.

$$\begin{aligned}
\Delta x\Delta y\Delta z\frac{\partial c}{\partial t} &= -\Delta y\Delta zD_x\left.\frac{\partial c}{\partial x}\right|_x - \left(-\Delta y\Delta zD_x\left.\frac{\partial c}{\partial x}\right|_{x+\Delta x}\right)\\
&= -\Delta x\Delta zD_y\frac{\partial c}{\partial y}|_y - \left(-\Delta x\Delta zD_y\left.\frac{\partial c}{\partial y}\right|_{y+\Delta y}\right)\\
&= -\Delta x\Delta yD_z\left.\frac{\partial c}{\partial z}\right|_z - \left(-\Delta x\Delta yD_z\left.\frac{\partial c}{\partial z}\right|_{z+\Delta z}\right)
\end{aligned} \tag{A1.2}$$

Here we have used Fick's first law for mass diffusion (or Fourier's first law for heat conduction) to give the diffusion fluxes, q_x, q_y, q_z:

$$q_x = -D_x\frac{\partial c}{\partial x}, \tag{A1.3a}$$

$$q_y = -D_y\frac{\partial c}{\partial y}, \tag{A1.3b}$$

$$q_z = -D_z\frac{\partial c}{\partial z}. \tag{A1.3c}$$

Equation (A1.2) states that the net rate of accumulation (or depletion) of the analyte (discussed in Chapter 2), with concentration c, in the incremental volume $\Delta x \Delta y \Delta z$, expressed as the LHS derivative in t, equals the net rate of diffusion of the analyte into (or out of) the incremental volume, expressed as the differences of RHS terms in x, y, z. This is the mass balance on the analyte. If the LHS derivative in t is positive, the analyte is accumulating; that is, its concentration c is increasing with t. If the LHS derivative in t is negative, the analyte is being depleted; that is, its concentration c is decreasing with t.

$u(x, y, z, t)$ is the dependent variable of eqs. (A1.2) and (A1.3), and x, y, z, t are the independent variables; D_x, D_y, D_z are the diffusivities in the x, y, z directions, respectively; they do not necessarily have to be equal if the medium in which the diffusion takes place is anisotropic (direction dependent). The minus in the RHS of eqs. (A1.3) is required, since the diffusion will be in the direction of decreasing concentration. In other words, the fluxes q_x, q_y, q_z are vectors with a direction as well as a magnitude. If these fluxes are positive, they denote mass diffusion in the positive x, y, z directions. But the gradients $(\partial c/\partial x), (\partial c/\partial y), (\partial c/\partial x)$ will be negative, so the minus is required for the LHS and RHS of eqs. (A1.3) to have the same sign.

More generally, diffusion in direction i can take place as a result of a concentration gradient in direction j. For this case, the diffusivity requires a double subscript, D_{ij}; there would then be nine diffusivities in three dimensional space, $D_{ij}; i = 1, 2, 3; j = 1, 2, 3$; these nine components comprise the 3×3 diffusivity tensor; here we use only $D_{ij}; i = j$, that is the diagonal elements of the diffusivity tensor. Further, we could use different coordinate systems, e.g., Cartesian, cylindrical, spherical. These more general cases are considered in [5], Appendix 1.

An analysis of the units in eqs. (A1.2) and (A1.3) also is instructive. First, for eq. (A1.3a), the LHS and RHS fluxes have the units

$$\frac{\text{mol}}{\text{m}^2 - \text{s}} = \frac{\text{m}^2}{\text{s}} \frac{\text{mol}/\text{m}^3}{\text{m}}.$$

Then, for eq. (A1.2) the LHS and RHS terms have the units

$$\text{m}^3 \frac{\text{mol}/\text{m}^3}{\text{s}} = (\text{m}^2)(\text{m}^2/\text{s}) \frac{\text{mol}/\text{m}^3}{\text{m}}.$$

Note in particular the use of the incremental areas perpendicular to the diffusion fluxes. For example, with $q_x = -D_x(\partial c/\partial x)$ from eq. (A1.3a), the total diffusion through the area or face $\Delta y \Delta z$ in the first RHS term is $(\Delta y \Delta z)(-D_x(\partial c/\partial x))$. Then when eq. (A1.2) is divided by the incremental volume $\Delta x \Delta y \Delta z$, the area $\Delta y \Delta z$ cancels, leaving Δx in the RHS denominator, which forms a derivative in the limit $\Delta x \longrightarrow 0$.

This process is illustrated by a straightforward rearrangement of eq. (A1.2).

$$\frac{\partial c}{\partial t} = \frac{D_x \left.\dfrac{\partial c}{\partial x}\right|_{x+\Delta x} - D_x \left.\dfrac{\partial c}{\partial x}\right|_{x}}{\Delta x} + \frac{D_y \left.\dfrac{\partial c}{\partial y}\right|_{y+\Delta y} - D_y \left.\dfrac{\partial c}{\partial y}\right|_{y}}{\Delta y} + \frac{D_z \left.\dfrac{\partial c}{\partial z}\right|_{z+\Delta z} - D_z \left.\dfrac{\partial c}{\partial z}\right|_{z}}{\Delta z}. \tag{A1.4}$$

Note the cancellation of the three areas in the RHS of eq. (A1.4). In the limit $\Delta x, \Delta y, \Delta z \longrightarrow 0$, eq. (A1.4) becomes

$$\frac{\partial c}{\partial t} = \frac{\partial\left(D_x \dfrac{\partial c}{\partial x}\right)}{\partial x} + \frac{\partial\left(D_y \dfrac{\partial c}{\partial y}\right)}{\partial y} + \frac{\partial\left(D_z \dfrac{\partial c}{\partial z}\right)}{\partial z}. \tag{A1.5a}$$

Note that in comparing eqs. (A1.4) and (A1.5a), we have made use of the notion that a partial derivative pertains to a change in one independent variable while the other independent variables do not change. For example, the first RHS term of eq. (A1.4),

$$\frac{D_x \left.\dfrac{\partial c}{\partial x}\right|_{x+\Delta x} - D_x \left.\dfrac{\partial c}{\partial x}\right|_{x}}{\Delta x}$$

has a change in x (x to $x + \Delta x$) while the other spatial variables, y and z, remain constant. This idea is expressed with the notation for the corresponding derivative in x

$$\frac{\partial\left(D_x \dfrac{\partial c}{\partial x}\right)}{\partial x}.$$

In other words, this partial derivative pertains to a change in x with y,z constant. This basic idea is also used when approximating partial derivatives to compute solutions to PDEs numerically.

For the case of constant diffusivities, eq. (A1.5a) is

$$\frac{\partial c}{\partial t} = D_x \frac{\partial^2 c}{\partial x^2} + D_y \frac{\partial^2 c}{\partial y^2} + D_z \frac{\partial^2 c}{\partial z^2}. \tag{A1.5b}$$

Equation (A1.5b) is Fick's second law for mass diffusion (or Fourier's second law for heat conduction). For the case $D_x = D_y = 0, D_z = D$, eq. (A1.5b) is eq. (1.18) and eq. (2.1).

In the application of balances or transport equations such as eq. (A1.1), a challenging requirement is the estimation of the transport coefficients, such as the diffusivity D. This is generally done by either of two methods:

1. Correlations of transport coefficients such as D are available based on experimental data. The main issue in using a correlation is whether it is based on data taken under conditions that closely resemble the experimental system of interest. In other words, the correlations have to be relevant and reliable.
2. Experiments are performed in which the dependent variable (in the 1D case) such as $c(z,t)$ is measured as a function of z and t; comparison of the solution of the PDE (in the form of the computed $c(z,t)$ as demonstrated in Chapter 1) with the experimental data gives a value of D. This procedure is usually termed parameter estimation or identification; it is also called the inverse problem since experimental and calculated solutions of the transport equations are compared to estimate the transport coefficients

rather than the forward process of using given values of the transport coefficients in the computed solution to arrive at a predicted concentration field (a term usually applied to a distribution in time and space, such as the $c(z,t)$ distribution in t and z in the case of eq. (A1.1), i.e., eq. (A1.1) can be considered a field equation).

In other words, the reliable estimation of the transport coefficients in a mathematical model may be the most challenging aspect of the use of the model. This same conclusion applies to the requirement for reliable thermodynamic, kinetic, and biological parameters. Typically experiments are required to measure or identify the model parameters, although just using estimates in the model equations can often provide valuable insights into the characteristics of the modeled system, and additionally can identify the parameters that are most sensitive in determining the characteristics of the modeled system and which may therefore require further refinement through experiments. Of course, experiments may be difficult to impossible, e.g., if performed on living systems, in which case it is necessary to settle on just estimated values. In any case, it is important to keep in mind the reliability of the model parameters in interpreting and judging the validity of the solutions to the model equations; perhaps the solutions to the model equations have substantial uncertainty because of uncertainty in the parameters used to compute the solutions.

To this point, we have used c as the PDE-dependent variable in this appendix since the PDEs were derived through conservation of mass (and thus the use of concentration, c, was logical). However, in the PDE literature, the dependent variable is usually designated as u, which we used throughout most of the preceding chapters. We will now use this convention.

Equation (A1.5a) can be expressed in vector–tensor notation (vectors and tensor expressed in boldface) as

$$\frac{\partial u}{\partial t} = \nabla \cdot (\mathbf{D} \cdot \nabla u), \tag{A1.6}$$

where $\cdot$ denotes a vector–vector or vector–tensor dot product. For example, for two vectors, $\mathbf{a}, \mathbf{b}$, the dot product is

$$\mathbf{a} \cdot \mathbf{b} = |a|\,|b| \cos(\theta)$$

and θ is the angle between $\mathbf{a}$ and $\mathbf{b}$, $\nabla\cdot$ is the divergence applied to a vector, and ∇ is the divergence applied to a scalar, also denoted *div* and *grad*, respectively. For example,

$$\nabla = \mathbf{i}\frac{\partial}{\partial x} + \mathbf{j}\frac{\partial}{\partial y} + \mathbf{k}\frac{\partial}{\partial z} \tag{A1.7a}$$

and $\mathbf{i}$, $\mathbf{j}$, and $\mathbf{k}$ are unit vectors in Cartesian coordinates. Then the grad of a scalar u is

$$\nabla u = \mathbf{i}\frac{\partial u}{\partial x} + \mathbf{j}\frac{\partial u}{\partial y} + \mathbf{k}\frac{\partial u}{\partial z} \tag{A1.7b}$$

and the div of the resulting vector is

$$\nabla \cdot \nabla u = \frac{\partial^2 u}{\partial x^2} + \frac{\partial^2 u}{\partial y} + \frac{\partial^2 u}{\partial z^2}, \tag{A1.7c}$$

where $\nabla \cdot \nabla = \nabla^2$ is termed the Laplacian operator (also denoted as $\triangle$); in Cartesian coordinates it is

$$\nabla \cdot \nabla = \text{div grad} = \nabla^2 = \frac{\partial^2}{\partial x^2} + \frac{\partial^2}{\partial y} + \frac{\partial^2}{\partial z^2}, \tag{A1.7d}$$

where we have used the dot product between the orthogonal unit vectors, that is for example, $\mathbf{i} \cdot \mathbf{i} = 1, \mathbf{i} \cdot \mathbf{j} = 0$. If the RHS of eq. (A1.7c) equals zero, the result is Laplace's equation.

The use of vector–tensor notation has the advantages of: (1) a compact notation and (2) independence from the coordinate system, that is, the PDE is general and can be specialized for any particular coordinate system. A discussion of the use of vector–tensor notation in various coordinate systems is given in [5], Appendix 1.

A1.2 Approximations of derivatives

When using an equation such as eq. (A1.1), we should keep in mind that we are using mathematics that is a human creation, and in particular, derivatives in ordinary and partial differential equations (ODE/PDEs), such as the partial derivatives in eq. (A1.1); we will term this continuous mathematics, since usually we analyze situations in which the solutions to the model equations are continuous and therefore the derivatives are well-defined and well-behaved (there are important exceptions to this smoothness requirement for ODE/PDE solutions, but we will not consider these here).

But computers, at least at their most fundamental level of digital arithmetic, do not naturally handle continuous mathematics, and it is therefore necessary to bridge this gap of expressing mathematics that human beings understand with equivalent mathematics that computers can "understand"; that is, they can work with some form of mathematics that basically does not go beyond digital arithmetic; we will term this type of computer-oriented mathematics discrete mathematics (for reasons that will become clearer as we proceed). This bridging of human and computer analysis is an essential step if we are going to use computers to study mathematical models, and in particular, models based on ODE/PDEs. As we might expect, this process of putting mathematical models on computers has been a major research activity for many years, and here we can only offer some basic ideas, but they will be sufficient for the computer analysis of partial differential equations applied to biomedical engineering, the central topic of this book.

As a specific example of formulating some mathematics that we can put on a computer, we must somehow express eq. (A1.1) in a way that it can be programmed for a computer using only digital arithmetic (since computers do not naturally handle partial derivatives), in other words, basically, addition, subtraction, multiplication, and division, but done very fast and reliably by computers. The basic tool we will use for human analysts to communicate with computers is the Taylor series.

Equation (A1.1) has two partial derivatives that have important differences. The independent variable t in $(\partial u/\partial t)$ is an initial value variable defined over the interval $0 \leq t \leq \infty$, while z in $(\partial^2 u/\partial z^2)$ is a boundary value variable defined over the interval $0 \leq z \leq h$ (as illustrated by eq. (2.3)). Numerical integration of these two derivatives is generally accomplished through application of the Taylor series. In the case of derivatives in t, library initial value integrators such as `ode15s` based on the Taylor series are well-established and therefore we will simply use them (for example, by calling `ode15s` in the main program of Listing 2.2). For derivatives in z, the Taylor series is used to construct approximations to the derivatives that can then be programmed for a computer.

To illustrate this process, we consider an approximation to a first derivative in z (which will be used in BC (2.2)). If we consider the grid in z illustrated in Fig. 2.2, the dependent variable at $z-\Delta z$ and $z+\Delta z$, $u(z-\Delta z,t)$ and $u(z+\Delta z,t)$, respectively, can be expressed through a Taylor series.

$$u(z+\Delta z,t) = u(z,t) + \frac{\partial u(z,t)}{\partial z}\frac{\Delta z}{1!} + \frac{\partial^2 u(z,t)}{\partial z^2}\frac{\Delta z^2}{2!} + \frac{\partial^3 u(z,t)}{\partial z^3}\frac{\Delta z^3}{3!} + \cdots, \tag{A1.8a}$$

$$u(z-\Delta z,t) = u(z,t) + \frac{\partial u(z,t)}{\partial z}\frac{(-\Delta z)}{1!} + \frac{\partial^2 u(z,t)}{\partial z^2}\frac{(-\Delta z)^2}{2!} + \frac{\partial^3 u(z,t)}{\partial z^3}\frac{(-\Delta z)^3}{3!} + \cdots. \tag{A1.8b}$$

If eq. (A1.8b) is subtracted from eq. (A1.8a) (the idea is to cancel the $u(z,t)$ and $(\partial^2 u(z,t)/\partial z^2)((-\Delta z)^2/2!)$ terms and retain the derivative of interest, $(\partial u(z,t)/\partial z)$, in the first order term),

$$u(z+\Delta z,t) - u(z-\Delta z,t) = 2\frac{\partial u(z,t)}{\partial z}\frac{\Delta z}{1!} + 2\frac{\partial^3 u(z,t)}{\partial z^3}\frac{\Delta z^3}{3!} + \cdots,$$

or solving for $(\partial u(z,t)/\partial z)$,

$$\frac{\partial u(z,t)}{\partial z} = \frac{u(z+\Delta z,t) - u(z-\Delta z,t)}{2\Delta z} + O(\Delta z^2). \tag{1.14, 2.12a, A1.9}$$

We can note the following details about this result.

- The approximation of eq. (A1.9) is a two point, centered, second order finite difference (FD) for a first derivative. These terms are explained as:
  - Two point: The approximation uses two values of the dependent value, $u(z+\Delta z,t)$ and $u(z-\Delta z,t)$.
  - Centered: These two points are centered or symmetric with respect to the point z that is the center or base for the approximation of $(\partial u(z,t)/\partial z)$.
  - Second order: The approximation of eq. (A1.9) is second order correct as denoted by $O(\Delta z^2)$. This order condition results from the third order derivative term in eqs. (A1.8), $(\partial^3 u(z,t)/\partial z^3)((\pm\Delta z)^3/3!)$, which is then divided by Δz to arrive at eq.

(A1.9). This second order term reflects the truncation error of eq. (A1.9) that results from the truncation of the two Taylor series of eqs. (A1.8) after the cubic term. Note that this order condition pertains to the accuracy of the FD approximation and not to the order of the derivative that is being approximated, which in this case is first order.
  - Finite difference: The approximation of eq. (A1.9) is based on the difference $u(z+\Delta z,t)-u(z-\Delta z,t)$ over the finite interval $2\Delta z$.

- The FD of eq. (A1.9) does not depend on $u(z,t)$, which is generally the case for centered FD approximations of odd order derivatives (first order in this case).
- The Taylor series approximations of eqs. (A1.8) are a special case of a two dimensional Taylor series in z and t. However, we are considering only changes in z so that the terms involving changes in t (with various partial derivatives in t) do not appear in the Taylor series.

This same procedure for the first derivative can be applied to give a FD approximation of a second derivative. In this case, eqs. (A1.8) are added (rather than subtracted). Note that the first and third derivative terms, $(\partial u(z,t)/\partial z)(\pm\Delta z/1!)$ and $(\partial^3 u(z,t)/\partial z^3)(\pm(\Delta z)^3/3!)$, now drop out and the second order term with the derivative $(\partial^2 u(z,t)/\partial z^2)$ remains,

$$u(z+\Delta z,t)+u(z-\Delta z,t)=2u(z,t)+2\frac{\partial^2 u(z,t)}{\partial z^2}\frac{\Delta z^2}{2!}+\cdots,$$

or

$$\frac{\partial^2 u(z,t)}{\partial z^2}=\frac{u(z+\Delta z,t)-2u(z,t)+u(z-\Delta z,t)}{\Delta z^2}+O(\Delta z^2). \tag{A1.10}$$

Equation (A1.10) is used in the MOL approximation of eq. (2.1) according to eq. (2.13a). The approximation of eq. (A1.10) is a three point, centered, second order FD for a second derivative. Note that the center point $u(z,t)$ is now used in the approximation in contrast with eq. (A1.9). Also, the order $O(\Delta z^2)$ follows in the same way as for eq. (A1.9).

A1.3 Approximation of boundary conditions

The approximation of BC (2.3) as discussed in Chapter 2, eqs. (2.12), involved the use of a fictitious point. We mention here that the use of fictitious points can be avoided by the use of noncentered approximations. For example, the three point, noncentered, second order FD approximations for a first derivative at the left and right boundaries are ([6], p100)

$$\frac{\partial u(z,t)}{\partial z}=\frac{-3u(z,t)+4u(z+\Delta z,t)-u(z+2\Delta z,t)}{2\Delta z}+O(\Delta z^2), \tag{A1.11a}$$

$$\frac{\partial u(z,t)}{\partial z}=\frac{3u(z,t)-4u(z-\Delta z,t)+u(z-2\Delta z,t)}{2\Delta z}+O(\Delta z^2). \tag{A1.11b}$$

Note that in eq. (A1.11a), only the boundary point at z and the interior points at $z+\Delta z, z+2\Delta z$ are used to calculate the first derivative at the left boundary z. Similarly, eq. (A1.11b) requires only the right boundary value at z and the two interior points at $z-\Delta z, z-2\Delta z$. Thus, if eqs. (A1.11) are used to approximate Neumann BCs (with a first derivative), fictitious points can be avoided.

The combination of eqs. (A1.9) and (A1.11) can be considered as a way of calculating first derivatives at the boundary and interior points in z that can be summarized through their weighting coefficients. For example, eq. (A1.9) has the weighting coefficients -1, 0, 1 applied to $u(z-\Delta z,t), u(z,t), u(z+\Delta z,t)$, respectively. The weighting coefficients for eqs. (A1.9) and (A1.11) can be summarized in a 3×3 differentiation matrix,

$$\frac{1}{2\Delta z}\begin{bmatrix} -3 & 4 & -1 \\ -1 & 0 & 1 \\ 1 & -4 & 3 \end{bmatrix}.$$

This differentiation matrix can then be applied to a vector of dependent value variables $\mathbf{u}(z,t)$ (defined on a spatial grid as in Fig. 2.2) to produce a vector of first derivatives, $(\partial \mathbf{u}(z,t)/\partial z)$ (here we use a bold face to denote a vector).

$$\frac{\partial \mathbf{u}(z,t)}{\partial z} = \frac{1}{2\Delta z}\begin{bmatrix} -3 & 4 & -1 \\ -1 & 0 & 1 \\ 1 & -4 & 3 \end{bmatrix}\mathbf{u}(z,t) + O(\Delta z^2), \tag{A1.12a}$$

where the first row of weighting coefficients is applied to $\mathbf{u}(z,t)$ at the left boundary, the last row of weighting coefficients is applied to $\mathbf{u}(z,t)$ at the right boundary and the center row of coefficients is applied to $\mathbf{u}(z,t)$ at all of the interior points (see eqs. (A1.9) and (A1.11) for how these weighting coefficients are used).

Two additional details can be noted about the differentiation matrix:

- The coefficients in any given row sum to zero. This is required for the correct differentiation of a constant function (to zero). Although this is a rather obvious requirement, it can be a useful check in the development of new differentiation formulas and matrices.
- The coefficients of the third row are antisymmetric with the respect to the first row in the sense of an interchange of positions in the rows and a change of sign. This is a general feature of differentiation matrices for odd order derivatives (such as first order), and also explains the zero in the second row.
- The weighted sums for the derivatives from the three rows is divided by $2\Delta z$; in particular, Δz to the first power in the denominator is expected when considering the units of a first derivative.

The idea of a differentiation matrix can be extended to higher order matrices. Thus, the 5×5 matrix for the first derivative is stated in eq. (A1.12b) below ([6], p 108).

$$\frac{\partial \mathbf{u}(z,t)}{\partial z} = \frac{1}{4!\Delta z}\begin{bmatrix} -50 & 96 & -72 & 32 & -6 \\ -6 & -20 & 36 & -12 & 2 \\ 2 & -16 & 0 & 16 & -2 \\ -2 & 12 & -36 & 20 & 6 \\ 6 & -32 & 72 & -96 & 50 \end{bmatrix}\mathbf{u}(z,t) + O(\Delta z^4). \tag{A1.12b}$$

Note again: (1) the coefficients in a given row sum to zero, (2) the coefficients are antisymmetric with respect to the center 0, and (3) a division by Δz as expected for a first derivative. Also, the derivatives computed according to eq. (A1.12b) are fourth order correct ($O(\Delta z^4)$).

Just to complete the discussion of eq. (A1.12b), the first row of coefficients is applied to the vector $\mathbf{u}(z,t)$ at the left boundary, the second row is applied to $\mathbf{u}(z,t)$ at Δz to the right of the left boundary, the fourth row is applied at Δz to the left of the right boundary, the fifth row is applied at the right boundary, and the third row is applied to all other interior points. Thus, the first derivative at the left boundary is given by

$$\begin{aligned}\frac{\partial u(z,t)}{\partial z}&\\ &= \frac{-50u(z,t)+96u(z+\Delta z,t)-72u(z+2\Delta z,t)+32u(z+3\Delta z,t)-6u(z+4\Delta z,t)}{4!\Delta z}\\ &\quad +O(\Delta z^4).\end{aligned} \tag{A1.12c}$$

Note again that fictitious points are not required in computing this first derivative. Also, parenthetically, although more computation is required in using the 5×5 matrix of eq. (A1.12b) than the 3×3 matrix of eq. (A1.12a) (multiplication by five coefficients followed by the summing of five terms, rather than three), usually this effort is well worthwhile since the resulting derivative will be fourth order correct rather than second order (an example of how this increase in FD order substantially reduces the error is given in [5], pp 82–87). Higher order differentiation matrices (e.g., 6×6, 8×8, etc.) are readily available from the Fornberg algorithm ([2]). Also, differentiation matrices of order two, four, ..., ten are implemented in library differentiation routines ([5]) and are available online ([3, 4]).

To return briefly to the earlier discussion of continuous and discrete mathematics, eq. (A1.12c) has continuous mathematics in the LHS (a derivative) and discrete mathematics in the RHS (involving the dependent variable $u(z,t)$ at discrete points in z). Note that the RHS requires only arithmetic, that is, multiplication by five weighting coefficients, addition of the five resulting terms, and division by $4!\Delta z$. These are the operations that a computer can perform with amazing speed and accuracy. Thus, through the use of equations like (A1.12c), we can perform mathematics while taking advantage of modern high speed computers; this provides an enormous advantage in applying mathematics to realistic physical problems.

To conclude this discussion of FD approximations, differentiation matrices for higher order derivatives are available from the Fornberg algorithm ([2]). Equation (A1.10) is an example of a line from a differentiation matrix for a second derivative with the weighting coefficients 1, −2, 1. Differentiation matrices of order two, four, ..., ten for second derivatives, with Dirichlet and Neumann BCs, are implemented in library differentiation routines ([5]) and are available online ([3, 5]).

This brief discussion of FD approximations, which permit the mathematical operation of differentiation to be performed with a computer, could be extended to cover other methods, such as the finite element, finite volume, spectral, and meshfree methods for implementing PDEs numerically on a computer. However, we conclude the discussion here with the intention of providing only an introduction to computer-based, approximate mathematics; the reader can then explore the literature pertaining to this important element of the PDE analysis of biomedical engineering systems.

A1.4 Derivation of a convection-diffusion-reaction PDE

We conclude this appendix with a derivation of diffusion equation (2.1) extended to include convection and reaction, a convection-diffusion-reaction (CDR) equation. This extension is accomplished by adding convection and reaction terms to eq. (A1.2).

A1.4.1 Cartesian coordinates

$$
\begin{aligned}
\Delta x \Delta y \Delta z \frac{\partial u}{\partial t} = & -\Delta y \Delta z D_x \left.\frac{\partial u}{\partial x}\right|_x - \left(-\Delta y \Delta z D_x \left.\frac{\partial u}{\partial x}\right|_{x+\Delta x}\right) \\
& - \Delta x \Delta z D_y \left.\frac{\partial u}{\partial y}\right|_y - \left(-\Delta x \Delta z D_y \left.\frac{\partial u}{\partial y}\right|_{y+\Delta y}\right) \\
& - \Delta x \Delta y D_z \left.\frac{\partial u}{\partial z}\right|_z - \left(-\Delta x \Delta y D_z \left.\frac{\partial u}{\partial z}\right|_{z+\Delta z}\right) \\
& + \Delta y \Delta z \left(v_x u|_x - v_x u|_{x+\Delta x}\right) \\
& + \Delta x \Delta z \left(v_y u|_y - v_y u|_{y+\Delta y}\right) \\
& + \Delta x \Delta y \left(v_z u|_z - v_z u|_{z+\Delta z}\right) \\
& - \Delta x \Delta y \Delta z k_r u^p. \qquad \text{(A1.13a)}
\end{aligned}
$$

Here we have used the diffusion flux, a vector with the components of eqs. (A1.3), and the convection flux, a vector with the components

$$w_x = v_x u; \; w_y = v_y u; \; w_z = v_z u.$$

We can note the following details about eq. (A1.13a).

- The convective terms have the three velocities v_x, v_y, v_z; these velocities are positive for flow in the direction of increasing x, y, z. The first term in each convective group, e.g., $v_x u|_x$, is the flow into the incremental volume $\Delta x \Delta y \Delta z$, while the second term, e.g., $v_x u|_{x+\Delta x}$, is the flow out of the incremental volume (note the signs of these terms).

- Each of these convective terms has units (again, with $u(z,t)$ interpreted as a concentration with units mol/m^3)

$$(\text{cm}^2)\left(\frac{\text{m}}{\text{s}}\right)\left(\frac{\text{mol}}{\text{m}^3}\right)=\frac{\text{mol}}{\text{s}},$$

  that is, the net (mol/s) flowing into or out of the incremental volume. Note that these are also the units of the LHS derivative in t and the first RHS diffusion terms.
- The reaction term includes the volumetric reaction rate constant, k_r. The order of the reaction is p. For a first order reaction, $p=1$ and k_r has the units s^{-1}, so that the net units of the reaction term are (mol/s). Since the term has a minus sign, this rate can be interpreted as a consumption due to the chemical reaction.

Division of eq. (A1.13a) by the incremental volume $\Delta x\Delta y\Delta z$ followed by the limit $\Delta x\to 0$, $\Delta y\to 0$, $\Delta z\to 0$ gives the PDE

$$\frac{\partial u}{\partial t}=\frac{\partial\left(D_x\frac{\partial u}{\partial x}\right)}{\partial x}+\frac{\partial\left(D_y\frac{\partial u}{\partial y}\right)}{\partial y}+\frac{\partial\left(D_z\frac{\partial u}{\partial z}\right)}{\partial z}-\frac{\partial\left(v_x u\right)}{\partial x}-\frac{\partial\left(v_y u\right)}{\partial y}-\frac{\partial\left(v_z u\right)}{\partial z}-k_\text{r}u^p. \tag{A1.13b}$$

If terms in z only are retained, and $D_z=D$ and $v_z=v$ are constant, eq. (A.13b) reduces to

$$\frac{\partial u}{\partial t}=D\frac{\partial^2 u}{\partial z^2}-v\frac{\partial u}{\partial z}-k_\text{r}u^p. \tag{A1.13c}$$

For $D=k_\text{r}=0$, eq. (A1.13c) reduces to the advection equation, eq. (1.1). For $v=k_\text{r}=0$, eq. (A1.13c) reduces to the diffusion equation, (1.18) and (2.1). Equation (A1.13c) is the CDR of eq. (1.28) (with $p=1$).

A1.4.2 Cylindrical coordinates

The corresponding derivation in cylindrical coordinates, (r,θ,z), follows from a mass balance on an incremental volume $r\Delta r\Delta\theta\Delta z$.

$$\begin{aligned}r\Delta r\Delta\theta\Delta z\frac{\partial u}{\partial t}=&-r\Delta\theta\Delta z D_r\left.\frac{\partial u}{\partial r}\right|_r-\left(-(r+\Delta r)\Delta\theta\Delta z D_r\left.\frac{\partial u}{\partial r}\right|_{r+\Delta r}\right)\\&-\Delta r\Delta z\frac{D_\theta}{r}\left.\frac{\partial u}{\partial\theta}\right|_\theta-\left(-\Delta r\Delta z\frac{D_\theta}{r}\left.\frac{\partial u}{\partial\theta}\right|_{\theta+\Delta\theta}\right)\\&-r\Delta r\Delta\theta D_z\left.\frac{\partial u}{\partial z}\right|_z-\left(-r\Delta r\Delta\theta D_z\left.\frac{\partial u}{\partial z}\right|_{z+\Delta z}\right)\end{aligned}$$

$$
\begin{aligned}
&+ r\Delta\theta\,\Delta z v_r u|_r - (r+\Delta r)\Delta\theta\,\Delta z v_r u|_{r+\Delta r} \\
&+ \Delta r \Delta z v_\theta u|_\theta - \Delta r \Delta z v_\theta u|_{\theta+\Delta\theta} \\
&+ r\Delta r \Delta\theta v_z u|_z - r\Delta r\Delta\theta v_z u|_{z+\Delta z} \\
&- r\Delta r\Delta\theta\,\Delta z k_{\mathrm{r}} u^p. \qquad \text{(A1.14a)}
\end{aligned}
$$

Here we have used the diffusion flux, a vector with the components

$$
q_r = -D_r \frac{\partial u}{\partial r},\; q_\theta = -\frac{D_\theta}{r}\frac{\partial u}{\partial \theta},\; q_z = -D_z \frac{\partial u}{\partial z},
$$

and the convection flux, a vector with the components

$$
w_r = v_r u,\; w_\theta = v_\theta u,\; w_z = v_z u.
$$

Division of eq. (A1.14a) by $r\Delta r\Delta\theta\,\Delta z$ and minor rearrangement gives

$$
\begin{aligned}
\frac{\partial u}{\partial t} = {} & \frac{1}{r}\frac{(r+\Delta r)D_r \left.\dfrac{\partial u}{\partial r}\right|_{r+\Delta r} - rD_r \left.\dfrac{\partial u}{\partial r}\right|_r}{\Delta r} \\
& + \frac{1}{r^2}\frac{D_\theta \left.\dfrac{\partial u}{\partial \theta}\right|_{\theta+\Delta\theta} - D_\theta \left.\dfrac{\partial u}{\partial \theta}\right|_\theta}{\Delta\theta} \\
& + \frac{D_z \left.\dfrac{\partial u}{\partial z}\right|_{z+\Delta z} - D_z \dfrac{\partial u}{\partial z}|_z}{\Delta z} \\
& - \frac{1}{r}\left(\frac{(r+\Delta r)v_r u|_{r+\Delta r} - r v_r u|_r}{\Delta r}\right) \\
& - \frac{1}{r}\left(\frac{v_\theta u|_{\theta+\Delta\theta} - v_\theta u|_\theta}{\Delta\theta}\right) \\
& - \left(\frac{v_z u|_{z+\Delta z} - v_z u|_z}{\Delta z}\right) \\
& - k_{\mathrm{r}} u^p. \qquad \text{(A1.14b)}
\end{aligned}
$$

For $\Delta r \to 0, \Delta\theta \to 0, \Delta z \to 0$, eq. (A1.14b) becomes

$$
\begin{aligned}
\frac{\partial u}{\partial t} = {} & \frac{1}{r}\frac{\partial\left(rD_r \dfrac{\partial u}{\partial r}\right)}{\partial r} + \frac{1}{r^2}\frac{\partial\left(D_\theta \dfrac{\partial u}{\partial \theta}\right)}{\partial \theta} + \frac{\partial\left(D_z \dfrac{\partial u}{\partial z}\right)}{\partial z} \\
& - \frac{1}{r}\frac{\partial\,(r v_r u)}{\partial r} - \frac{1}{r}\frac{\partial\,(v_\theta u)}{\partial \theta} - \frac{\partial\,(v_z u)}{\partial z} - k_{\mathrm{r}} u^p \qquad \text{(A1.14c)}
\end{aligned}
$$

For the special case of constant diffusivities and velocities, eq. (A1.14c) becomes

$$\frac{\partial u}{\partial t}=\frac{D_r}{r}\frac{\partial\left(r\frac{\partial u}{\partial r}\right)}{\partial r}+\frac{D_\theta}{r^2}\frac{\partial^2 u}{\partial\theta^2}+D_z\frac{\partial^2 u}{\partial z^2}$$
$$-\frac{v_r}{r}\frac{\partial(ru)}{\partial r}-\frac{v_\theta}{r}\frac{\partial u}{\partial\theta}-v_z\frac{\partial u}{\partial z}-k_r u^p, \tag{A1.14d}$$

or after differentiating the product terms in r,

$$\frac{\partial u}{\partial t}=D_r\left(\frac{\partial^2 u}{\partial r^2}+\frac{1}{r}\frac{\partial u}{\partial r}\right)+\frac{D_\theta}{r^2}\frac{\partial^2 u}{\partial\theta^2}+D_z\frac{\partial^2 u}{\partial z^2}$$
$$-v_r\left(\frac{\partial u}{\partial r}+\frac{u}{r}\right)-\frac{v_\theta}{r}\frac{\partial u}{\partial\theta}-v_z\frac{\partial u}{\partial z}-k_r u^p. \tag{A1.14e}$$

Experience has indicated that the expanded form of the r terms in eq. (A1.14e) leads to MOL numerical solutions more reliably than using the r terms in eq. (A1.14d). Additionally, product terms such as in r in eq. (A1.14d) are commonplace and expanding them through differentiation is generally recommended before attempting a numerical solution.

We can note the following details about eqs. (A1.14).

- Again, with $u(z,t)$ interpreted as a concentration with units mol/m^3, each of the terms in the equations with the LHS $(\partial u/\partial t)$ has the units (mol/m^3 s) (as a practical matter, consistency of units throughout any of these equations should be checked before they are used).
- Equation (A1.14a) is based on a mass balance for the incremental volume in cylindrical coordinates $r\Delta r\Delta\theta\Delta z$ (note the LHS and the RHS reaction term). With this incremental volume in mind, each RHS term for convection or diffusion is based on an incremental area that is transverse (perpendicular) to a vector for convection or diffusion. This is illustrated with the following terms.
  - For diffusion in the r direction modeled as

$$-r\Delta\theta\Delta z D_r\left.\frac{\partial u}{\partial r}\right|_r-\left(-(r+\Delta r)\Delta\theta\Delta z D_r\left.\frac{\partial u}{\partial r}\right|_{r+\Delta r}\right)$$

    the transfer area is (increment in θ)(increment in z) = $(r\Delta\theta)(\Delta z)$.
  - For diffusion in the θ direction modeled as

$$-\Delta r\Delta z\frac{D_\theta}{r}\left.\frac{\partial u}{\partial\theta}\right|_\theta-\left(-\Delta r\Delta z\frac{D_\theta}{r}\left.\frac{\partial u}{\partial\theta}\right|_{\theta+\Delta\theta}\right)$$

    the transfer area is (increment in r)(increment in z) = $(\Delta r)(\Delta z)$.
  - For diffusion in the z direction modeled as

$$-r\Delta r\Delta\theta D_z\left.\frac{\partial u}{\partial z}\right|_z-\left(-r\Delta r\Delta\theta D_z\left.\frac{\partial u}{\partial z}\right|_{z+\Delta z}\right)$$

the transfer area is (increment in r)(increment in θ) = $(\Delta r)(r\Delta\theta)$.

– For convection in the r direction modeled as

$$+r\Delta\theta\Delta z v_r u|_r - (r+\Delta r)\Delta\theta\Delta z v_r u|_{r+\Delta r}$$

the transfer area is (increment in θ)(increment in z) = $(r\Delta\theta)(\Delta z)$.

– For convection in the θ direction modeled as

$$-\Delta r\Delta z v_\theta u|_\theta - (-\Delta r\Delta z v_\theta u|_{\theta+\Delta\theta})$$

the transfer area is (increment in r)(increment in z) = $(\Delta r)(\Delta z)$.

– For convection in the z direction modeled as

$$+r\Delta r\Delta\theta v_z u|_z - r\Delta r\Delta\theta v_z u|_{z+\Delta z}$$

the transfer area is (increment in r)(increment in θ) = $(\Delta r)(r\Delta\theta)$.

- Equations (A1.14b) to (A1.14e) have terms of the form $(1/r)$, which can cause computational problems if $r = 0$ is in the (r,θ,z) solution domain. This singularity is usually handled in one of the following ways:
  - L'Hospital's rule is applied to remove the indeterminant form, (0/0).
  - At $r = 0$, the Laplacian $\nabla^2 u$ is approximated in Cartesian coordinates (which does not involve $(1/r)$) while for $r \neq 0$, cylindrical coordinates are used.
  - The PDE is integrated numerically in Cartesian coordinates (which again does not involve $(1/r)$) and the curved boundaries that are handled conveniently in cylindrical coordinates are accommodated by meshfree (meshless) methods.

- Generally, eqs. (A1.14) are a starting point for modeling a physical system with cylindrical geometry. This approach has been used extensively in numerical studies of convection-diffusion-reaction systems. The $(1/r)$ singularity may require special care, as discussed above.

A1.4.3 Spherical coordinates

The corresponding derivation in spherical coordinates, (r,θ,ϕ), follows from a mass balance on an incremental volume $(\Delta r)(r\Delta\theta)(r\sin(\theta)\Delta\phi)$ (θ is the angle with respect to the z axis and ϕ is the angle with respect to the x axis in the $x-y$ plane ([1], pp 826–828)).

$$(\Delta r)(r\Delta\theta)(r\sin(\theta)\Delta\phi)\frac{\partial u}{\partial t} =$$

$$-(r\Delta\theta)(r\sin(\theta)\Delta\phi)D_r\left.\frac{\partial u}{\partial r}\right|_r - \left(-((r+\Delta r)\Delta\theta)((r+\Delta r)\sin(\theta)\Delta\phi)D_r\left.\frac{\partial u}{\partial r}\right|_{r+\Delta r}\right)$$

$$
\begin{aligned}
&-(\Delta r)(r\sin(\theta)\Delta\phi)D_\theta \left.\frac{\partial u}{r\partial\theta}\right|_\theta - \left(-(\Delta r)(r\sin((\theta+\Delta\theta))\Delta\phi)D_\theta \left.\frac{\partial u}{r\partial\theta}\right|_{\theta+\Delta\theta}\right)\\
&-(\Delta r)(r\Delta\theta)D_\phi \frac{1}{r\sin(\theta)}\left.\frac{\partial u}{\partial\phi}\right|_\phi - \left(-(\Delta r)(r\Delta\theta)D_\phi \frac{1}{r\sin(\theta)}\left.\frac{\partial u}{\partial\phi}\right|_{\phi+\Delta\phi}\right)\\
&+(r\Delta\theta)(r\sin(\theta)\Delta\phi)v_r u|_r - ((r+\Delta r)\Delta\theta)((r+\Delta r)\sin(\theta)\Delta\phi)v_r u|_{r+\Delta r}\\
&+(\Delta r)(r\sin(\theta)\Delta\phi)v_\theta u|_\theta - (\Delta r)(r\sin((\theta+\Delta\theta))\Delta\phi)v_\theta u|_{\theta+\Delta\theta}\\
&+(\Delta r)(r\Delta\theta)v_\phi u|_\phi - (\Delta r)(r\Delta\theta)v_\phi u|_{\phi+\Delta\phi}\\
&-(\Delta r)(r\Delta\theta)(r\sin(\theta)\Delta\phi)k_r u^p. \qquad \text{(A1.15a)}
\end{aligned}
$$

Here we have used the diffusion flux, a vector with the components

$$
q_r = -D_r\frac{\partial u}{\partial r};\; q_\theta = -\frac{D_\theta}{r}\frac{\partial u}{\partial\theta};\; q_\phi = -\frac{D_\phi}{r\sin(\theta)}\frac{\partial u}{\partial\phi};
$$

and the convection flux, a vector with the components

$$
w_r = v_r u;\; w_\theta = v_\theta u;\; w_\phi = v_\phi u.
$$

Division of eq. (A1.15a) by $(\Delta r)(r\Delta\theta)(r\sin(\theta)\Delta\phi)$ and minor rearrangement gives

$$
\begin{aligned}
\frac{\partial u}{\partial t} = {}& \frac{(r+\Delta r)^2 D_r \left.\frac{\partial u}{\partial r}\right|_{r+\Delta r} - r^2 D_r \left.\frac{\partial u}{\partial r}\right|_r}{\Delta r}\\
&\times\left(\frac{1}{r^2\sin(\theta)}\right)\frac{\sin(\theta+\Delta\theta)D_\theta \left.\frac{\partial u}{\partial\theta}\right|_{\theta+\Delta\theta} - \sin(\theta)D_\theta \left.\frac{\partial u}{\partial\theta}\right|_\theta}{\Delta\theta}\\
&\times\left(\frac{1}{r^2\sin^2(\theta)}\right)\frac{D_\phi \left.\frac{\partial u}{\partial\phi}\right|_{\phi+\Delta\phi} - D_\phi \frac{\partial u}{\partial\phi}|_\phi}{\Delta\phi}\\
&-\left(\frac{1}{r^2}\right)\frac{(r+\Delta r)^2 v_r u|_{r+\Delta r} - r^2 v_r u|_r}{\Delta r}\\
&-\left(\frac{1}{r}\right)\frac{\sin(\theta+\Delta\theta)v_\theta u|_{\theta+\Delta\theta} - \sin(\theta)v_\theta u|_\theta}{\Delta\theta}\\
&-\left(\frac{1}{r\sin(\theta)}\right)\frac{v_\phi u|_{\phi+\Delta\phi} - v_\phi u|_\phi}{\Delta\phi} - k_r u^p. \qquad \text{(A1.15b)}
\end{aligned}
$$

For $\Delta r \to 0, \Delta\theta \to 0, \Delta\phi \to 0$, eq. (A1.15b) becomes

$$\begin{aligned}\frac{\partial u}{\partial t} = {} & \frac{1}{r^2}\frac{\partial\left(r^2 D_r \dfrac{\partial u}{\partial r}\right)}{\partial r}\frac{1}{r^2\sin(\theta)}\frac{\partial\left(\sin(\theta)D_\theta \dfrac{\partial u}{\partial\theta}\right)}{\partial\theta}\frac{1}{r^2\sin^2(\theta)}\frac{\partial\left(D_\phi \dfrac{\partial u}{\partial\phi}\right)}{\partial\phi}\\ & -\frac{1}{r^2}\frac{\partial\left(r^2 v_r u\right)}{\partial r}\\ & -\frac{1}{r\sin(\theta)}\frac{\partial\left(\sin(\theta)v_\theta u\right)}{\partial\theta}\\ & -\frac{1}{r\sin(\theta)}\frac{\partial\left(v_\phi u\right)}{\partial\phi} - k_r u^p. \end{aligned} \quad \text{(A1.15c)}$$

For the special case of constant diffusivities and velocities, eq. (A1.15c) becomes

$$\begin{aligned}\frac{\partial u}{\partial t} = {} & \frac{D_r}{r^2}\frac{\partial\left(r^2\dfrac{\partial u}{\partial r}\right)}{\partial r} + \frac{D_\theta}{r^2\sin(\theta)}\frac{\partial\left(\sin(\theta)\dfrac{\partial u}{\partial\theta}\right)}{\partial\theta} + \frac{D_\phi}{r^2\sin^2(\theta)}\frac{\partial\left(\dfrac{\partial u}{\partial\phi}\right)}{\partial\phi}\\ & -\frac{v_r}{r^2}\frac{\partial\left(r^2 u\right)}{\partial r} - \frac{v_\theta}{r\sin(\theta)}\frac{\partial\left(\sin(\theta)u\right)}{\partial\theta} - \frac{v_\phi}{r\sin(\theta)}\frac{\partial u}{\partial\phi} - k_r u^p, \end{aligned} \quad \text{(A1.15d)}$$

or after differentiating the product terms in r and θ,

$$\begin{aligned}\frac{\partial u}{\partial t} = {} & D_r\left(\frac{\partial^2 u}{\partial r^2} + \frac{2}{r}\frac{\partial u}{\partial r}\right) + \frac{D_\theta}{r^2\sin(\theta)}\left(\sin(\theta)\frac{\partial^2 u}{\partial\theta^2} + \cos(\theta)\frac{\partial u}{\partial\theta}\right) + \frac{D_\phi}{r^2\sin^2(\theta)}\frac{\partial^2 u}{\partial\phi^2}\\ & - v_r\left(\frac{\partial u}{\partial r} + \frac{2}{r}u\right) - \frac{v_\theta}{r\sin(\theta)}\left(\sin(\theta)\frac{\partial u}{\partial\theta} + \cos(\theta)u\right) - \frac{v_\phi}{r\sin(\theta)}\frac{\partial u}{\partial\phi} - k_r u^p. \end{aligned}$$
(A1.15e)

Again, experience has indicated that the expanded form of the r and $\sin(\theta)$ terms in eq. (A1.14e) leads to MOL numerical solutions more reliably than using the r and $\sin(\theta)$ terms in eq. (A1.14d). Additionally, product terms such as in r and $\sin(\theta)$ in eq. (A1.14d) are commonplace and expanding them through differentiation is generally recommended before attempting a numerical solution.

We can note the following details about eqs. (A1.15).

- Again, with $u(z,t)$ interpreted as a concentration with units mol/m^3, each of the terms in the equations with the LHS $(\partial u/\partial t)$ has the units (mol/m^3 s) (as a practical matter, consistency of units throughout any of these equations should be checked before they are used).
- Equation (A1.15a) is based on a mass balance for the incremental volume in spherical coordinates $(\Delta r)(r\Delta\theta)(r\sin(\theta)\Delta\phi)$ (note the LHS and the RHS reaction term). With this incremental volume in mind, each RHS term for convection or diffusion is based on an incremental area that is transverse (perpendicular) to a vector for convection or diffusion. This is illustrated with the following terms.

– For diffusion in the r direction modeled as

$$-(r\Delta\theta)(r\sin(\theta)\Delta\phi)D_r\left.\frac{\partial u}{\partial r}\right|_r-\left(-((r+\Delta r)\Delta\theta)((r+\Delta r)\sin(\theta)\Delta\phi)D_r\left.\frac{\partial u}{\partial r}\right|_{r+\Delta r}\right)$$

the transfer area is (increment in θ)(increment in ϕ) = $(r\Delta\theta)(r\sin(\theta)\Delta\phi)$.

– For diffusion in the θ direction modeled as

$$-(\Delta r)(r\sin(\theta)\Delta\phi)D_\theta\left.\frac{\partial u}{r\partial\theta}\right|_\theta-\left(-(\Delta r)(r\sin((\theta+\Delta\theta))\Delta\phi)D_\theta\left.\frac{\partial u}{r\partial\theta}\right|_{\theta+\Delta\theta}\right)$$

the transfer area is (increment in r)(increment in ϕ) = $(\Delta r)(r\sin(\theta)\Delta\phi)$.

– For diffusion in the ϕ direction modeled as

$$-(\Delta r)(r\Delta\theta)D_\phi\frac{1}{r\sin(\theta)}\left.\frac{\partial u}{\partial\phi}\right|_\phi-\left(-(\Delta r)(r\Delta\theta)D_\phi\frac{1}{r\sin(\theta)}\left.\frac{\partial u}{\partial\phi}\right|_{\phi+\Delta\phi}\right)$$

the transfer area is (increment in r)(increment in θ) = $(\Delta r)(r\Delta\theta)$.

– For convection in the r direction modeled as

$$+(r\Delta\theta)(r\sin(\theta)\Delta\phi)v_r u|_r-((r+\Delta r)\Delta\theta)((r+\Delta r)\sin(\theta)\Delta\phi)v_r u|_{r+\Delta r}$$

the transfer area is (increment in θ)(increment in ϕ) = $(r\Delta\theta)(r\sin(\theta)\Delta\phi)$.

– For convection in the θ direction modeled as

$$+(\Delta r)(r\sin(\theta)\Delta\phi)v_\theta u|_\theta-(\Delta r)(r\sin((\theta+\Delta\theta))\Delta\phi)v_\theta u|_{\theta+\Delta\theta}$$

the transfer area is (increment in r)(increment in ϕ) = $(\Delta r)(r\sin(\theta)\Delta\phi)$.

– For convection in the ϕ direction modeled as the transfer area is

$$+(\Delta r)(r\Delta\theta)v_\phi u|_\phi-(\Delta r)(r\Delta\theta)v_\phi u|_{\phi+\Delta\phi}$$

the transfer area is (increment in r)(increment in θ) = $(\Delta r)(r\Delta\theta)$.

- Equations (A1.15b) to (A1.15e) have terms of the form $(1/r)$ and $(1/\sin(\theta))$, which can cause computational problems if $r=0$ or $\theta=n\pi, n=0,1,\cdots$ is in the (r,θ,ϕ) solution domain. These singularities are usually handled in one of the following ways:
  - L'Hospital's rule is applied to remove the indeterminant form (0/0).
  - At $r=0$, or $\theta=n\pi, n=0,1,\cdots$, the Laplacian $\nabla^2 u$ is approximated in Cartesian coordinates (which does not involve $(1/r)$ or $(1/\sin(\theta))$) while for $r\neq 0$, $\theta\neq n\pi$, spherical coordinates are used.
  - The PDE is integrated numerically in Cartesian coordinates (which again does not involve $(1/r)$ or $(1/\sin(\theta))$) and the curved boundaries that are handled conveniently in spherical coordinates are accommodated by meshfree (meshless) methods.
- Generally, eqs. (A1.15) are a starting point for modeling a physical system with spherical geometry. This approach has been used extensively in numerical studies

of convection-diffusion-reaction systems. The $(1/r)$ and $(1/\sin(\theta))$ singularities may require special care, as discussed above.

References

[1] Bird, R. B., Stewart, W. E. and Lightfoot, E. N. (2002), *Transport Phenomena*, 2nd edn., New York: John Wiley and Sons

[2] Fornberg, B. (1998), Calculation of weights in finite difference formulas, *SIAM Rev.*, **40**, (3), September, 685–691

[3] Hamdi, S., Schiesser, W. E. and Griffiths, G. W. (2007), Method of lines, *Scholarpedia*, **2**, (7), 2859; www.scholarpedia.org/article/method_of_lines (Part II has the routines; Part I discusses basic concepts)

[4] Schiesser, W. E. and Griffiths, G. W. (2007–2011), *Analysis of Partial Differential Equations Using MATLAB and Maple*; www.pdecomp.net (a library of differentiation routines can be downloaded from the `DSS` folder)

[5] Schiesser, W. E. and Griffiths, G. W. (2009), *A Compendium of Partial Differential Equations*, NY: Cambridge University Press

[6] Schiesser, W. E. (1991), *The Numerical Method of Lines Integration of Partial Differential Equations*, San Diego: Academic Press

Appendix 2 Stiffness and eigenvalue analysis of ODE systems

In Chapter 1, Section (1.2.3.3), we briefly considered a 2×2 ODE system, and in particular, the stiffness (ratio of the largest to smallest eigenvalues). The general conclusion from that discussion is that as the stiffness increases, explicit integration algorithms become increasingly inefficient, and for stiff ODE systems (large stiffness ratios), implicit algorithms should be used. We now consider some additional mathematical background, particularly basic linear algebra and its association with ODEs.

A2.1 Linear algebraic eigenvalue problem

We now extend the discussion of Section (1.2.3.3), starting with the derivation of the analytical solution of the following 2×2 ODE test problem by two methods: (1) exponential functions and (2) the Laplace transform. These solution procedures lead us to a consideration of some basic concepts in linear algebra.

$$\begin{aligned} \frac{du_1}{dt} &= a_{11}u_1 + a_{12}u_2 \quad u_1(0) = u_{10}, \\ \frac{du_2}{dt} &= a_{21}u_1 + a_{22}u_2 \quad u_2(0) = u_{20}. \end{aligned} \tag{A2.1}$$

Generally linear, constant coefficient ODEs such as eqs. (A2.1) have as solutions exponential functions of the independent variable (t), so as a starting point, we assume

$$\begin{aligned} u_1(t) &= c_1 e^{\lambda t}, \\ u_2(t) &= c_2 e^{\lambda t}, \end{aligned} \tag{A2.2a}$$

where c_1, c_2, and λ are constants to be determined. Substitution of eqs. (A2.2a) in eqs. (A2.1) gives

$$\begin{aligned} c_1 \lambda e^{\lambda t} &= a_{11} c_1 e^{\lambda t} + a_{12} c_2 e^{\lambda t}, \\ c_2 \lambda e^{\lambda t} &= a_{21} c_1 e^{\lambda t} + a_{22} c_2 e^{\lambda t}. \end{aligned} \tag{A2.2b}$$

Cancellation of $e^{\lambda t}$ gives a system of algebraic equations (this is the reason why assuming exponential solutions works in the case of linear, constant coefficient ODEs – note that the exponential will in general not be zero so this division is possible):

$$\begin{aligned} c_1 \lambda &= a_{11} c_1 + a_{12} c_2, \\ c_2 \lambda &= a_{21} c_1 + a_{22} c_2, \end{aligned}$$

or

$$\begin{aligned}(a_{11}-\lambda)c_1+a_{12}c_2&=0,\\ a_{21}c_1+(a_{22}-\lambda)c_2&=0.\end{aligned} \tag{A2.3}$$

Equations (A2.3) are the 2×2 case of the linear algebraic eigenvalue problem. In other words, this discussion illustrates the relation between linear, constant coefficient ODEs, and linear algebraic equations.

Equations (A2.3) can be stated in general vector–matrix notation as

$$(\mathbf{A}-\lambda\mathbf{I})\mathbf{c}=\mathbf{0}, \tag{A2.4}$$

where

$$\mathbf{A}=\begin{bmatrix} a_{11} & a_{12} & \cdots & a_{1n}\\ a_{21} & a_{22} & \cdots & a_{2n}\\ \vdots & & \ddots & \vdots\\ a_{n1} & a_{n2} & \cdots & a_{nn}\end{bmatrix},$$

$$\mathbf{I}=\begin{bmatrix} 1 & 0 & \cdots & 0\\ 0 & 1 & \cdots & 0\\ \vdots & & \ddots & \vdots\\ 0 & 0 & \cdots & 1\end{bmatrix},$$

$$\mathbf{c}=\begin{bmatrix} c_1\\ c_2\\ \vdots\\ c_n\end{bmatrix},$$

$$\mathbf{0}=\begin{bmatrix} 0\\ 0\\ \vdots\\ 0\end{bmatrix}.$$

We use a bold faced symbol for a matrix or a vector, and in the case of eqs. (A2.1), $n=2$.

The preceding matrices and vectors are

$\mathbf{A}$	$n \times n$ coefficient matrix,
$\mathbf{I}$	$n \times n$ identity matrix,
$\mathbf{c}$	$n \times 1$ solution vector,
$\mathbf{0}$	$n \times 1$ zero vector.

Note that in specifying a vector to be $n \times 1$, we mean n rows and one column. In other words, the first dimension is the row dimension and the second dimension is the column dimension, which is in accordance with the usual notation for vectors and matrices (and a vector is a one dimensional matrix). The reader should confirm that the matrices and vectors in eq. (A2.4) have the correct dimensions for all of the indicated operations (e.g., matrix additions, vector–matrix multiplications).

As a specific example, eq. (A2.4) applied to eqs. (A2.3) gives

$$\mathbf{A}=\begin{bmatrix} a_{11} & a_{12} \\ a_{21} & a_{22} \end{bmatrix},$$

$$\mathbf{I}=\begin{bmatrix} 1 & 0 \\ 0 & 1 \end{bmatrix},$$

$$\mathbf{c}=\begin{bmatrix} c_1 \\ c_2 \end{bmatrix},$$

$$\mathbf{0}=\begin{bmatrix} 0 \\ 0 \end{bmatrix}.$$

Substitution in eq. (A2.4) gives

$$\left(\begin{bmatrix} a_{11} & a_{12} \\ a_{21} & a_{22} \end{bmatrix}-\lambda\begin{bmatrix} 1 & 0 \\ 0 & 1 \end{bmatrix}\right)\begin{bmatrix} c_1 \\ c_2 \end{bmatrix}=\begin{bmatrix} 0 \\ 0 \end{bmatrix},$$

$$\begin{bmatrix} a_{11}-\lambda & a_{12} \\ a_{21} & a_{22}-\lambda \end{bmatrix}\begin{bmatrix} c_1 \\ c_2 \end{bmatrix}=\begin{bmatrix} 0 \\ 0 \end{bmatrix}.$$

The two LHS matrices can be multiplied (using the rows × columns rule)

$$\begin{bmatrix} (a_{11}-\lambda)c_1+a_{12}c_2 \\ a_{21}c_{21}+(a_{22}-\lambda)c_2 \end{bmatrix}=\begin{bmatrix} 0 \\ 0 \end{bmatrix}$$

This result is the previous system of two linear algebraic equations, eqs. (A2.3).

Note that eq. (A2.4) is a linear, homogeneous algebraic system (homogeneous means that the RHS is the zero vector). Thus, eq. (A2.4), or its 2 × 2 counterpart, eqs. (A2.3), will have nontrivial solutions ($\mathbf{c} \neq \mathbf{0}$) if and only if (iff) the determinant of the coefficient matrix is zero, i.e.,

$$|\mathbf{A}-\lambda\mathbf{I}|=0. \tag{A2.5}$$

Equation (A2.5) is the characteristic equation for eq. (A2.4) (note that it is a scalar equation). The values of λ that satisfy eq. (A2.5) are the eigenvalues of eq. (A2.4). For the 2 × 2 problem of eqs. (A2.3), eq. (A2.5) is

$$\begin{vmatrix} a_{11}-\lambda & a_{12} \\ a_{21} & a_{22}-\lambda \end{vmatrix}=0,$$

or

$$(a_{11}-\lambda)(a_{22}-\lambda)-a_{21}a_{12}=0. \tag{A2.6}$$

Equation (A2.6) is the characteristic equation or characteristic polynomial for eqs. (A2.3); note that since eqs. (A2.3) constitute a 2 × 2 linear homogeneous algebraic system, the characteristic equation (eq. (A2.6)) is a second order polynomial (in λ). Similarly, since eq. (A2.4) is an $n \times n$ linear homogeneous algebraic system, its characteristic equation is a nth order polynomial.

Equation (A2.6) can be factored by the quadratic formula

$$\lambda^2 - (a_{11} + a_{22})\lambda + a_{11}a_{22} - a_{21}a_{12} = 0,$$

$$\lambda_1, \lambda_2 = \frac{(a_{11} + a_{22}) \pm \sqrt{(a_{11} + a_{22})^2 - 4(a_{11}a_{22} - a_{21}a_{12})}}{2}. \tag{A2.7}$$

Thus, as expected, the 2×2 system of eqs. (A2.3) has two eigenvalues. In general, the $n \times n$ algebraic system, eq. (A2.4), will have n eigenvalues, $\lambda_1, \lambda_2, \cdots, \lambda_n$ (that may be real or complex conjugates, distinct or repeated).

A2.2 Exponential solutions

Since eqs. (A2.1) are linear constant coefficient ODEs, their general solution will be a linear combination of exponential functions, one for each eigenvalue

$$\begin{aligned} u_1(t) &= c_{11}e^{\lambda_1 t} + c_{12}e^{\lambda_2 t}, \\ u_2(t) &= c_{21}e^{\lambda_1 t} + c_{22}e^{\lambda_2 t}. \end{aligned} \tag{A2.8}$$

This addition or superposition of solutions is a distinguishing feature of linear differential equations and follows from substituting eqs. (A2.8) in eqs. (A2.1).

$$\frac{du_1}{dt} = c_{11}\lambda_1 e^{\lambda_1 t} + c_{12}\lambda_2 e^{\lambda_2 t} = a_{11}\left[c_{11}e^{\lambda_1 t} + c_{12}e^{\lambda_2 t}\right] + a_{12}\left[c_{21}e^{\lambda_1 t} + c_{22}e^{\lambda_2 t}\right],$$

$$\frac{du_2}{dt} = c_{21}\lambda_1 e^{\lambda_1 t} + c_{22}\lambda_2 e^{\lambda_2 t} = a_{21}\left[c_{11}e^{\lambda_1 t} + c_{12}e^{\lambda_2 t}\right] + a_{22}\left[c_{21}e^{\lambda_1 t} + c_{22}e^{\lambda_2 t}\right],$$

or

$$[(a_{11} - \lambda_1)c_{11} + a_{12}c_{21}]e^{\lambda_1 t} + [(a_{11} - \lambda_2)c_{12} + a_{12}c_{22}]e^{\lambda_2 t} = 0,$$

$$[(a_{22} - \lambda_1)c_{21} + a_{21}c_{11}]e^{\lambda_1 t} + [(a_{22} - \lambda_2)c_{22} + a_{21}c_{12}]e^{\lambda_2 t} = 0.$$

Each of the terms in square brackets in this last result is zero from eqs. (A2.3) for the two cases $\lambda = \lambda_1, \lambda_2$.

Equations (A2.8) have four constants that occur in pairs, one pair for each eigenvalue. Thus, the pair $[c_{11}\ c_{21}]^T$ is the eigenvector for eigenvalue λ_1 while $[c_{12}\ c_{22}]^T$ is the eigenvector for eigenvalue λ_2. In general, the $n \times n$ system of eq. (A2.4) will have an $n \times 1$ eigenvector for each of its n eigenvalues. Note that the naming convention for any constant in an eigenvector, c_{ij}, is the ith constant for the jth eigenvalue. We can restate the two eigenvectors for eq. (A2.8) (or eqs. (A2.3)) as

$$\begin{bmatrix} c_{11} \\ c_{21} \end{bmatrix}_{\lambda_1}, \begin{bmatrix} c_{12} \\ c_{22} \end{bmatrix}_{\lambda_2}. \tag{A2.9}$$

Finally, the four constants in eigenvectors (A2.8) are related through the initial conditions of eqs. (A2.1) and either of eqs. (A2.3)

$$\begin{aligned} u_{10} &= c_{11}e^{\lambda_1 0} + c_{12}e^{\lambda_2 0}, \\ u_{20} &= c_{21}e^{\lambda_1 0} + c_{22}e^{\lambda_2 0}. \end{aligned} \tag{A2.10}$$

As in Chapter 1, Section (1.2.3.3), we can simplify the analysis somewhat by considering the special case $a_{11} = a_{22} = -a, a_{21} = a_{12} = b$, where a and b are constants. Then from eq. (A2.7), we have two real eigenvalues,

$$\lambda_1, \lambda_2 = \frac{-2a \pm \sqrt{(2a)^2 - 4(a^2 - b^2)}}{2} = -a \pm b = -(a-b), -(a+b). \tag{A2.11}$$

The relationships of eqs. (A2.11) between the eigenvalues λ_1, λ_2 and the constants a, b in eqs. (A2.1) will facilitate the subsequent analysis.

From the first of eqs. (A2.3) for $\lambda = \lambda_1$

$$(a_{11} - \lambda_1)c_{11} + a_{12}c_{21} = 0,$$

or

$$(-a + (a-b))c_{11} + bc_{21} = 0,$$

$$c_{11} = c_{21}.$$

Similarly, for $\lambda = \lambda_2$

$$(a_{11} - \lambda_2)c_{12} + a_{12}c_{22} = 0,$$

or

$$(-a + (a+b))c_{12} + bc_{22} = 0,$$

$$c_{12} = -c_{22}.$$

Substitution of these results in eqs. (A2.10) gives

$$u_{10} = c_{11} - c_{22},$$

$$u_{20} = c_{11} + c_{22},$$

or

$$c_{11} = \frac{u_{10} + u_{20}}{2} = c_{21},$$

$$c_{22} = \frac{u_{20} - u_{10}}{2} = -c_{12}.$$

Finally, the solution from eqs. (A2.8) is

$$\begin{aligned} u_1(t) &= \frac{u_{10} + u_{20}}{2}e^{\lambda_1 t} - \frac{u_{20} - u_{10}}{2}e^{\lambda_2 t}, \\ u_2(t) &= \frac{u_{10} + u_{20}}{2}e^{\lambda_1 t} + \frac{u_{20} - u_{10}}{2}e^{\lambda_2 t}. \end{aligned} \tag{A2.12}$$

Equations (A2.12) can easily be checked by substitution in eqs. (A2.1) (with $a_{11} = a_{22} = -a, a_{21} = a_{12} = b$) and application of the initial conditions at $t = 0$:

$$
\begin{array}{ll}
\dfrac{du_1}{dt} & \lambda_1 \dfrac{u_{10} + u_{20}}{2} e^{\lambda_1 t} - \lambda_2 \dfrac{u_{20} - u_{10}}{2} e^{\lambda_2 t} \\
 & = -(a-b)\dfrac{u_{10} + u_{20}}{2} e^{\lambda_1 t} + (a+b)\dfrac{u_{20} - u_{10}}{2} e^{\lambda_2 t} \\
+au_1 & +a\left(\dfrac{u_{10} + u_{20}}{2} e^{\lambda_1 t} - \dfrac{u_{20} - u_{10}}{2} e^{\lambda_2 t}\right) \\
-bu_2 & -b\left(\dfrac{u_{10} + u_{20}}{2} e^{\lambda_1 t} + \dfrac{u_{20} - u_{10}}{2} e^{\lambda_2 t}\right) \\
= & = \\
0 & 0 \\
\dfrac{du_2}{dt} & \lambda_1 \dfrac{u_{10} + u_{20}}{2} e^{\lambda_1 t} + \lambda_2 \dfrac{u_{20} - u_{10}}{2} e^{\lambda_2 t} \\
 & = -(a-b)\dfrac{u_{10} + u_{20}}{2} e^{\lambda_1 t} - (a+b)\dfrac{u_{20} - u_{10}}{2} e^{\lambda_2 t} \\
+au_2 & +a\left(\dfrac{u_{10} + u_{20}}{2} e^{\lambda_1 t} + \dfrac{u_{20} - u_{10}}{2} e^{\lambda_2 t}\right) \\
-bu_1 & -b\left(\dfrac{u_{10} + u_{20}}{2} e^{\lambda_1 t} - \dfrac{u_{20} - u_{10}}{2} e^{\lambda_2 t}\right) \\
= & = \\
0 & 0
\end{array}
$$

For the initial conditions of eqs. (A2.1),

$$u_{10} = \frac{u_{10} + u_{20}}{2} e^{\lambda_1 0} - \frac{u_{20} - u_{10}}{2} e^{\lambda_2 0} = u_{10},$$

$$u_{20} = \frac{u_{10} + u_{20}}{2} e^{\lambda_1 0} + \frac{u_{20} - u_{10}}{2} e^{\lambda_2 0} = u_{20}.$$

as required.

For $u_{10} = 0, u_{20} = 2$, eqs. (A2.12) are

$$
\begin{aligned}
u_1(t) &= e^{\lambda_1 t} - e^{\lambda_2 t}, \\
u_2(t) &= e^{\lambda_1 t} + e^{\lambda_2 t}.
\end{aligned}
\qquad \text{(A2.13)}
$$

Equations (A2.13) are investigated subsequently for various values of the stiffness ratio (λ_2/λ_1).

A2.3 Laplace transform solutions

The Laplace transform is another general approach to the solution of systems of linear, constant coefficient ODEs such as eqs. (A2.1); it can also be applied to other types of ODE/PDE systems, but the equations must be linear.

If we define the Laplace transforms

$$U_1(s) = L\{u_1(t)\} = \int_0^\infty u_1(t)\mathrm{e}^{-st}\mathrm{d}t; \quad U_2(s) = L\{u_2(t)\} = \int_0^\infty u_2(t)\mathrm{e}^{-st}\mathrm{d}t,$$

eqs. (A2.1) transform to

$$sU_1 - u_{10} = a_{11}U_1 + a_{12}U_2, \tag{A2.14a}$$

$$sU_2 - u_{20} = a_{21}U_1 + a_{22}U_2. \tag{A2.14b}$$

Equations (A2.14) are two linear algebraic equations in the two unknowns U_1, U_2; they can be solved by Cramer's rule

$$U_1(s) = \frac{\begin{vmatrix} -u_{10} & a_{12} \\ -u_{20} & a_{22}-s \end{vmatrix}}{\begin{vmatrix} a_{11}-s & a_{12} \\ a_{21} & a_{22}-s \end{vmatrix}}, \tag{A2.15a}$$

$$U_2(s) = \frac{\begin{vmatrix} a_{11}-s & -u_{10} \\ a_{21} & -u_{20} \end{vmatrix}}{\begin{vmatrix} a_{11}-s & a_{12} \\ a_{21} & a_{22}-s \end{vmatrix}}, \tag{A2.15b}$$

where we have now used || to denote a determinant. Note that eqs. (A2.15) require

$$\begin{vmatrix} a_{11}-s & a_{12} \\ a_{21} & a_{22}-s \end{vmatrix} = (a_{11}-s)(a_{22}-s) - a_{12}a_{21} \neq 0, \tag{A2.16}$$

to avoid a division by zero (since in general the numerators of eqs. (A2.15) will not be zero). Equation (A2.16) is the opposite of eq. (A2.6) with regard to the RHS. This difference occurs because eqs. (A2.6) are homogeneous (zero RHS) while eqs. (A2.14) are nonhomogeneous (nonzero RHS – the ICs u_{10}, u_{20} are not both zero).

Equation (A2.16) can be written in factored form

$$(a_{11}-s)(a_{22}-s) - a_{12}a_{21} = s^2 - (a_{11}+a_{22})s + a_{11}a_{22} - a_{12}a_{21} = (s-r_1)(s-r_2), \tag{A2.17a}$$

where

$$r_1, r_2 = \frac{a_{11} + a_{22} \pm \sqrt{(a_{11} + a_{22})^2 - 4(1)(a_{11}a_{22} - a_{12}a_{21})}}{2}. \tag{A2.17b}$$

Note that eqs. (A2.7) and (A2.17b) are the same and we can therefore expect that r_1, r_2 are the eigenvalues of the 2×2 ODE system of eqs. (A2.1).

Equations (A2.15) can then be stated as a partial fraction expansion

$$U_1(s) = \frac{-(a_{22} - s)u_{10} + a_{12}u_{20}}{(s - r_1)(s - r_2)} = \frac{c_{11}}{s - r_1} + \frac{c_{12}}{s - r_2}, \tag{A2.18a}$$

$$U_2(s) = \frac{-(a_{11} - s)u_{20} + a_{21}u_{10}}{(s - r_1)(s - r_2)} = \frac{c_{21}}{s - r_1} + \frac{c_{22}}{s - r_2}, \tag{A2.18b}$$

where $c_{11}, c_{12}, c_{21}, c_{22}$ are constants to be determined by the usual method for partial fractions. Thus, if eq. (A2.18a) is multiplied by $s - r_1$, then $s = r_1$,

$$c_{11} = \frac{-(a_{22} - r_1)u_{10} + a_{12}u_{20}}{r_1 - r_2}. \tag{A2.19a}$$

Similarly,

$$c_{12} = -\frac{-(a_{22} - r_2)u_{10} + a_{12}u_{20}}{r_1 - r_2}, \tag{A2.19b}$$

$$c_{21} = \frac{-(a_{11} - r_1)u_{20} + a_{21}u_{10}}{r_1 - r_2}, \tag{A2.19c}$$

$$c_{22} = -\frac{-(a_{11} - r_2)u_{20} + a_{21}u_{10}}{r_1 - r_2}. \tag{A2.19d}$$

From the Laplace transform pair

$$L\{e^{at}\} = \frac{1}{s - a},$$

eqs. (A2.18) invert to

$$u_1(t) = \{U_1(s)\}^{-1} = c_{11}e^{r_1 t} + c_{12}e^{r_2 t}, \tag{A2.20a}$$

$$u_2(t) = \{U_2(s)\}^{-1} = c_{21}e^{r_1 t} + c_{22}e^{r_2 t}. \tag{A2.20b}$$

Equations (A2.19) and (A2.20) are the general solution to eqs. (A2.1).

For the special case considered previously, $a_{11} = a_{22} = -a, a_{12} = a_{21} = b$, from eq. (A2.17b),

$$r_1 = \frac{-2a + \sqrt{(-a - a)^2 - 4(1)[(-a)(-a) - (b)(b)]}}{2} = -(a - b), \tag{A2.21a}$$

$$r_2 = \frac{-2a - \sqrt{(-a - a)^2 - 4(1)[(-a)(-a) - (b)(b)]}}{2} = -(a + b), \tag{A2.21b}$$

$$r_1 - r_2 = 2b,$$

$$c_{11} = \frac{-(-a + (a - b))u_{10} + bu_{20}}{2b} = \frac{u_{10} + u_{20}}{2}, \tag{A2.22a}$$

$$c_{12} = -\frac{-(-a + (a + b))u_{10} + bu_{20}}{2b} = \frac{u_{10} - u_{20}}{2}, \tag{A2.22b}$$

$$c_{21} = \frac{-(-a + (a - b))u_{20} + bu_{10}}{2b} = \frac{u_{10} + u_{20}}{2}, \tag{A2.22c}$$

$$c_{22} = -\frac{-(-a + (a + b))u_{20} + bu_{10}}{2b} = \frac{-u_{10} + u_{20}}{2}, \tag{A2.22d}$$

and eqs. (A2.20) become

$$u_1(t) = \frac{u_{10} + u_{20}}{2} e^{r_1 t} + \frac{u_{10} - u_{20}}{2} e^{r_2 t}, \tag{A2.23a}$$

$$u_2(t) = \frac{u_{10} + u_{20}}{2} e^{r_1 t} + \frac{-u_{10} + u_{20}}{2} e^{r_2 t}, \tag{A2.23b}$$

which are eqs. (A2.12) (with $r_1 = \lambda_1, r_2 = \lambda_2$).

With $u_{10} = 0, u_{20} = 2$, eqs. (A2.23) are

$$u_1(t) = e^{r_1 t} - e^{r_2 t}, \tag{A2.24a}$$

$$u_2(t) = e^{r_1 t} + e^{r_2 t}, \tag{A2.24b}$$

which are eqs. (A2.13) (with $r_1 = \lambda_1, r_2 = \lambda_2$).

Additional information about initial value ODEs and stiff ODEs is available from the articles by Shampine and Thompson [2, 3] and from [1], Appendix C.

A2.4 Numerical eigenvalue analysis

We now consider some numerical values of the eigenvalues λ_1, λ_2 of eqs. (A2.13). For $a_{11} = a_{22} = -a, a_{21} = a_{12} = b$ in eqs. (A2.1), from eqs. (A2.11)

$$\lambda_1, \lambda_2 = -a \pm b = -(a - b), -(a + b).$$

We now consider the stiffness ratio (λ_2/λ_1) for some specific values of a, b see Table A2.1. Consider the maximum Euler step for the stiff case (see also Section 1.2.3.3). If $\lambda_2 = -(a + b) = -1\,000\,000$, the maximum stable step is given by $|\lambda h| = 2$ or $h = 2/1\,000\,000 = 0.000\,002$. However, $\lambda_1 = -(a - b) = -1$, and to compute a complete solution, we require a final t given approximately by $\lambda_1 t \approx -10$ (or $t = 10$ so that $e = \exp^{-10}$ in eqs. (A2.24) has decayed to insignificance). Thus, we must take $10/0.000\,002 = 5 \times 10^6$ steps! If this doesn't seem like a large number of steps, consider $a = 500\,000\,000.5, b = 499{,}999{,}999.5$ for which the ratio (|largest eigenvalue|/|smallest eigenvalue|) =$(|\lambda_{max}|/|\lambda_{min}|)$ = $(|\lambda_2|/|\lambda_1|) = 10^9$ and

Table A2.1. Some stiffness ratios

Values of a, b	Values of λ_1, λ_2	$(\lvert\lambda_2\rvert/\lvert\lambda_1\rvert)$ and description
Case 1		
$a = 50.5$	$\lambda_2 = -100$	$(\lvert\lambda_2\rvert/\lvert\lambda_1\rvert) = 100$
$b = 49.5$	$\lambda_1 = -1$	Nonstiff
Case 2		
$a = 500.5$	$\lambda_2 = -1000$	$(\lvert\lambda_2\rvert/\lvert\lambda_1\rvert) = 1000$
$b = 499.5$	$\lambda_1 = -1$	Moderately stiff
Case 3		
a=500 000.5	$\lambda_2 = -1\,000\,000$	$(\lvert\lambda_2\rvert/\lvert\lambda_1\rvert) = 1\,000\,000$
b=499 999.5	$\lambda_1 = -1$	Stiff

5×10^9 steps would be required to compute a complete solution (physical problems in which this stiffness ratio = $(|\lambda_{max}|/|\lambda_{min}|) = 10^{12}$ to 10^{15} are not unusual).

Thus, if we require the solution to a system of stiff ODEs, we should not use the Euler method (because of the stability limit $|\lambda h| = 2$ and the resulting large number of integration steps to achieve a stable solution). We might consider a higher order method, e.g., the modified Euler method of `meuler` (Listing 1.4) or the classical fourth order RK method of `rk4` (Listing 1.5), but if we try a stability analysis, we arrive at a stability limit that is not much better than for the Euler method. For example, for the fourth order RK method, the stability limit is $|\lambda h| = 2.7$. Thus, higher order explicit methods give higher accuracy, but do very little for improved stability. Therefore, an implicit integrator should be used for stiff ODEs.

To conclude this discussion of stiffness, we can also note that:

- If an ODE system is nonlinear, it does not necessarily mean that it is stiff (a common misconception) in the sense that an implicit integrator has to be used to compute a numerical solution.
- In other words, we should not always start out using a stiff integrator for a nonlinear ODE system. Rather, if a nonstiff integrator computes a solution with reasonable effort, it should be used since the computational effort could be significantly less than with a stiff integrator.

References

[1] Lee, H. J. and Schiesser, W. E (2004), *Ordinary and Partial Differential Equation Routines in C, C++, Fortran, Java, Maple and MATLAB*, Boca Raton FL: CRC Press

[2] Shampine, L. F. and Thompson, S. (2007), Initial value problems, *Scholarpedia*, **2** (3), 2861; www.scholarpedia.org/article/Initial_value_problems

[3] Shampine, L. F. and Thompson, S. (2007), Stiff systems, *Scholarpedia*, **2** (3), 2855; www.scholarpedia.org/article/stiff_systems

Index